D0878197

Just Fine

Unmasking Concealed
Chronic Illness and Pain

Carol Sveilich, MA

Avid Reader Press

Austin, Texas

Published by Avid Reader Press, Austin, Texas   www.AvidReaderPress.com

Copyright © 2005 Carol Sveilich   www.WriteFaceForward.com

All photographs by Carol Sveilich. Exceptions listed below.
The photograph of Peter S. was taken by Chris Penrod. The photographs of Robert
B. and Tim C. are personal submissions.

The information in this book is based on the experiences and research of the author.
The material is for informational purposes only. The publisher and author are not
engaged in rendering medical services or advice. If expert assistance is required, the
services of a competent professional should be sought. No liability is assumed for
damages resulting from the use of the information herein. If you cannot accept these
conditions, please return your book to the place of purchase.

All rights reserved. No part of this book shall be reproduced, stored in a retrieval
system, or transmitted by any means, electronic, mechanical, photocopying, recording, or otherwise, without express written permission from the publisher. Printed in
the United States of America.

09 08 07 06 05   5 4 3 2 1

Library of Congress Cataloging-in-Publication Data

Sveilich, Carol, 1954-
Just fine : unmasking concealed chronic illness and pain / Carol Sveilich.—
1st ed.
p. cm.
Includes bibliographical references and index.
ISBN 0-9700150-3-8 (hardback) — ISBN 0-9700150-4-6 (pbk.)
1. Sick—Attitudes. 2. Chronically ill—Psychology. 3. Chronically ill—
Biography. 4. Chronic pain. 5. Body language—Evaluation. I. Title.

R726.5.S845 2005
616'.0472—dc22
2004011393

For his encouragement, contagious wit,
and reverence for f-stops and bebop,
this book is dedicated to my father,
Joseph Sveilich.

Be kind, for everyone you meet

is fighting a hard battle.

—Plato (c. 427–347BC)

Contents

Foreword

This is an amazing book, researched and compiled by a remarkable author. Although I suspect that *Just Fine* will be a wonderful support source for patients, this book also should be required reading in every medical school, and practicing physicians should avail themselves of this unique opportunity to better understand a major subset of their patients.

The practice of medicine is exactly that: an attempt for physicians to continuously enhance their medical and scientific awareness, technical competence, and compassion. Most of us never completely achieve our personal goals in these areas. Some fall behind more than others.

One of the greatest challenges to any physician is any apparent disconnect between patients' medical histories and their appearances. Although remarkably few patients purposely attempt to dupe their physicians, healthcare professionals seem to have a morbid fear of possible malingerers. As a result, physicians, when confronted by the kinds of patients that are so well described in this book, find it exceptionally difficult to achieve empathy and compassion. Such just fine individuals are very common and often terribly depressed and discouraged due to the fact that the medical profession frequently fails to meet their very real needs.

Doctors can be prisoners of numbers. If their physical examinations and favorite diagnostic tests seem to be normal, the patient's symptoms must somehow be imagined. Of course, the converse is almost universally true. In fact, the patient who describes serious symptoms without any immediately diagnosable malady is almost always correct in appraising the true state of their own health. Physicians who tell such patients that their illness must be due to stress or that their symptoms are all in their heads are almost always dead wrong. The wise physician must often admit an inability to define a diagnosis at a particular moment in time. Nevertheless, patients know their own bodies best of all, and they should always be assumed to be correct when they describe their symptoms.

Many of the patients in this wonderful book are strangely familiar to me since my own practice has included multiple replicas of their poignant stories. Despite my own best efforts, I have not always been as supportive, understanding, and helpful as my own patients have deserved. I wish that I could have done much better. Gastroenterologists see a great many patients with disabling disorders such as Crohn's disease, ulcerative colitis, and severe irritable bowel syndrome. Many of these patients look as healthy as can be, and most have had negative experiences with multiple health professionals.

Even the most modern and highly trained physicians often have little knowledge permitting them to successfully diagnose, treat, and support these patients who appear just fine. The medical graduates of the twenty-first century are the most scientifically aware in history, and their heads are full of esoteric diagnoses and explicit management approaches to dire disorders of all sorts. However, many are absolutely stumped by the healthy appearing person who describes symptoms that seem monstrously out of proportion to his or her demeanor. Physicians are driven by many impulses other than the simple desire to care for their patients. We live in a litigious era, and managed care organizations and insurance companies are vigorously upholding tight cost controls. As a result, there is much pressure to minimize diagnostic testing and to have such testing guided mostly by objective findings rather than symptoms. The patients who suffer the most from such managed care constraints are the just fine individuals who would seem able to survive nicely without expensive testing or treatment.

Although I am not naïve enough to think that all doctors will buy this book and read it, still, I hope that many will do so. If they do, it will make them better doctors. Whether healthcare professionals read the book and learn these precepts or not, this book is certain to be a godsend to a great many patients. If nothing else, they will learn that they are in very good company indeed. We all must be indebted to the patients who were willing to bare their souls in order that others understand the mysteries of patients who are ill but who appear to be just fine.

Dr. Malcolm Robinson, MD, FACP, FACG
Gastroenterologist, Clinical Professor of Medicine
Medical Director of the Oklahoma Foundation for Digestive Research, with thirty-four years as a clinical investigator of gastrointestinal illnesses

My advice to people who live with chronic pain or illness and those who love them: read this book! Another book on pain and other chronic symptoms? you ask. The answer is an emphatic, Yes, and thank God! as well as a reverberating, No. . . a thousand times no! This is not just another cognitive book about chronic pain and illness.

Just Fine takes a compassion-provoking look at the unseen trauma and untold trials of those who look good but feel bad much of the time. It not only provides insight into the emotional chaos that badgers chronic illness and pain sufferers, but it also offers numerous practical strategies for coping and compensating in a world that is driven by energetic human doers rather than frail human beings.

As a physician whose life is devoted to restoring health, I have discovered that patients who feel heard, understood, and respected are more apt to respond to treatment than those who don't have the support of a caring doctor. I also recognize that the patient-physician relationship is built on trust. Therefore, I trust the complaints of my patients. When medicine fails, it is my job to help patients accept the new physical reality of their illnesses by providing them with a means of adapting. The book you are holding is a crucial tool for those who want to adjust their lives and live without dread.

Just Fine is a healing therapy for those who feel alone in their pain and other chronic symptoms. It is also a practical instrument for coping and connecting in the midst of a medical malaise. I urge you to secure copies of this book to share with anyone who is suffering through a chronic illness. In doing so, you will be offering an authentic hope that will radically change their lives.

Wishing you the best of health.

Bill McCarberg, MD FABPM
Founder and Director, Chronic Pain Management Program
Kaiser Permanente, San Diego, California

Preface

A Personal Journey

I used to maintain an extraordinarily clean house. My kitchen, in particular, was kept spotless and in order. The counters were always scrubbed, and there was never a crumb left in the microwave. The spoons never caroused with the forks in the silverware drawer. Like dutiful soldiers, they remained in their proper positions at all times. They knew their assignment was never to mingle with the other utensils or they would be court-martialed. . . by me. Perhaps there was a little obsessive-compulsive spin to my housekeeping, but that was the way I had always been and assumed I always would be. The only area of my home that was allowed to be in disarray was the kitchen junk drawer, where rusty scissors and expired grocery coupons lived in harmony with assorted thumbtacks and misplaced car keys.

The 1980s were a time of social turbulence as well as complacency. This decade would become known as the Reagan Era, featuring a ten-year span of teased hair, long skirts, Cabbage Patch dolls, Pac-Man games, colossal shoulder pads, Rubik's Cubes, and the close of the Cold War. But for me, it was a time of ignoring, battling, and finally accepting the debilitating symptoms of my own health challenges.

Throughout that decade, my physical condition steadily declined. At the time, I was working as a counselor in a large university and enjoying my days interacting with students and faculty. I regularly handled numerous tasks at once—simultaneously spinning many plates in the air without letting one of them drop. However, annoying physical symptoms began to interfere with daily activities and grew increasingly difficult to ignore. The worse these symptoms became, the harder I had to work at minimizing them. As I went on with my life, I became quite skilled at ignoring the pain and physical dysfunction as if they were foes I refused to acknowledge. I became convinced they were false signals, and I simply was not going to heed their call. Toughen up, I insisted to myself. It's all in your head. Pull yourself up by your bootstraps. These were just some of the messages parading through my mind nearly every day.

Ultimately, there was a diagnosis of several serious, but easily concealed illnesses. They led me directly to the hospital without passing GO or collecting two hundred dollars. Having lost a great deal of blood, I managed to hit a wall of fatigue that was unlike anything I had ever experienced. I quickly shifted from a highly energetic and productive person to one who could barely crawl out of bed to take her medication or splash water on her face. The fallout from the side effects of medication and the foreign body in which I found myself residing left me bewildered and scared on the inside. On the outside, however, I looked as I always did—perfectly healthy, energetic, and just fine.

Having my life impacted by a chronic illness was like having someone come into my neat little kitchen and turn all of the drawers upside down. The plates were no longer stacked in an orderly pile. The counters refused to remain crumb-free and the rest of my kitchen started to look like the junk drawer—it was in serious disarray. My life was littered with obstacles. Everything was in chaos, and I could not seem to put it back in order. I no longer had the resilience. I felt like Humpty Dumpty. All the wise doctors and all my willpower could not put me back together again.

The fatigue and pain filtered in, keeping me from my household chores, social life, and job responsibilities. My mind started to feel as weary as my body. It was no longer clear or capable of functioning at warp speed. Spinning ten plates in the air, as I had always done at the office and at home, was no longer my strong suit. I had to learn to let some plates fall and break. I had to let some things slip to the ground and accept that they would not always be as I had intended them to be. I had to recognize that there was a new set of rules in place, and I had to make peace with them and let loose of previous plans.

I did not know how to manage my life with all of the new lifestyle rules and diet restrictions. My stamina had declined so dramatically that I felt as though I had aged several decades in a few weeks. After four long months of recuperation, I headed back to work and to my previous position as a college counselor. I easily fell into a state of denial about my own health dilemmas. Plowing ahead seemed the most practical way to survive. Taking care of everyone else's needs helped divert attention from my own symptoms and pain. I thought if I ignored my symptoms and pretended nothing ever happened, perhaps the pains and other symptoms would vanish.

My old self, the one whose skin I had always felt comfortable in, had departed. A new self was taking over my old territory and I had to uncover a way to make peace with her. The challenge came in trying to force my old way of functioning into this new body and weakened state. This new self, the one that was struggling with fatigue, chronic pain, malfunctioning organs, and sleep deprivation, seemed to be affecting and infecting my career and personal relationships. The journey of the next ten years would include some rocky roads, a few moments of clarity, a time of mourning for the body and the life I was forced to abandon, several soaring moments of exhilaration, and numerous instances of compassion I had not felt prior to my diagnoses of Crohn's disease, fibromyalgia, and Ménière's disease.

The time had come to seek out some form of support. I had to learn to cope with a malfunctioning body that did not seem to want to cooperate. In searching my hometown for information and support groups, I found few resources. Over the next several months, I decided to take matters into my own hands and plant the seeds of a support group in my community. At that time, I had no idea how many other people were living with the same concealed symptoms and fears. Feeling isolated and different from the masses around me, I imagined only a handful of people were in the same sorry boat that I found myself in.

Several people responded with great enthusiasm, so I moved ahead and scheduled the first meeting in my small living room. These meetings focused on a range of different topics. As we continued to meet on a monthly basis, the personality of the group shifted with the entrance of each new member. Useful information and experiences were exchanged, and we shared many laughs and light moments. Sooner than I expected, the number of attendees grew from 8 people to 158. Needless to say, we were quickly forced to stop meeting in my cramped living room and moved to a large, donated office space.

The group continued to meet for the next nine years. I started an Internet support and newsgroup that drew together people across the country and throughout the world. The goal continued to be the exchange of resources and feelings on concealed chronic illness and pain. No matter the age, gender, or ethnicity of the many contributors, we all spoke the same language as we all lived with similar concerns. Many caring individuals contributed a vast amount of information on these Internet groups regarding health issues, medical advances, personal concerns, and coping mechanisms. Medical professionals occasionally chimed in with helpful information on the latest research and treatments. For a ten-year span, I had the joy of co-creating and distributing a worldwide newsletter for people with these chronic disorders. I always gained more from these ventures than I could give. When people come together for a common goal, immense strength and healing are generated from the sheer pleasure and power of connectivity.

A common thread began to emerge from my work with the support group, Internet site, and newsletter publication. People with these physical conditions and challenges were dealing with two major issues: the physical symptoms of the illness and the emotional impact of looking like they *should* be okay, but feeling far from it. Numerous members of this group expressed the same sentiment on a recurrent basis: We are the healthiest looking bunch of sick people around. It was true. We all appeared perfectly healthy, even while dealing with a host of debilitating and chronic symptoms. The dissimilarity between appearance and reality was one of the factors that led to my exploration of concealed chronic illness, not only with words, but also through pictures.

Even after years of living with a concealed chronic disability, a person can appear healthy, lively, and on top of their game. This can become a mixed blessing. The person who enjoys looking healthy and does not want to be perceived as weak or sickly can begin to doubt or belittle legitimate illness or pain.

Should people who are ill or in pain always try to look their best, even though their life has turned as messy as that proverbial junk drawer? Should they dispense with grooming, stop dressing attractively or don a sorry expression in order for others to realize they are not feeling well? Or do these sorts of choices simply damage one's own self image? These are just some of the questions and topics explored in the profiles featured in *Just Fine*.

About the Portraits and Participants

Although there are many good books on the topic of coping with chronic illness, there is an absence of resources that examine an individual's outward appearance and how it runs contrary to their pain, symptoms, and inner world. This juxtaposition is the cornerstone of *Just Fine*.

For each person who thought this book would be an excellent vehicle for telling the true tale of concealed chronic illness, a dozen more discouraged the project for one explicit reason. They felt that no one would want to reveal their face, or their illness in such a public forum, let alone discuss them in a candid and detailed manner. Much to my delight, the reaction from the community of people who live with concealed symptoms was just the opposite. I had more volunteers who wanted an opportunity to tell their story than I had pages available. Numerous participants informed me that the interview sessions were cathartic and healing (and the photo sessions painless and pleasant). Each person seemed to gain a great deal of personal insight and growth through their involvement in this book, and each expressed gratitude for the opportunity to participate in such a telling project.

The uniqueness of this book is that the truth of concealed illness and cloaked symptoms is revealed through the potent coupling of words and pictures. In the interviews, participants discuss their personal challenges, coping mechanisms, feelings, and experiences. Each portrait reveals how the person appears to the outside world: healthy, vibrant, and just fine. However, their words reveal the true story and the daily struggle of living with a concealed illness or hidden pain. As one participant reported, "It seems unbelievable to me that I can feel so ill, as if I am dying, but I look just fine."

Affliction, whether emotional, physical, or spiritual—or all three simultaneously—can be a doorway to transformation and growth. Participants were encouraged to break their silences and open themselves to the truth of their situation and share what they had lived and learned.

The people who reveal their feelings and experiences in the second half of this book are at various stages of acceptance and growth. Some of the questions and dilemmas explored include:

• How do you cope with the uncertainties and the challenges of your concealed illness or pain?
• How do you hide your symptoms from those around you?
• Do you hide your symptoms from yourself?
• Do you withdraw from the world?
• Do you become a master of illusion and disguise? (Most people with

concealed symptoms become incredibly effective actors!)
- Have you acquired some valuable coping tools along the way?
- How has this concealed illness or chronic pain impacted your life?

The chapters ahead will examine the best time for someone to disclose their disease or condition. The initial sting of diagnosis and how others have responded to their illness will be explored, as well as the doubt from others and self that often accompanies a concealed disorder. I will examine medical care from traditional to complementary medicine, the hidden impact of symptoms on loved ones and coworkers, and the fickle nature of flare-ups. Finally you will see the special problems of intimacy, self-care, and learning to embrace a more realistic pace.

I wrote this book from the perspective of the person who is living with a body or mind that no longer functions as effectively as it once did. Although there are many medical and mental health professionals, as well as alternative and complementary health practitioners cited in *Just Fine,* this is not a medical book and is not intended to be used as such. Rather, it uniquely explores those individuals whose internal lives runs contrary to their outward appearances.

All of the individuals profiled in the book are featured with a first name (or a pseudonym) and the first initial of their last name only. You will meet Mike E., a young comedian who hides his own kidney disorder and bowel disease from those he works with. He carries a heavy secret and reveals some of the challenges of maintaining an undercover existence. Nancy G. was an active and hardworking social worker, but since a life-changing auto accident, she has been unable to continue her career or even manage to get a decent night's rest. However, her challenges have led her life in a new and exciting direction of placing specially trained animals with people in pain. Lisa V. is a young woman in her early twenties who lives with systemic lupus erythematosus, an inflammatory, autoimmune disorder that affects various parts of the body including the joints, blood, and kidneys. This disease derailed her modeling career, altered her friendships, and impacted her ability to travel. Even so, she considers herself fortunate and discusses why in the following pages. These people and many others have learned not to define themselves by the illness or condition that exists in their body. They have a disease, but they are not the disease.

No one knows where their particular passport in life will ultimately take them. Just weeks before turning in this manuscript to my publisher, I was interviewed by a writer in her late fifties. She was researching and writing an article for a prestigious university newsletter geared to physicians, medical researchers, and nurses. The article would focus on what it was like to live with unremitting physical symptoms. In her fifty-nine years, she had not experienced chronic pain or illness in her own body. After we chatted for awhile, and I discussed a bit about my own dietary and physical restrictions and the chronic nature of my symptoms, she sat back against the couch cushion, paused for a long while, and finally spoke. "You and I live in different countries," she said. Initially, I was taken aback by her comment. I wasn't quite sure what she meant by this abrupt observation. "Your days and concerns are so different from mine, and other healthy people," she said with an intense, but compassionate gaze. She was right. She awoke each morning with very different concerns, priorities, and anticipations than I did. We looked at each other, laughed, and talked for another hour about how true this statement was for countless others. I had become grateful for many things that she was not generally aware of during the course of a day. On the other hand, she could enjoy activities that now seemed out of my reach. In sharing more details about our own "countries," we learned a great deal about one another and learned a new appreciation for things in our respective worlds that we hadn't reflected upon in a long while. Ultimately, we had both traveled a road very different from the one we had intended on venturing along. However, a change in scenery and a shift in destination are not necessarily bad things. New expeditions can open our eyes to promising horizons and new ways of seeing life.

This book is a salute to a very special, but ever-growing group of individuals who live in this very different country, where chronic symptoms greet them in the morning and tuck them in at night. This book places a spotlight on the people who live with concealed chronic illness or pain, the challenges they face, and the facades they must wear to camouflage themselves in the world of normalcy and good health. Beyond the medical elements included in the introductory discussion of chronic disorders, the intimacy of experiences and the feelings exposed and expressed by the participants themselves will raise the collective consciousness of friends, relatives, and coworkers who live with, or know someone who lives with, concealed chronic illness or pain.

There is a spectrum of fear and confusion that medical tests and medications cannot address or measure. This is where shared human strength, insight, and experience are needed. The power in knowing you are not alone is immense and as necessary as medical treatment. It can keep your spirits from sinking into a dark place of isolation and despair.

The message relayed by the images and essays in this book is "not one of pity overdue for those who find themselves living with chronic illness or pain," as Dr. Margaret Elizondo, a physician with a thriving private practice in family medicine, observes: "In the face of uncertainty, sacrifice, chronic struggle, and recurrent setbacks, the individuals in this book and in my medical practice have endeavored to persist. Their tenacious resolve should be an inspiration to us all." [1]

Although the term invisible illness has been used in the past to describe particular illnesses and conditions, I have fashioned the phrase concealed chronic illness and pain in *Just Fine* to describe the wide variety of conditions and diseases of the body that easily hide from view. My greatest hope is that the profiles featured here will help to inspire and educate others while illuminating the shadows of fear and self-doubt that often accompany these concealed disorders.

Note to Reader: Various forms of healing were researched and explored for *Just Fine* because many of those who live with chronic disorders seek relief through complementary, as well as conventional medical care. A comprehensive list of the practitioners interviewed is featured in the Resources section located at the back of this book.

Acknowledgements

This book is a jigsaw puzzle made up of many pieces, each of them unique, and each of them essential to the completion of the mission. I am pleased to have the opportunity to express in writing my heartfelt thanks to the many people who have helped make this book possible and who helped me complete this intricate puzzle. First and foremost, I owe an enormous debt of gratitude to the courageous men and women featured in these pages who have so openly and selflessly shared intimate details of their lives in the hopes of reaching and benefiting others who are fighting their own battles with concealed chronic illness or pain. Their candor and courage to share the defeats, as well as the victories, are what bind the pages of this book. I also wish to thank the members of the support group I facilitated for nearly a decade. We exchanged so much healing and humor, grief, and joy, and finally, a camaraderie that only soldiers of a common battle can come to know. The extraordinary benefit of getting to know each one of these individuals is something I will always treasure.

A special note of appreciation to a select group of physicians, nurses, and mental health professionals for allowing others to benefit from their knowledge and insights: Malcolm Robinson, M.D.; Bill McCarberg, M.D.; Margaret Elizondo, M.D.; Geneé Jackson, Ph.D.; Michael Wrobel, Ph.D.; Marie Zadravec, R.N.; Hollie Ketman, L.P.N.; Daniel Kalish, D.C.; Jan Yaffe, M.F.T.; and Bejai Higgins, M.F.T. An additional note of gratitude is offered to the complementary health professionals who generously shared their knowledge and experiences in these pages.

A message of thanks to Rolf Benirshke, former placekicker for the San Diego Chargers, for embodying an encouraging example of a life lived with courage, resilience, and inspiration. I'd like to offer a personal note of appreciation to Marsha Patinkin, Grandma Doralee Patinkin-Rubin, Gail Hawkins, Dave and Marilyn Koster, Trisha Stewart, Carol Westover, Iris Kenney, Diane Jepsen, and Mel Billik for their dear friendship and keen eyesight. A special word of gratitude to Lee Silber, an author born to inspire other writers to march toward their goal with unwavering determination, and to Sudie Moran, for her assistance with the book's website. A personal thank you to three special angels: Margaret West, Barbara Watkins, and Alicia Avila Outcalt, who forged with me through the darkest hours of my own illness and pain.

And last, but certainly not least, a heartfelt expression of gratitude and love to my husband, Don Kenney, for cheering me up and cheering me on as I continue to navigate a challenging obstacle course called concealed chronic illness.

Introduction

Has someone ever said to you, "You look great!" while inside you felt ill, fatigued, or were in profound pain? Imagine facing the dilemma of appearing a certain way, yet feeling quite another, nearly every day. People who live with a concealed illness or hidden condition do just that. However, even if they are not visually apparent, these illnesses and symptoms are most certainly real.

Just Fine: Unmasking Concealed Chronic Illness and Pain reveals, through words and pictures, how the special population of people who live with these unseen illnesses and chronic conditions often conceal their physical challenges and project themselves to the world in a particular manner that is contrary to the way they feel. These individuals choose to wear the mask of normalcy and often appear just fine, despite having to contend with a host of invisible and difficult challenges.

Since not all illnesses manifest themselves outwardly, people sometimes have a difficult time believing that a person with a healthy appearance and lively demeanor can have so many symptoms and limitations. Several years ago, actor David Lander (Squiggy, from the *Laverne and Shirley* television show) announced that he had been living with the symptoms of multiple sclerosis for a number of years. In 2002, actress Teri Garr revealed she had been living with multiple sclerosis for nearly two decades. People were shocked when they heard these reports because she, like David Lander, still appeared healthy. There were no telltale signs of illness or difficulty with function. Michelle Akers, an Olympic gold medalist, became the world's best soccer player while battling chronic fatigue syndrome. She always appeared perfectly healthy. So did former Miss Pennsylvania-USA for 2001, Jennifer Watkins, who has talked openly about her diagnosis of fibromyalgia, a painful condition that affects more than 2% of Americans.

Anchor and news reporter, Cynthia McFadden, has suffered for many years with a serious illness of the digestive system called Crohn's disease. There is nothing in her appearance or manner that divulges her illness. She appears energetic and in perfect health. Nicole Johnson, Miss America (1999), became an inspiring role model for people living with diabetes, which currently affects 17 million Americans—almost one out of every ten adults. Laura Hillenbrand, the author of *Seabiscuit,* is a young woman who suffers from chronic fatigue syndrome, which leaves her with vertigo, weakness, and other difficult symptoms. It took nearly four grueling years to research and write her book because she often was forced to go for long stretches where she was unable to emerge from bed. Her persistence during the exhausting years she wrote *Seabiscuit* is a testament to the strength of her spirit, even during the most debilitating days of her challenging illness. Susan Olsen, the cheerful youngest sister on the television show *The Brady Bunch* suffered from chronic migraines when she was a child. Actress and talk-show host, Rosie O'Donnell, put a face on the illness of clinical depression. Ironically, it looks like the same face she had before she revealed her illness. Rolf Benirschke, former placekicker for the San Diego Chargers, suffered for years with ulcerative colitis, and more recently was diagnosed with hepatitis C. He appears robust and stays active with his wife, four children, and a demanding career in finance. We all know the story of actor Michael J. Fox. He spoke openly about his battle with Parkinson's disease, but only years after his initial diagnosis. In the years immediately following his diagnosis, Fox appeared healthy with no change in appearance or noticeable physical struggles. He still made us laugh. He still had a spirited and boyish appearance. We never suspected that anything could be physically awry or that he was living with difficult and debilitating symptoms.

A person with concealed chronic illness or pain can look great while feeling miserable. However, this appearance of looking just fine can be both a blessing and a curse. The family of concealed illnesses and conditions includes, but is not limited to: diabetes, lupus, endometriosis, Crohn's disease, fibromyalgia, post-polio syndrome, epilepsy, narcolepsy, chronic fatigue syndrome, hepatitis, thyroid disorders, multiple sclerosis, arthritis, Sjogren's syndrome, ulcerative colitis, nephrotic syndrome, migraines, polymyalgia, Raynaud's disease, hearing and vocal disorders, asthma, bipolar affective disorder, interstitial cystitis, hypertension, alcoholism, polycystic ovary syndrome, Ménière's disease, certain forms of cancer, chronic pain, chemical sensitivities, and environmental illness. Most of these illnesses and conditions are represented in this book.

No instruction book exists to guide people living with concealed but often challenging illnesses and conditions. The symptoms of fatigue and pain that are present in most of these disorders are difficult if not impossible to see. People who live with chronic symptoms must learn to adapt to new limitations. There was a time in their lives when they would promptly recover after being sick or feeling poorly. But now they find themselves riding a wave of symptoms that wax and wane and never quite go away. This is a tricky ride to maneuver, especially for someone who is accustomed to having good health and a prompt and reliable recovery.

The average person becomes ill and waits for recovery from whatever ails him. Renewed health may not come quickly but eventually does arrive. Those with a chronic, but concealed, illness or pain have to redefine this portion of the illness because chronic translates into a roller-coaster ride that doesn't end. The ride often goes from calamity to calm, but never comes to a screeching stop. A chronic disorder never resolves and recovery doesn't occur in the typical sense. One may recover from the shock of illness but not from the illness itself. This is where it is essential to develop and utilize new skills.

Personal and career-related goals that once seemed reasonable become out of reach. Former goals must be replaced with more attainable ones, and new lifestyle rules must be developed and adhered to. Days are often filled with doctor visits, new medications, and medical tests. Social activities and trips are either rescheduled or canceled. Jobs are difficult to maintain and are sometimes lost. Relationships are affected and forever altered. First the body and then the spirit take beatings as the person adjusts to a new and unpredictable way of living. However, the news is not all bad. There are also benefits to this upheaval. New skills such as flexibility, wisdom, and compassion are learned, and a new resilience and strength can emerge as a result of these disruptions and challenges.

The terms concealed illness and concealed condition refer to those chronic disorders that do not necessarily influence how a person appears to the outside world. These sorts of health challenges offer no visible evidence of suffering or pain. In short, individuals who live with concealed chronic illness or pain look like everyone else. However, the unpredictability of their symptoms and the invisibility of the associated disability often lead to complex challenges. Family members, friends, and coworkers are often affected as well, and their lives are changed in a variety of ways.

Chronic or concealed symptoms twist and turn a person's fate. Routines, once taken for granted, soon become rattled, and goals remain just out of reach. Since the symptoms of these disabilities often flare-up and then calm down, planning activities days or weeks ahead of time is very difficult. Activities sometimes have to be canceled or postponed. Attending a job or school can become especially challenging and can cause persistent anxiety or depression.

Hidden symptoms can impact a person's quality of life, restrict a long-standing lifestyle, and leave the ill person feeling defensive, stigmatized, and at times, misunderstood. As symptoms wax and wane, there can be a sense of loss. This includes loss of body control and loss of control over income, job, and relationships. Life itself spins out of control.

"The worst part of this illness," reported one person in the book, is "not having control over whether or not I will have a nice day." It is impossible to make plans, commit to vacations, or even take a trip to see a movie. This lack of control over symptoms can leave a person feeling as though they live within the body of an unpredictable stranger. For people who are in the habit of planning a month or a year in advance, simply making plans for activities the next day becomes a challenge and a frustration.

Well-meaning acquaintances, family members, and friends, who say, "But you *look* fine," can often unleash a sense of anger or compound feelings of isolation in the person who lives with multiple challenges that are hidden from view. The person with a concealed disability would much rather hear, "I cannot imagine the difficulties you experience and still manage to live a productive and meaningful life. You are incredible!" Our visually oriented society seldom takes the time to look beyond the appearance. People tend to believe what they see; and if an illness or condition cannot be seen, it does not exist.

Most individuals who live with an invisible illness or well-concealed disorder do not give in to it. When faced with strenuous situations, they tend to push themselves beyond their comfort levels. They know from experience that their limitations are not perceived, understood, or even accepted by those around them. Therefore, why should they limit themselves? As a result, they pay a high price for overexertion, which often aggravates the condition or illness. Symptoms may worsen for days or even weeks. Sometimes, having a good day is simply having a day that is realistically paced.

Honoring limitations is one of the most difficult challenges a person with a concealed disability must learn to do. These people tend to move beyond their comfort levels into more psychologically comfortable spaces so that they appear normal and perfectly capable. Over time, they must learn the fine art of managing their illnesses and learning to say no to many of the activities and chores most people take for granted.

"One of the disadvantages of having an invisible health challenge," reports Trish G., a school nurse, "is that your behavior is frequently mistaken for negative personality traits, such as laziness, being a complainer, and not being a team player at work." Trish lives with inflammatory bowel disease. "I leave my job early sometimes and take sick leave at other times. I'm sure many people think that I'm just lazy. It's difficult for people to understand how I can feel great one minute and incapacitated or exhausted the next."

Later in this book, you will meet Marie Z., a registered nurse, who was diagnosed with systemic lupus erythematosus. Marie and many others who appear healthy, but feel quite fatigued and symptomatic much of the time, believe that people who have a visibly apparent illness or condition tend to be believed more easily than those with concealed illness or pain. Marie's friends look at her and see the same person they always knew. They do not take her health challenges seriously because she appears just fine.

"I feel that living with a hidden condition is much different and more difficult than contending with one that is more noticeable," reports Shawna F. who lives with the severe pain of endometriosis. "It is quite disheartening and frustrating to be in the emergency room in the middle of the night, doubled over in pain, and the guy next to you with a bad knee is taken in first. People see the visual signs of his pain with the obvious swelling and discoloration and have more sympathy, while the source of my pain is not obvious."

Maria D., who lives with the fatigue and symptoms of hepatitis C, no longer tries to act tougher than she is. Beyond the extreme fatigue, she experiences fever, nausea, and stomach pain. "I used to plan big days and then be miserable because I couldn't keep up. I don't feel normal, even if I look normal. I have to plan all of my activities now. For instance, today I have a yoga class, and I need to pick up my medications and shop for vegetables. I am worried because I don't know how I will do it all. I get so frustrated when I can't even shop and clean my house in the same day."

Prior to a serious injury, Kathleen H. was a bright young court reporter. Her life felt very much in control. "Until this figurative train wreck in the middle of my life, I had no problem living and working within certain expectations of myself. Now, and quite suddenly, all control is gone. I'm not living the way I had planned, and I don't know how to fix it so that I can." I noticed that Kathleen seldom smiled during our first meeting together. The train wreck, as she called it, had taken a tremendous toll not only on her independence, but also on her psyche.

"I notice how people act when someone who has a noticeable physical challenge passes them on the street," says Laurie E., a tall woman with striking features who could easily be mistaken for a fashion model. "You can see that their reaction is based on the physical demonstration of an illness or disability. When you live with something that is not easily seen, or not seen at all, you don't get those reactions, and I often think that people doubt what I am saying about my illness. It is as if they think I am lying to them to gain sympathy. They seem to want me to be able to prove my illness or limitations to them so that they can see it with their own eyes."

Some people who have an undetectable chronic condition or illness spend much of the little energy they have trying to blend in with the crowd. "I just force myself to move and do whatever needs to be done when I am in public or at work," says Jill D. "Of course, when I get home I am totally exhausted and usually in a lot of pain. So, I pay for my charade. I am learning not to force myself to do this or that, but it is difficult."

"Sometimes I think I should just go into acting!" Shawna F. laughs. She lives with the painful symptoms of endometriosis and already feels like a seasoned actress. "I should win an award for some of the roles I've had to play in trying to hide my pain and symptoms from others."

Mike E. performs stand-up comedy routines on the road and often at a night club in a posh tourist town close to his home. His wife is a physician and they have a young son at home. Mike suffers from a chronic kidney disorder and has undergone a serious surgical procedure for ulcerative colitis where his entire large colon was removed. "If I appear healthy," says Mike E., "then the expectation is that I will be able to engage in all normal activities. Therefore, I must either lie about why I cannot participate, or reveal my hidden illness. In either case, I must respond to the expectations of others. None of this is easy. It seems that if people cannot see an illness, then it does not exist or is not valid. I often remind myself that just because someone looks healthy on the outside, that appearances do not always tell the entire story. My appearance certainly doesn't tell my story."

People who live with concealed symptoms try to control all that is within their control. These individuals must be smart about what they eat. If they have bladder or bowel problems, they should carry a change of clothing with them whenever they leave their house. They must remember to take medications at the proper time. "If people start limiting themselves because of what-if thinking," claims Bejai Higgins, a marriage and family therapist, "there is no end to asking that question. Pretty soon they will not even leave their bathroom, and no one is going to go in there and dig them out. It's their life and no one else's life. At some point the person has to realize this, grab the bull by the horns, and move on as best they can."

Some people who experience chronic symptoms and pain never receive a clear diagnosis. If a diagnosis is finally heard, the person may feel bombarded with a great number of questions such as:

- How will it change my life?
- What can I eat and not eat?
- What activities can I no longer participate in?
- Will this affect my mind, as well as my body?
- What side effects do the medications have?
- What treatments are available?

There is a tremendous amount of information to gather, which can become overwhelming. Going to educational seminars on a particular condition or seeking a support group where other people have similar symptoms can be worthwhile and comforting.

People sometimes treat individuals who have these concealed conditions as though they choose to have their illness or pain. They are unaware that the person with the disorder has lost many opportunities for achievement because of their symptoms and challenges. The portraits presented in this book, coupled with comments from the individuals themselves, will cast a new and more realistic light on the inner experiences and feelings behind the masks of normalcy. The combination of words and images in the last part of *Just Fine* will tell a more complete tale than if limited to one expression or the other. Coupling images with experiences and emotions will enlighten readers and connect them in a new and profound way to the vast community of individuals who live with concealed chronic health challenges.

Part One

Deception, Diagnosis,
Disclosure, and Deviation

One

Why Seeing is Not Always Believing

About Face

It may seem true that every picture tells a story. However, after further scrutiny, it is more precise to say that every picture, and in particular every portrait, has the ability to un-tell a story—either convey a false impression or reveal a mere fraction of the person it hopes to reveal. Photographer, Rollie McKenna, once stated, "There cannot be one definitive picture, since we human beings have many facets."[1] This is certainly true of the portraits in *Just Fine,* which present the guise that is normally revealed to the world. The illusion displayed through a pleasant and healthy appearance is at the heart of this book and the collection of images, where what you see is not necessarily what is true. One must read the accompanying text to discover what is actually going on behind the masks often worn by individuals who live with chronic illness or pain.

Human nature, for the most part, is visually oriented. We believe what we see and often make character judgments based solely on visual perception. But, what happens when the person who *appears* healthy, energetic, and just fine to family, friends, and coworkers, is quietly suffering from chronic pain or the challenges of an ongoing illness?

Most people feel divided as they wrestle with internal rifts. They often imagine they are split into two conflicted parts, with one representing genuine emotions and the other showing the facade they are compelled to project to others. The array of feelings and experiences within is not easily revealed. This is especially true for the person who is ill, yet appears to be perfectly healthy.

Linda F. is in her forties and has lived with diabetes since she was a little girl. However, most people express surprise when they learn this. Why? Because she looks healthy and does not seem to be suffering in any way. Other people do not see the injections she must self-administer throughout the day. They cannot detect the challenges of following a stringent diet plan for all meals consumed. "To wake up in the morning and lead a normal life must be wonderful," says Linda. "I begin my morning with insulin injections, followed by more of them throughout the day."

Imagine, on a daily basis, feeling as shaky and weak as you do when you have a bad case of the flu. People like Leslie W. don't have to imagine such debilitating and chronic symptoms. She lives with the ongoing exhaustion and pain of lupus, a disease in which misguided immune cells attack the body's

28

DNA, and fibromyalgia, a syndrome of widespread musculoskeletal pain and fatigue. "I know people have trouble accepting these illnesses and the fatigue that goes along with them. I look perfectly normal and just fine to others. They want me to stay the same, but on those days that I'm feeling bad, I cannot do the things they expect me to be able to do—the things I used to do so effortlessly."

Marilyn M. was brought up to do everything for herself. Independent by nature, she certainly does not like to admit that she needs help. "I'm sure I give the impression that I don't have a problem with pain, and that confuses people. On the one hand, I'm saying 'I hurt and am tired,' but if they look at me, they don't see the pain and fatigue. They certainly don't see the beaten spirit that has emerged as a result of my chronic symptoms."

Society is not attuned to the needs of people with hidden disabilities. While many feel compelled to help someone with an obvious physical challenge, they may respond negatively when asked to help or provide special accommodations to someone who appears healthy and looks just fine. Yet, a growing segment of the population is dealing with the profound limitations and challenges associated with concealed illness or pain. "It's discouraging and demoralizing to be in pain every single day," says Peggy S., who lives with the chronic symptoms of fibromyalgia. It is one of many heterogeneous illnesses; meaning that each person may experience the same disorder in a variety of ways. "Sometimes I become overwhelmed with the pain. It wears me down and takes a lot of explaining because most people cannot relate to being in pain all of the time."

"I often wonder why I have to deal with it and why I haven't gotten better," says Laurie E. who lives in chronic pain. "I have asked, begged, pleaded, and demanded to be better and to be healthy again. As each day goes by and I'm still dealing with my illness, the core of who I am feels shaken. On the other hand, my spiritual base is stronger. Somehow, I find the strength to get through each day. I still have glimpses of a normal life here and there, and this affords me the ability to cope and to face each new day. I have developed such strong coping mechanisms that I am now able to face trials in life in a way that my friends can only imagine. I watch others who are unable to cope with the small events in their lives and this makes me feel thankful for the new inner resources I have developed."

Leslie W. becomes more irritable when her symptoms worsen. "I don't explain anything to anyone. I just keep to myself." As far as her friends and family can see, she is perfectly healthy. She used to care about doing everything well. "Now, I don't try to do my best as often. Just getting through each day takes enormous planning and effort."

Steve B. has a deep-seated love of music and was once employed as a disk jockey. He recently suffered a diabetic-related stroke. Steve struggles with his words as he recounts how this last episode left him discouraged and unable to do the things he has always enjoyed. "I try to do things that I used to do, like play the guitar, or try to repair something, but I fail. Abilities such as walking and physical sensations such as touch are diminished. When I had my stroke, the left side of my face and my speech were affected. As a former radio broadcaster, this had an impact on not only my mood, but on my very essence—my spirit. I thought that I would never talk on the radio again. A couple of years later, after regaining my speech, I finally did go back to work on the radio doing news and traffic reports. That was a small, but significant, victory for me."

Ken L. is a young man who plays in a rock band. However, his chronic pain and concealed illness have shaken his foundation. "I went from being a guy who lifted weights, trained in karate, rode a mountain bike, and did computer graphics, to someone unable to do any of those things." Ken is now twenty-nine years old and has moved in with his parents to try to make ends meet. He can no longer do computer work, sit very long, or drive for more than an hour. He cannot carry anything. "Nothing sends me into hard-core pain faster than computer work," reports Ken. Unfortunately, his livelihood depended on it. Now, he must secure employment that does not require him to use his upper body in any repetitive manner. "It's like becoming a dependent child. It's very disheartening and embarrassing, and leaves me feeling ashamed." On the other hand, Ken has found other forms of strength in his new challenges. "I have no alternative but to accept the new cards that have been dealt to me and to rise above my circumstances and challenges. I believe that will happen. It may take years, but there are many others who suffer much more than I do. I always try to remind myself of that."

Carol C. is a young woman who has undergone a liver transplant and lives with a serious chronic disease of the colon. She has been reminded, in a most profound way, the importance of taking time to smell the roses. "I do not take life for granted anymore," says Carol. "In addition to appreciating what being alive means and how precious each day is, I try to remind others who are in dire straits that better days do come."

Despite appearing healthy, people who live with a concealed chronic illness or condition often suffer greatly, but quietly. They may have to contend with unrelenting pain, loss of bodily functions, limited exposure to sun or physical activities, debilitating fatigue, and other chronic symptoms. An otherwise strong-willed individual may be tested repeatedly, and as a result, their enthusiasm for life may be impacted. Some become too ill to work and are forced to abandon vital activities and careers that had long been a source of profound joy and fulfillment.

Many times, an illness can go undiagnosed for years, which can leave the person feeling depressed and frustrated. They cannot understand why their body no longer "cooperates" in one way or another. Similarly, perplexed physicians are at a loss. Medical schools focus little on the unique challenges associated with the treatment of patients with no observable symptoms and inconclusive test results. There appears to be a desperate need in this country to train physicians to care for people with chronic, but concealed, disorders. "This is the most important arena for many, if not most, physicians in their everyday professional lives," says Dr. Malcolm Robinson, a noted gastroen-terologist and medical director of the Oklahoma Foundation for Digestive Research. "Physicians are often poorly equipped by training or personality to deal with invisible illnesses and hidden conditions. This needs to be rem-edied at all stages of medical education."[2]

The Quiet Storm

Most people with concealed illness or pain do not gracefully surrender. They valiantly do battle with their symptoms and yearn for their previous life. They fondly recall a time when a flight of stairs didn't seem akin to climbing Mount Everest. They long for a good night's sleep and a pain-free awakening. They remember easier times that didn't involve a perennial quest for a restroom. They miss earlier days when travel was not fraught with unpredictable symp-toms.

This battle to evade a new life with challenging obstacles usually persists until the body forces individuals to concede and make significant allowances for their symptoms. "The biggest adjustment that I've had to make is learning to accept my limitations in spite of my intense, highly competitive personal-ity," says Shawna F. "I was an all-state, tri-sport athlete and had to turn down three scholarships because my body just couldn't keep up with my mind any-more. It is very frustrating when you are raised to be active, and you have talent, but you are no longer able to do the things that you enjoy."

People with chronic illness or pain are survivors, and accepting limita-tions is in conflict with the code that survivors live by. No one wants to be sick. No one chooses to give up those things in life that bring joy. Yet at some point, people with chronic disorders need to learn to say no to many things that have always been a part of their lives. Being told to look on the bright side by well-meaning friends and family members simply adds insult to in-jury. Positive platitudes and quick-fix suggestions trivialize pain and symp-toms and cheapen the impact of these difficult and relentless challenges.

Chronic pain is real. Yet it becomes difficult to talk to friends and family members about it. Not only do people want to be free of chronic pain, they do not want to feel like a burden. "It's a large part of who I am. I just don't want to be pitied by my friends or be known as 'the suffering one' to those I love or the people I work with," says Donna L. "Everyone becomes tired of hearing about how much I hurt, including myself! Some people think I am making it up or exaggerating my symptoms. But chronic pain is very real. Even the medical community doesn't always take my pain seriously."

Pain management is at the vortex of incompatible agendas among gov-ernment watchdogs, insurance companies, doctors, and patients. Fear of ad-diction is the key issue. Concerned that patients will become addicted, doctors are sometimes hesitant to prescribe painkillers. However, individuals with chronic pain, or those who require significant pain management, rely on anal-gesics just as a diabetic depends on insulin. Erica D., a mother of three, counts herself fortunate. "I now have a good doctor who does not shy away from the issue of pain management. He prescribes the appropriate medication when needed and necessary. I go about my life, but when the disease acts up, I'm not afraid to medicate and then move on."

Some people who live with painful conditions feel the need to be stoic about their plight. They see their pain as a sign of weakness, or feel their character is being disparaged because of their suffering, and thus refuse to manage their symptoms with effective medication. They deprive themselves of the relief that may allow them to regain a better quality of life.

When people who appear in robust health receive disability insurance payments because they no longer have the stamina to meet a job's demands, they often must contend with suspicious coworkers, supervisors, the disability system, and even family members. "What do you do all day?" is a frequent question asked of those who find themselves unable to work. After all, they appear as if they should be able to work. Some observers actually feel envious and often decide that an illness-based hiatus is an undeserved vacation. They imagine that someone with a disability enjoys copious free time with unlimited opportunities for fun and extracurricular pursuits. In the overwhelming majority of cases, nothing could be further from the truth. Healthy appearances notwithstanding, those who live in the cradle of disability benefits are usually profoundly ill. On most days, the disease takes center stage and requires 'round the clock management. In fact, disability insurance recipients usually deal with a raft of debilitating symptoms on a daily basis. Oftentimes, they are chronically fatigued because they don't get the rest they need. They spend their days wrestling with intractable pain, cognitive problems, and the side effects of medication. They are so busy trying to appear able-bodied that they spend a full day attempting to accomplish the things that a well person can easily achieve in an hour. If people with the disorder are able to simply clear away their morning dishes or take a short walk to the mailbox, they experience a sense of great accomplishment.

Before her illness, Leslie W. enjoyed a fast-paced life. Now, she derives peace and fulfillment from the completion of small tasks. Even so, she can still become frustrated by her new, slow-paced life. "What used to take two hours, such as cleaning the house, now takes two days!" The house-bound world of the seriously ill person is quite small. These individuals must use their strength to maneuver through the medical world of doctors and tests, drug side effects, and the trial and error of both successful and unsuccessful treatments. A very precious commodity, energy must be reserved for the most important activities. Therefore, those who are very ill must forego many of the simple tasks and pleasures that people with healthy bodies take for granted.

People who live with concealed chronic illness or pain often need to revise their expectations of themselves. They must learn to redefine their notion of achievement because the old definitions cannot be relied upon to offer a sense of feeling worthwhile or skilled. "I help clients accept the concept of a new normal. And within this realm they can make decisions to live a life with meaning," says Jan Yaffe, a psychotherapist for twenty-seven years.[3]

Yaffe helps her clients, many of them cancer patients, appreciate their new uniqueness so that they can embrace their illness as just one part of themselves.

Jill V., who lives with chronic fatigue syndrome, used to enjoy strolling through art shows and attending neighborhood concerts. "I no longer go to crowded gatherings such as street fairs or concerts or malls, because all the stimuli wear me out. I don't drive very far anymore, because freeway driving is too much for my nerves." She also cannot sit through classes anymore, which is especially difficult for this young woman who loves to learn and would like to further her education. "I have not been able to read since this illness began because I have trouble concentrating."

Steve B. lives with his wife, his two daughters, and his strange new bedfellow, diabetes. The illness has turned his world upside down. Diabetes is a progressive disease that may take years for symptoms to develop. For that reason, it sometimes is referred to as a hidden or concealed disease. Steve was warned early in his life that he was prone to diabetes, but since there were no signs of the illness, he continued to eat and enjoy everything on his plate. As happens all too often, Steve's illness has become quite serious over time. A short list of his disease's significant complications includes toe amputations, heart problems, a stroke, and severe depression. Now on insulin, he suffers from impotence and feels much older than his years.

As mentioned, Steve B. loves music and used to play the electric guitar. Music was much more than a hobby; it provided an outlet for his feelings—his joys and his sorrows. "I was never great at it, but I entertained myself. I definitely used to be better at it than I am now. Because of a diabetes-related stroke in 1990, I am unable to form certain musical chords on the guitar. That is very frustrating, and this frustration destroys my desire to sit down and play." In addition, Steve used to like to fiddle with and repair electronic gizmos. "Electronics used to be somewhat of a hobby with me, but because of diabetic retinopathy, my eyesight does not allow me to see details clearly any longer, and soldering the wrong wires together is definitely a bad idea!"

Daily lifestyle adjustments for diabetes include rigid adherence to scheduled meals, testing blood glucose levels, and self-injecting insulin or taking oral medications, depending on the disease's severity. Steve's illness has had a radical impact on his diet, all of his activities, and most importantly, his zest for life. However, his supportive wife, who is a nurse, and two daughters keep him going. His wife's nursing skills certainly come in handy with his diabetic ups and downs. But Steve is a self-proclaimed rebel. He knows that better eating habits and attitude could have a more positive impact on his disease, but sometimes he refuses to play by the new rules. There are periods when the anger and resentment of having to live with a chronic health disorder persist for a long while.

Steve was once at the top of his game. His career was flourishing and his spirits were high. He now drifts in and out of hospital stays and finds himself in temporary jobs which afford far less stature and satisfaction. Diabetes, a disease whose complications present microscopically over a long period of time, attacks the cells of every body component. He notes, "I've had to make adjustments for every physical attribute (especially in dietary habits) and for emotional stability as well." Steve discussed diabetes' catch-22, one that characterizes a variety of other chronic conditions. "Exercise is a major factor in the control of diabetes, but exercise is difficult when you are walking impaired." People who live with chronic fatigue syndrome, lupus, or fibromyalgia also have trouble getting enough exercise, even though physical fitness is critically important for their general health and mental outlook. "My doctor keeps telling me to exercise five days a week," says Nancy G., whose muscles continually ache from the pain of fibromyalgia. "But how can I do that when I feel like I have the flu seven days a week? I feel guilty for not doing more, but. . . I just can't."

Guilt is a wasted emotion, but people with a concealed illness or condition spend a good portion of their time generating heavy doses of it. They feel guilty if they are sick too often or if they feel tired all of the time. They spend an inordinate amount of time obsessing, berating themselves, and generating self-destructive, wide-ranging litanies that chronicle their shortcomings: "I don't help with the kids as much as I should; I don't feel as sexual as I should; I'm not earning as much money as I once did; I'm not saving enough money; I'm too moody; I don't do as much shopping as my spouse; others do more for me than I do for them."

"Even though I did nothing to cause my diabetes," says Steve B., "I am the only one who can control it. Guilt has become my constant companion. Frustration is also ever-present, because of the things I can no longer do. Anger is not only a way of life, but a detriment to my health. Along with diabetes comes high blood pressure. Ironically, my anger about having this disease raises my blood pressure!"

Adjusting to a new disorder impacts the internal and external life in a multitude of ways. People who live with a concealed illness must refresh and embrace their spirituality in a way that releases the angst they feel towards the illness, even if the lift is temporary. They face an overwhelming range of challenges as they wrestle with guilt and self-blame. They must assign new roles to family members and to themselves. They must learn a new set of rules for their lifestyle, one that involves simplification, rationing out their energy for the most important daily tasks, and pacing themselves through the ups and downs of chronic symptoms. They must somehow learn to accept all of the emotions surrounding their new limitations and challenges. But first, they have to learn what those limitations are.

Leslie W. has lupus and fibromyalgia, neither of which affects her healthy appearance and energetic demeanor. She is just beginning to be mindful of her reduced capacity. "When my fibromyalgia acts up, I slow down. The lupus forces me to rethink my daily activities, so I'm constantly restructuring my days. It's like learning to ride a bicycle again. I'm learning to change the speed on my bike to slow!"

At some point, people who live with concealed illnesses or painful conditions stop trying to cure themselves or fight the disorder and instead work toward a peaceful co-existence with their disorder. "I say 'no' to a lot of people now," says Jill V. "I used to hate canceling for fear of appearing 'flaky.' All this has changed. I realize now that I have only a certain amount of energy, and I have to be very picky about where I spend it."

Frequently, there is a dichotomy between image and reality. The line between who appears disabled and who is disabled is a ragged one. Most of us are guilty of drawing sweeping conclusions based on appearance. Though this is only natural as we assess someone's abilities, it is important to realize just how deceiving looks can be. Someone in a wheelchair may be perfectly capable of grocery shopping, cooking, and driving the city streets, whereas another who appears fit and able-bodied may have trouble walking to the end of the block or gathering enough stamina to prepare a simple meal.

"Many who suffer with chronic illness struggle to maintain a degree of normalcy in their lives," says Dr. Margaret Elizondo, a family physician who sees an array of chronically ill patients throughout the day. "If the malady does not affect the person's outside appearance, that person has the opportunity to keep the beast hidden from others. We all want to buy into the image of good health, and we want others to buy into it as well. For some, putting their symptoms on the backburner and ignoring their limitations is an expression of denial; for others, it is a survival mechanism."

It's staggering to grasp the most recent statistics that show fourteen million to twenty-two million Americans, mostly women, are currently contending with autoimmune disorders. They include lupus, fibromyalgia, Raynaud's syndrome, rheumatoid arthritis, Crohn's disease, and many others. These perplexing illnesses and conditions strike approximately three times as many women as men, possibly because of the effects of female hormones on the immune system. Many times, the role of mother and the ability to sustain a career become elusive goals which leaves women vulnerable in the prime of their life, and in their reproductive years.[4]

Having a chronic illness or living with chronic pain changes not only how you do things but who you are. In the face of extraordinary physical challenges, some have an easier time than others honing in on the strength and hearty wisdom necessary to reinvent a different life and new vision for the future. Inevitably, a former self, as well as a previous way of being in the world, fall away and give rise to a new way of functioning and embracing life.

Two
The Crisis of Diagnosis

Learning to Change the Rules

Crises revolve around disruption. A radical change can separate one's present life from the past and introduce a new and puzzling set of life rules. People who suddenly face an onslaught of chronic symptoms feel severed from their past. They are fired, like a cannon ball, from a familiar setting into unknown territory. To the people around them, nothing appears to have changed because appearances have not been altered. However, behind the mask of normalcy exists an inner world of shifts, fears, losses, and rediscoveries taking place. This disruption doesn't merely threaten the body's comfort level, it threatens an established way of life that has disappeared. It disrupts the everyday self.

A disabling illness or pain can hit suddenly or crawl slowly into one's path, disassembling a person's routine. What was once taken for granted and easily accomplished is now a constant stream of uphill battles and obstacles. Responsibilities in relationships may need to shift, lifestyles may have to be modified, and moods may fluctuate more frequently. Others who have been available in the past may slowly, but surely, pull away. There will always be people who are threatened by illness or fearful of people who are different from them because it reminds them of their own potential helplessness. However, new acquaintances who understand the importance of support and the special challenges of chronic symptoms may suddenly appear and take on important and supportive roles. Resources abound. They include community support groups and online chat rooms that focus on a particular condition or illness. Eventually, a few important and significant relationships may develop. Old friendships may shift and family relationships may either strain or become richer and more defined. Having to relearn how to live one's own life is not an easy chore.

"The biggest hurdle in having a concealed disorder is finding out what it is," says Michael N., who spent many frustrating months running from one specialist to another trying to find out what was causing his pain and other symptoms. How do most people react to their initial diagnosis of a chronic illness or condition? For some, that reaction is shock and fear; for others, it is disbelief. For Michael, however, there was a sense of relief and validation that a name had finally been connected with his array of symptoms. A diagnosis confirmed his suspicion that something was wrong. "Patients appreciate being able to deal with the known as opposed to the unknown, and therefore appreciate a specific diagnosis," says nurse Marie Zadravec. "But, if they don't know what to expect, there is also an element of fear."

When Leslie W. received her diagnosis of lupus, her initial reaction was one of validation. "Finally, all of this had a name. Next came fear. No one could explain exactly what lupus was. They could only say it is incurable and fatal unless properly treated. The fear began to set in when I was advised that I was in the final stages of the illness. I cried a lot. I felt alone. Nobody could possibly understand how alone you feel when going through the initial diagnosis. Other people's lives would go on, but mine looked like it was ending. I felt so alone."

"When I was first diagnosed," says Mike E., "there was a feeling of 'why me?' because I had always taken good care of myself. It was hard to accept that, while others smoked and drank, I was the one who had become ill. It seemed so unfair. I was constantly envious of the vigor of others around me."

Jaye B. was working as a nurse when she received her diagnosis of inflammatory bowel disease, a serious digestive disorder marked by abdominal pain, diarrhea, weight loss, and an array of other disabling problems. Inflammatory bowel diseases include Crohn's disease and ulcerative colitis. Even though Jaye B. worked in the medical field for years, her reaction was one of absolute horror. "I must have looked like a deer in the headlights. In the x-ray department, I saw the terminal ileum in my digestive system on the screen and, because I am a nurse, I recognized the disease. The doctor later confirmed what I had seen and already knew. My parents were at my house when I got home that day and I was able to tell them the name of the disease, but I didn't elaborate on the seriousness of it. I didn't want to alarm them. Basically, I think that I was numb. Later, I realized that I was relieved to know that my signs and symptoms were based on an actual disease process instead of being all in my head."

David K. is a school teacher in his fifties who felt enormous relief—mixed with a bit of confusion—at the diagnosis of his illness. "The first thought when I heard that I had Crohn's disease was that this is the best news that I have heard in a long time. My next thought was, what the heck is that? I had never heard of Crohn's disease. I had spent about twenty years with misdiagnoses of my symptoms—generally being told that my problems were 'all in my head.' Then the doctors decided that I had advanced cancer of the colon. They told me that they were sure it was terminal. The first time I heard the correct diagnosis of Crohn's disease, I was being wheeled out of the operating room. I heard my wife's voice yelling to me, 'It's not cancer. It's Crohn's disease!' and I felt a huge sigh of relief."

Once people hear a diagnosis, after they have endured long, arduous diagnostic testing where it was difficult to determine the root of their symptoms, they feel relief. They finally have an anchor to which they can ground their worries, fears, and anxieties. Based in reality, their situation suddenly becomes focused. "People tend to be more frightened when they have very little knowledge or information about the diagnosed condition," says psychologist Dr. Geneé Jackson, whose practice focuses primarily on treating those with chronic illness and pain.[1]

Living with a concealed chronic illness conveys a unique set of issues. Often, people with these disorders feel isolated and different from friends and family. Their easily concealed symptoms can elicit not only the suspicions of others, but the ill person's own doubts about whether the condition is real or valid. To fuel the fire, many of these types of disorders resist proper diagnosis for months, and sometimes years, because of their hidden nature. "My first diagnosis was that I had a psychosomatic illness," reports one man living with a serious autoimmune disorder. "I kept trying to change my thought patterns and relax in order to relieve my symptoms! Fortunately, I now have the correct diagnosis."

Nancy G. was in her mid-forties when she was diagnosed with fibromyalgia. Her initial reaction to the diagnosis was utter confusion. "I had never heard of it!" She became horrified as she realized the impact it would have on her career and social life. Her fear was that she would ultimately be unable to work and would have to resort to living on Social Security disability income. After pushing herself beyond her physical limits for a significant period of time, Nancy reluctantly filed for State disability benefits. Ultimately, her fears of being unable to work and having to live on disability income materialized, but Nancy's world did not end. She did, however, have to make considerable adjustments in her daily life and scale down her material requirements and housing needs.

Marilyn K. and David K. have been married for over three decades. Each lives with a different chronic illness that carries its own unique set of challenges and symptoms. They claim, quite emphatically, that their separate conditions have actually brought them closer. "Both of us have a chronic illness and it has been an interesting journey for the thirty-five years we have been married. Most of the time, we have been lucky that our individual flare-ups have happened at separate times so that one of us has always been able to keep things going in the household."

For some people, the crisis following a diagnosis can feel like a brutal slap in the face. Sometimes it is possible to diminish the fear and anxiety that accompany a new diagnosis by learning relaxation techniques or sharing feelings about the disorder. A person may feel overwhelmed and may wonder how to cope with all of the symptoms and adjustments. However, instead of asking "What if I cannot cope?" the question should be "How can I cope?" Even so, how does one regain a sense of self-worth and accomplishment when an illness makes it impossible to do the numerous things that were once easily achieved?

Dr. Geneé Jackson works closely with people who face a variety of chronic health challenges. The task, she says, is to redefine and broaden the person's identity so that the previous sense of self extends beyond the usual social roles. "This kind of personal work can be very challenging, depending on how someone has been socialized. Those whose self-value has been based on their ability to serve others, to please others, or take care of others, will have to stretch the most. What I help people do is shift their thinking in such a way that they view their own needs, comfort, and happiness as equally important as those of anyone else. For example, I will ask a hard-core caregiver-type to imagine themselves as being a child, friend, or family member in need that is looking to them for protection and nurturance. At any given moment, they have to ask themselves, What can I do for this person that would be most helpful? What is in their best interest? Is this person sad, hungry, tired, or overwhelmed? How could I help this person be more comfortable or feel better? Now imagine that person in need is you."[2] The person with the concealed disorder must learn to listen and respond to their own needs, just as they would listen and respond to the needs of others. It may take a little practice, but these skills can be developed over time.

People with a chronic, but concealed, illness or condition must learn to become their own best ally. Dr. Michael Wrobel, a medical psychologist who works with the growing population faced with chronic illness or pain, tries to reinforce several important concepts to his clients, including that they are dealing with extremely difficult situations. He tries to help them understand that real meaning and worth do not derive from what a person used to do. He also tries to help people get in touch with the feelings of self-worth that existed before they were stricken by illness. "They are still there now," says Wrobel. "People need to grieve the loss of things they can no longer do and find activities that remain doable." This important first step in the healing process takes place in the psyche.[3]

"Like any loss," adds psychotherapist Jan Yaffe, "there is often denial, numbness, shock, anger, bargaining, depression, and hopefully, acceptance. I let my clients tell their story, and I listen empathetically. I validate their feelings—all of them—because all their feelings are real for them at this moment. Clients need to know that they are not alone. I assure them that I will do everything I can for them, that I will walk with them through this journey and help them discover other resources: support groups, books, articles, doctors, alternative treatments, friends, and family. What does my client need at this point to feel grounded, to accept their illness, and to move along with it? The real question is, given the givens, how can I help them find meaning in life in a new way?"[4]

The onset of a chronic illness or condition is the beginning of a new adventure that often involves the loss of many familiar aspects of one's previous life. Goals, control, flexibility, energy, and independence can all be impacted. "Sometimes, I will just begin crying because I do not feel I have a future anymore," says one of this book's participants. Faith in a better future often has to be turned a bit to reassert itself: Tomorrow may be easier. If not, there is always the next day. The person new to chronic illness or pain must slowly begin to do several things: rearrange priorities, become more realistic, recognize new limitations as well as new goals, and hone new strengths. Accepting yourself as a mix of strengths, as well as weaknesses, becomes a vital life lesson for those who live with chronic symptoms and new limitations.

Good Grief

Feeling constant pain or living with a concoction of debilitating symptoms is not on anyone's wish list, and grief is a natural response to these unwelcome visitors. But the loss accompanying chronic illness or chronic pain can be different from the anguish that surrounds a terminal illness. The nature of chronic illness is that you can be in remission and feel relatively normal one day only to be catapulted back to raging symptoms the next. It is difficult, and quite different, for those who lament losses that generate unrelenting problems than for those who mourn one defining loss.

Diane M. has lived with chronic fatigue syndrome and migraine headaches for over a decade. She spends the mornings in bed resting and sleeping while her husband gets their daughter ready for school. Like many people who live with chronic fatigue syndrome or fibromyalgia, deep sleep is elusive at night. Many people try to capture a few moments of rest here and there during the day to make up for the missed hours of deep, restful nighttime slumber. As Diane struggles to come to terms with the chronic nature of her illness, her anger bubbles to the surface. She often asks herself, "What did I do to deserve this?" Eventually, she realized that she had done nothing that had ignited her condition. "But, sometimes," she adds, "it just feels good to rail at something."

When people get stuck in their anger, they can become annoyed and at odds with everyone and everything. "I've taken good care of myself. I've always exercised, eaten right, and had checkups with my doctor. I prayed to God every night. I went to church on Sunday. I took good care of my kids. It just is not fair." They see the people around them—family members, friends and coworkers—living idyllic lives. Sometimes, people with illness or pain resent those who tell them what to eat or what they should or cannot do. "They act as if I am already knocking on heaven's door." If people remain like this, bitterness can displace all of their energy, and anger can begin to eclipse the enjoyment of just about everything life has to offer.

This year has been particularly difficult for Judy R., a young single woman who has lived with the ups and downs of Crohn's disease for most of her adult life. Normally an upbeat and gregarious person, she just emerged from her tenth intestinal resection surgery and says that she feels she is at the end of her rope. "Going under the knife is usually no big deal for us veterans of surgery," Judy says with a slight smile, "but this last one was difficult, not only on my body, but on my very spirit. I am still here, so I won the battle, but I feel as though I'm losing the war."

Judy and others who endure multiple surgeries sometimes begin to feel helpless, hopeless, and depressed. And as each scar replaces the previous one, even the hardiest souls begin to perceive themselves as damaged goods. The depression that accompanies such repeated physical challenges can damage self-esteem. "This illness leaves me feeling like I'm defective—not just physically, but emotionally." When she is quite ill, Judy and many others have difficulty remembering what good times and pleasant thoughts felt like. Conversely, remissions have an amnesiac quality and enable people like Judy to forget the frightening and depressing periods. Remissions blessedly provide shelter from painful memories and sensations and transport those with serious chronic conditions to safer ground. Judy emerged from her last emergency surgery with feelings of helplessness and hopelessness. Her wonderful sense of humor and her ability to cope got lost in the haze of too many hospital procedures and a plentiful menu of medications. She sank into despair and a deep depression.

By working through grief and loss, however, people with concealed chronic illness move forward into their new life. They learn to reduce stress by lowering their expectations; by generating new, more attainable goals; and by minimizing or reprioritizing the must-do tasks in order to get through the day, the morning, or the hour. Sound decision making and the successful completion of chores and simple activities often translate to a greater sense of well-being.

"Write a letter to the pain," suggests psychotherapist Jan Yaffe.[5] "Talk to others and embrace who you are when you are with the pain. Instead of feeling trapped, boxed in, and helpless, locate a community support group for your particular condition or illness. There you will find solace, comfort, inspiration, and knowledge." If depression emerges, ask others who are in the same situation how they have coped. Individual therapy is also very helpful. It can provide a fresh perspective, an alternate look at the pain and symptoms, and can enable an individual to value life in new ways.

Diane M. spends most of her days in bed or working at her desk. She has become an avid writer as this is a form of expression that requires the power of the pen and not the entire muscular system. Diane's house is spacious and located in an upscale seaside community. She obviously adores her home but spoke sadly about having to put it up for sale. Diane was not able to continue her career as a social worker. The chronic nature of her symptoms made maintaining a large house and mortgage payments impossible. The loss of her income was becoming too great a challenge. Like most people who can no longer work because of an illness, something had to give; that something was this beautiful home that she had worked so hard to acquire, a home that all her family had come to love. This left her deeply immersed in a state of depression for some time.

There is no preordained schedule for moving from grief to acceptance. Often, emotions overlap. However, most people begin their journey of acceptance with feelings of denial. "Being on Social Security disability and having such an illness will never happen to me," thought Nancy G. "I still think I will get rid of it somehow." People who are newly diagnosed with a disease or condition are not prepared to deal with the loss of their good health. They may begin to doubt the doctor, the medical test results, and the seriousness of their health condition. A common response is to shield themselves from thoughts about the impact of a particular disease or condition. Filing these worries away and putting them on a shelf for another day is much easier. "It took me six years to stop working after the diagnosis," reports Nancy. She found herself stuck in denial and set up camp there for awhile. "It was extremely difficult to quit my business, and shelve my identity." Sometimes people use their denial to derive strength. "People tend to be very stoic at times and put their illness on the back burner," reports Hollie Ketman, a nurse who works for a rheumatologist. Ketman regularly sees patients who live with the painful symptoms and limitations of rheumatoid arthritis, osteoarthritis, and fibromyalgia. "They ignore it and downplay what is happening to them. It is their way of coping, and it works for awhile, but not forever."

Perhaps a person with diabetes or Crohn's disease might say, "I'm going to eat whatever I want. This condition is not going to take away my freedom to enjoy the foods I love." This type of denial is common to those who must adhere to a new set of dietary restrictions. Another person might say, "I may or may not take my medication. It's my decision and I don't have to if I don't want to."

Teenagers with chronic, but concealed, disorders are often legendary at denying their conditions. Since they don't want to accept reality, and friends cannot see their disabilities, why acknowledge it at all with diet restrictions and medications? Often an adult must intervene if teens veer too far off the pathway to remission or if they refuse to cooperate with their treatment plan. They still must go through the process of coming to terms with new limitations without giving up hope.

Knowledge is power, and when a person acquires information about their illness or condition, the need for denial and anger often dissipates. This puts the person and their emotions back in the driver's seat. Kim H. is a petite young woman in her mid-forties. She was diagnosed with Crohn's disease in 1970 when very little was known about helping patients maintain a decent quality of life. Treatments were limited and consisted primarily of steroids or surgery. "Living with this disease for many years has shown me that I must be an active participant in my own care. I have had numerous flare-ups, a few nice long remissions, and multiple surgeries. I have tried most of the drugs on the market with varying degrees of success. I have had four bowel resections, leaving me with twenty-one inches of small intestine and a condition known as short-bowel syndrome, which carries its own assortment of problems."

What has made the biggest difference has been Kim's attitude and willingness to make the necessary changes to achieve the best quality of life possible. "I have always pushed myself to live as normal a life as possible. If that meant taking prescription medicines, I did it gladly. If it meant giving up certain foods, I did that, too." To maintain her health at the highest level possible, Kim takes low doses of steroids, has given up dairy foods, salads, most roughage, and has limited sugar in her diet. "When I follow all of this, it works beautifully. Yet, I am like everyone else on any sort of diet. If I cheat, I pay the price."

Kim remained proactive when the odds were stacked against her, and this has paid off tenfold. Over many years of searching for a cure or a better approach to her illness, Kim traveled to many clinics that claimed to have the answer. They rarely did. She became discouraged after awhile as there was not a one-size-fits-all treatment for her disorder. Crohn's disease is as individual as the people who suffer from it, and people often experience varying degrees of success with treatments. Kim even traveled across the country to take part in a Federal Drug Administration clinical trial sponsored through Harvard University's Brigham and Women's Hospital to address the problems of short-bowel syndrome. Fortunately, she responded beautifully to their protocol. That is where she learned about diet modification, and she has stuck to her diet with great success.

Even while trying more holistic approaches, Kim never stopped taking her prescription medication. "If I decided to try a new alternative treatment, I did so while still taking my prescriptions. If I started to improve, the medication was altered with my doctor's assistance." Throughout a lifetime of trial and error, Kim grew dispirited now and then, but she never stayed down for long. She moved forward, stayed involved in her own treatment, maintained an attitude of determination, and eventually found a few things that worked well for her particular system and symptoms.

Those with concealed chronic illness may have to make not only financial adjustments, but drastic lifestyle changes. Although they once traveled without a second thought or ate whatever they desired without consequence, new restrictions now govern everyday life. Those with diabetes are limited not only by what they can eat, but also when they can *not* eat. "I adjust in the worst possible way," reports Steve B. "I ignore or deny it. My biggest problems revolve around my eating habits. A psychiatrist explained to me not too long ago that, since I am being deprived of so many ordinary functions, it's no wonder I'm depressed. Eating is the one last pleasure in life that I can still gain some momentary gratification from, even though what I eat can negatively affect my illness. My brother once asked me how I was able to quit a two-pack a day smoking habit cold turkey, but I am not able to control my eating. I told him that when you quit smoking or drinking, you quit, you don't just slow down. We all have to eat, so controlling it is harder. Sometimes you just do not want to."

"Friends, relatives, and even healthcare professionals will try to convince you not to feel sorry for yourself," states one man who lives with a chronic hidden condition. "I say screw 'em. You're damn right I'm going to feel angry and sorry for myself. I'd feel sorry for any other person who had to live with this, so why shouldn't I feel sorry for myself? The trick is to lament, cuss, be angry, or put your fist through a wall. Vent your anger, but don't let the anger consume you. Get it over with, pick yourself up, dust yourself off, and get on with the business of living."

The effects of illness are profound. As with any major life shift, there is a search for meaning. Why did I develop this condition or illness in the first place? Is there a rhyme or reason to its presenting itself right now, or did I simply become ill like so many others? There is also worry about what life is going to be like. "I am concerned that I will get to the point where I am not able to do much of what I enjoy doing," says Marsha S. When someone is diagnosed with a life-changing illness, there is always a reevaluation of the definition of life.

Marriage and family therapist Bejai Higgins says that her favorite aspect of counseling involves discussing with clients the shifts in life perception and self-worth. "I have had some wonderful conversations with people about what they think life is about and where they fit. Oftentimes, people will change their lives because of a chronic illness, mainly because they cannot work like they did before, just as I myself can't work as I could before I became ill with my own health issues. Some people find that what they did for a living before is impossible for them now. A client I had was very successful, but hated what he did for a living. He was an AIDS patient. When he found out that his life was going to be fundamentally different, he said, 'I don't want to do that anymore. That doesn't feel right to me anymore.' He decided to completely change his career. The last time I heard from him he was happy as a clam."[6]

Dave K. also has reevaluated his notion of success. He now derives a feeling of accomplishment as a father and husband, rather than from his career. "Many successful people have had to neglect their family, which can adversely affect their children," says Dave. "Seeing my children happy means more to me than a job, success, power, or material goods."

Fear is an integral part of living with a chronic illness or pain. There is often significant fear about the unknown future and how the physical disability will affect everyday life, relationships, jobs, family dynamics, self-image, and intimacy.

Linda F. has been a diabetic all of her life, so she is no stranger to fear. "Being alone and having an insulin reaction is a very frightening thought. I try to be very careful that this does not happen." For Steve B., who has adult onset diabetes, fear is a constant companion. "I experience fear of what will go wrong with me next; which function will I lose next; which function will become diminished? Will my children inherit my problem? I also feel sorrow for the normal life I might have led if it had not been for diabetes."

After a diagnosis come fundamental shifts. Living with a chronic illness often directs the person to look at life and decide what is important and then go after the top priorities. "They are no longer willing to wait for Friday night or two weeks in June to enjoy their lives," says Higgins. "This is the real strength of what happens when people are diagnosed. Priorities are clarified. New goals are set. New realizations are faced about what is truly important in their life."[7]

Higgins sees a lot of self-blame and anger in her clients with chronic illness. "A lot of people will say, 'What did I do to deserve this?' To this, I will always ask them, 'What's the worst thing you ever did?' I have never heard anything that would justify the kind of disability, embarrassment, and pain that these people experience. I usually tell them, 'Hey, that just doesn't sound bad enough to measure up. Maybe it isn't a punishment.' Only after coming to terms with their illness or pain can they help enlighten the people around them. Most of the people we're talking about are younger adults. I rarely see anyone over fifty years old. Most people who are sixty, seventy or eighty expect to be ill. But younger people with a chronic illness find that they not only have to deal with it themselves, they have to teach their entire support system how to be appropriate with them. And they are pissed off about that. 'Why do I have to tell them the right things to say to me?' they often ask. My response to this is, 'Well, you don't, but if you want them to know, that is the easiest way. You have to tell them because there isn't a course that someone can take about how to be a good caregiver.'"

Most people eventually reconcile themselves to their illness. They tolerate its intrusion into their lives. They manage the symptoms and rearrange their days as needed. In order to maintain some level of peace, they learn to hold the hand of pain and fatigue, not because they want to, but because they must befriend their symptoms.

An intrusive illness or condition leads one to feel out of control. The embarrassment of the inability to perform as well as they used to or the lack of productivity in their new life can lead someone to a new vision and a new way of defining who they are. People learn to embrace their good days and to tolerate the frustrating ones. As their daily regimen alters, they learn to catch the rhythm of a new set of rules. Eventually, an updated self can emerge from this new way of being. Embracing that new self can be the most significant success imaginable.

The Great Depression

Depression seems to tag along as an annoying side dish to chronic illnesses such as lupus, diabetes, hepatitis, Crohn's disease, multiple sclerosis, and many others. The rational question becomes, Who wouldn't be depressed if they were dealing with such persistent and debilitating symptoms? Depression is a reasonable response to what is happening to a person who lives with chronic illness or pain. There are a great number of changes and challenges to contend with, and most people would feel discouraged and experience some degree of depression if they had to try to navigate a medical system that seems to be at odds with their needs and a body that seems diametrically opposed to normal expectations.

Sadly, most people who live with chronic disease, pain, and suffering are not thinking proactively, yet they are often left to seek out mental health resources on their own. However, it is incredibly difficult to be resourceful when you are physically and psychologically debilitated. "I see antidepressants being prescribed to assist with fatigue," states Zadravec, "but with no mental health support or counseling adjunct therapy added. I feel that therapy is a piece of the puzzle that needs to be improved."[8]

Spending your days in waiting rooms or in hospital beds when you look perfectly healthy is no picnic. "I feel as though I am putting my life on hold when I am in the hospital," says Carol C., a young woman who has seen her share of hospital corridors. "I feel depressed, alone, and vulnerable in the hospital but try to remind myself it will pass and things will be better in time."

Depression is like being buried under an extraordinarily heavy blanket from which you cannot emerge. The poet John Keats once wrote of depression,

> I am in that temper
> that if I were under water,
> I would scarcely kick to come to the top.

Clearly, the weight of this depth of depression often goes hand in glove with chronic disorders.

"Depression is understandably the most common associated symptom of chronic pain and illness," says Dr. Geneé Jackson. "When depression follows the onset of the illness, it is typically related to a loss of physical mobility, cognitive functioning, social connections, and other lifestyle changes. When a person hurts all the time, an incredible amount of energy is used just living from one minute to the next, and the joy of living becomes lost in the haze of a painful existence. This sense of loss often starts early in the course of an illness or chronic pain condition, typically looks like grief or mourning, and can last for several years. The problem becomes much more complex with time as multiple areas of a person's life are affected. Depression can cause an increase in pain levels, sleep disturbances, appetite changes, and a host of other serious symptoms. It actually creates biochemical changes in the brain, which in turn can aggravate the original problem. As a psychologist, I recognize that a current depressive state can often be linked to, and fueled by other major losses. Treatment becomes more manageable when the person can recognize what has been triggered for them that may not even be directly related to the illness. One by one, we can examine the core issues that underlie the sadness and develop and identify needed resources, both internally and externally."

Frequently, the level of depression of people whose health is severely compromised can leave them feeling unwanted and unlovable. They may believe they are of no use to others and perhaps feel that their suffering is a sign that they deserve to be punished. Sometimes people can feel angry in a spiritual sense, and their core belief can be, "I have been unfairly punished." Without acknowledgement and appropriate constructive action, this type of anger often camouflages a depressive state. "This gets back to the issue of finding and creating meaning from experiences that involve hardship and difficulty," says Jackson. "This type of depression is often a general loss of faith in those things once seen as important. Depression can also be based primarily on biochemical components brought on by a drop in serotonin levels due to an ongoing pain that causes sleep deprivation. In these cases, the person can often be helped by antidepressant medication."

Dr. Jackson encourages people who live with chronic concealed illness or pain to try to reach out to others to help counteract the social isolation that typically occurs. People who live with chronic conditions need to know that they are not alone. They need to avail themselves of community resources such as support groups, pain clinics, and even day spas for relaxation or full body massages with someone who is knowledgeable about chronic pain and illness. Often, challenges with physical mobility can make leaving the house very difficult. One way to deal with this problem is to write letters, join online support groups, and make frequent phone calls to those who offer the greatest comfort. Nonverbal techniques such as creating artwork, doing simple dance movements or yoga in the comfort of your home, or playing a musical instrument, can also counteract feelings of isolation. Sometimes a simple craft project or a wild dance in the living room, accompanied by flailing arms and sweeping movements, can work wonders toward counteracting some of the most desperate and hopeless feelings.

Additionally, those with chronic concealed illness or pain must educate family and friends as much as possible about their condition or disease process. Clearly, contending with a chronic illness can be a full-time job with numerous responsibilities. No wonder fatigue and depression are part of the chronic illness and chronic pain picture.

As a clinical psychologist working primarily in an institutional healthcare setting, the majority of patients referred to psychologist Steven Hickman are individuals who have a dual diagnosis in the nontraditional sense. Traditionally, dual diagnosis is a label often applied to individuals who have a substance abuse problem along with a psychiatric diagnosis. In this situation, however, the dual diagnosis is typically a chronic physical illness in addition to a psychiatric diagnosis, and that psychiatric diagnosis can often be depression.

Dr. Hickman sees many individuals with chronic pain or chronic illness, who are also depressed and anxious about coping with both their illness and associated life issues. "I do the bulk of my clinical work in conjunction with a multidisciplinary chronic pain treatment program, so many of the patients I see have chronic pain. This can range from individuals with back pain due to a variety of causes (including trauma, disease and unexplained); to people with myofascial (muscle) pain due to fibromyalgia or other illnesses; abdominal pain due to gastrointestinal disorders; cancer pain and a large number of other etiologies."[9] Hickman also treats those about to undergo lifesaving liver and kidney transplants and patients with chronic diseases like diabetes, HIV, lupus, chronic fatigue syndrome, and many others. He sees himself as unique in the healthcare system, as he is often the only person not treating the specific medical diagnosis involved, but instead treats the person. They come to him, or are asked to see him, because they are manifesting symptoms of depression, anxiety, stress, or fear. While they often conclude that their physician has referred them because the physician believes the illness is "all in their head," this is typically not the case. "In the vast majority of cases referred to me," says Hickman, "the primary treating physician or specialist has recognized that the patient's psychological condition is not optimal and may be hindering the process of proper medical assessment, negatively impacting treatment, or preventing the person from improving his or her level of everyday functioning."

In the type of psychotherapy Dr. Hickman practices, the aim is to balance concerns about medical issues with coping skills and strategies. "I often end up playing the role of coach to some patients who have difficulty communicating in an assertive manner, helping them to formulate strategies to address their needs or questions regarding medical treatment. In other situations we are more focused upon life beyond the examining room and devising lifestyle changes such as exercise, healthy eating, sleep hygiene, relationship issues, and occupational concerns. The restoration of balance between medical illness and the rest of life is often crucial to patients. As they get more and more focused on their illness' symptoms such as pain, treatment, and functional limitations, they can easily lose perspective. They literally become their diagnosis and their identity revolves around having fibromyalgia, or chronic regional pain syndrome, or tinnitus or Crohn's disease. While this is certainly a prominent part of their situation at the time that I see them, they have often lost track of the fact that they are infinitely more than their diagnosis, despite how it feels at the time."

Dr. Hickman talks with patients about the familiar pain-level question that physicians often ask: "What is your pain on a scale of one to ten?" He points out that physicians and patients alike almost universally loathe that question. "Physicians dislike this question because it is not empirical and is too subjective (but in the absence of any blood test or x-ray that can quantify pain, a necessary one). Patients struggle with this question because they often see the pain as so overwhelming that they find it impossible to rate. Furthermore, patients often respond with numbers off the scale, e.g. fifteen, that exasperate physicians and nurses who believe the person is exaggerating their pain unnecessarily." Hickman, on the other hand, likes this scale (including the possibility that someone will rate their pain as fifteen) because he does not see it as a scale determined by a single factor: pain. "Specifically, I suggest that the rating is a composite of two subcomponents of pain: sensation and distress. Sensation is the actual neural impulse from the affected area going to the brain. It signals various sensations including burning, twisting, wrenching, tingling, searing, pulsing, etc. Distress, on the other hand, is the emotional component to the sensation. This can include fear, sadness, grief, anxiety, despair, hopelessness, helplessness, anger, etc. This component of the pain rating could also be called suffering. Thus, a person with a chronic back pain sensation of seven on a one–ten scale, who fears that they will lose their job, that their marriage is failing due to their physical limitations, and is feeling guilty over the accident that caused the initial injury, could have a distress component of eight, leaving a total of fifteen."

Mary N. lives with the unpredictable symptoms of an illness that leaves her looking perfectly healthy and fit most of the time. She also lives with an accompanying clinical depression. "It's a double-whammy," she says. "When my symptoms become intolerable and stop me in my tracks, I allow myself a couple of days of saying 'not again!' and 'why me?' Then I give myself a swift kick and tell myself that I cannot let it win. I give myself a limited amount of time to come to grips with my body's latest betrayal and do whatever I can to get back on my feet. I have found that the longer I stay down, the harder it is to get up and get going again. Our lives are every bit as valuable as people without these types of challenges. That is what I try to remind myself of as often as possible."

There are days when Mary can complete a lot of little tasks. "Other times I accomplish zilch. Sometimes when I'm really feeling down, I think to myself, there is probably someone who is equally as down. Sometimes when I need something, such as attention or a lift in my spirits, I call someone on the phone and talk to them and listen to the problems they are having. I try to give them a little bit of encouragement. That, in turn, encourages me. To get out of that inertia of being down in the dumps over this illness, I lie on the bed and chat with people for hours on the phone. Sometimes I have to force myself to do this because within myself, I guess I don't really want to. But once I get up, and speak up, it helps tremendously."

There is no doubt that chronic conditions can cause varying degrees of depression. In many ways, it is a natural and expected reaction to the challenge of living with chronic symptoms. However, most people eventually determine that if they are able to locate the seedling of who they are, apart from their body's piercing pain and profound suffering, they can rediscover their enjoyment and appreciation of simply being alive.

Three

The Sticky Door of Disclosure—
Poised at New Portals

If you decide to tell others about your illness, whom do you tell? Do you keep it hidden from the scrutinizing eyes of coworkers, supervisors, friends, and family? Whom can you trust with this profound secret? Will your health worsen if you tell others, or might it improve, absent a disguise of boundless energy and good health? Will you feel like a failure in their eyes if others know about your flaws? Will they reject you? Will they doubt you? After all, you look perfectly healthy and just fine to them. Also, if you do decide to tell, how much do you reveal? Should you remove the mask of illusion, or should it remain securely fastened? If you do not wish to be viewed as being a sick person, deciding whether or not to disclose your diagnosis or to disguise your limitations is very difficult.

There is little doubt that opening up to potential partners about your illness can be stressful and risky. Many people who live with a concealed chronic illness or condition often have to make a choice about if, when, and to whom to disclose their condition. And they have to repeatedly make this difficult choice. "In a sense," says psychologist Geneé Jackson, "this is akin to 'coming out of the closet' and can be hard for several reasons. Sometimes it is because of your own struggle with acceptance. You find it difficult to accept the limitations posed by the illness or to accept an identity for one's self that involves the label of being weak, helpless, needy, unusual, or even unworthy. To see yourself as someone who needs help, extra care, or stands out as different or strange, can be experienced across a continuum from uncomfortable to intolerable. You might actually be projecting your own internalized biases and stereotypical beliefs about what being a sick person means. The same social influences that helped create these biases in you form the same negative beliefs in others, coloring their perceptions of you. These people are often your family members, employers, friends, or professional colleagues."[1]

Depending on a person's situation, disclosing a chronic condition can sometimes mean a loss of advantages such as employment, insurance benefits, friendship, marriage, or the respect of colleagues. In truth, only those who live with physical pain or symptoms can determine what the true cost of disclosure would be to their well-being and whether they are ready and able to handle the outcome.

Diane M. says that she no longer tells people about her chronic fatigue syndrome or migraines. "I'm sick of thinking about having this illness, and I'm sure everyone I am close to is sick of it, too. I try to focus my life away from my illness as much as possible. I've had to make major adjustments, and within those, I just try to get on with things and be as happy as possible. I like the feeling that I am just a regular person, not a sick person who needs extra sympathy or who is complaining all the time. I did that for a long time because I had to share the burden of my illness. The constant misery was too much to carry alone. But now, I'm just trying to get on with my life."

Rick D. makes his living as an engineer, but he also served in the Gulf War. He currently suffers from a hearing loss that causes some embarrassment and anxiety in managing his work affairs. Rick recounted his bitter battle with the aftermath of the war that left him with an autoimmune condition. This disorder caused partial deafness and the loss of his fingernails. Rick still was unsure if the disorder was the result of a virus or something else that he had been exposed to. He only knew that his life had been turned upside down by persistent physical challenges. His outward appearance revealed no battle scars. When I first met him, he was in front of his suburban house, still panting from an early morning jog. His shirt was soaked with sweat, and the winter sun was fooling itself into thinking it was summer. It was eighty-two degrees at ten o'clock in the morning, but Rick showed no sign of slowing down because of the heat. He looked tan and fit with no signs of illness, depression, or the anger that had been impacting his life. He grabbed his mountain bike and was ready to go for a ride after our meeting. "I have difficulty bringing up the subject of my hearing impairment to strangers or coworkers," he says timidly. "Many business situations do not lend themselves to a time or situation where I can stop and explain my condition and request that people speak louder. I usually try to fake it instead."

"I feel awkward letting people know about my disease unless it's in a healthcare setting," says Jaye B., a former registered nurse who lives with both irritable bowel syndrome and inflammatory bowel disease. "When I ask for special accommodations, I don't elaborate, and usually, no one asks. For instance, I'll request an aisle seat at the theater. If I ever have any trouble, I'll simply cite the Americans with Disabilities Act and they will have to accommodate me. Fortunately, I haven't had to go that far yet."[2]

Disclosing a concealed illness or condition is quite different from revealing one that is, or will become, more obvious. After all, no one ever has to know, do they? They cannot see it, therefore, it does not have to be revealed. A visible disability does not permit a choice about whom to tell, how much to tell, or when to tell. When the illness is visible, information becomes public, rather than private, knowledge. Surprisingly, some people with a concealed illness or condition said they would opt for a visible condition over their concealed one. Why? So their limitations would be taken more seriously. "People don't readily see the problem and therefore they may not think a problem exists," reports Mary N. She lives with fibromyalgia, which is often accompanied by a variety of challenges such as sleep dysfunction, chronic pain, and cognitive problems. Mary's home has indeed become her castle, especially since she is housebound most of the time with the symptoms of fibromyalgia and profound clinical depression. Her husband danced in and out of the kitchen as she and I spoke about her years of pain. She had struggled for many years to keep the pain to herself. She spoke of her strong faith and of not wanting to bother other people with her own challenges. For someone who spends much of her time comforting others, she seldom feels comfortable letting people into her world of physical challenges. Mary was stoic in presentation and demeanor. She was not one to discuss her symptoms with friends or members of her church. She freely admitted that she had her share of dark days and suicidal ponderings. "People who know me at church would be surprised to learn just how deep my struggle has been. I don't talk about it. I don't want to trouble anyone with my own problems." Her deep religious beliefs helped to keep her afloat during the worst of times, and she restored and nourished her faith on her better days.

"When people think of illness in general," reports Sahar A., a young woman with inflammatory bowel disease, "they depend on seeing the results of that illness manifest in some visual way so they can compartmentalize it, justify it, and eventually accept it. Despite my medical test results, which are conclusive, I continually question what is making me ill on a daily basis. It is as if my mind cannot consider the disease as the culprit. If I am having this much difficulty accepting these parameters, I can only imagine the frustration my loved ones are having when trying to console me through my relapses of the illness. They themselves cannot visually see it, and therefore cannot comprehend it."

"People cannot see how weak I feel," reported Cindy V., who has lived with a chronic concealed illness since she was an infant. She now has babies of her own, works full-time, and tries to balance her daily responsibilities with an energy level that fluctuates with each passing hour.

Lisa V. is a single woman in her early twenties who lives with lupus, a serious chronic illness that often hits young people. She is nearly six feet tall and has distinct and lovely features. Lisa's smile never seemed to fade during our interview, as she explained how she used to be thin and was often offered modeling work, that is until the steroids she had to take puffed her cheeks and induced a rapid weight gain. Lisa's illness has turned her young life into a daily struggle with the side effects of medications and the illness' debilitating fatigue. Despite all of these challenges, Lisa continues to smile a big smile and wear the facade that is frequently worn by those who live with concealed, but chronic, symptoms. She believes that people have been conditioned to prejudge based solely on appearance. "Usually, the first idea that a person has in their head about someone is based on visual signs," she explains. "If you have a smile on your face or you have bothered to dress nicely, people have a hard time believing that you are chronically ill or in pain. There are so many invisible symptoms one might be experiencing at any given time: headaches, nausea, arthritic pain, fatigue, and depression, that an observer will be unaware of, unless of course, they are told."

Marie Z. is a registered nurse who also lives with lupus. "Most people in our society seem to feel more comfortable with visible evidence of illness or disability. It is harder for them to envision what they cannot readily see. I believe it may involve a trust component to accept what they are hearing, rather than what they are seeing. A visible illness is easier to accept because the visible evidence is harder to doubt."

"People never truly understand your limitations," says one woman, who has lived for many years with the easily concealed symptoms of chronic fatigue syndrome. "They may ask you to do something that is as impossible to you as walking is to a paraplegic or seeing is to a blind man. You have to keep reminding people what your limitations are. Many people cannot accept these limits and will badger you to just go for a walk or sit up long enough to do what they want you to do. They will tell you to quit whining or explain that they are tired, too, but still are doing things. Other people understand and do not expect more than you say is possible. But, having to remind them constantly is so tiresome. There are many who blame your limitations on a bad attitude or depression. The most ridiculous assumption is that, because the injuries to your body are inside and basically unseen, willpower, positive thinking, or prayer can heal them. People who tell me this think I am ridiculous when I say that is no different than trying to heal someone who just got run over by a train and has their leg severed. Will prayer reattach the leg? No, of course not. Nor would it rebuild the smaller sized cells that are badly damaged in my immune system, in my liver, and in my hypothalamus."

Nancy G., a social worker who is no longer able to maintain employment, feels that if her fibromyalgia were more visible, people would be more apt to believe the severity of her condition. "What they cannot see, they question as being real. They are also less compassionate if they have never experienced the pain themselves."

"How are you doing?" or "How are things going?" are two of the most difficult questions to respond to if you look healthy but are suffering with an array of concealed symptoms. These are simple questions that were once answered very easily without even thinking about them. However, once you have lived with a chronic illness or chronic pain, finding the correct response is complicated and confusing. Do you really feel fine or do you simply say that to avoid a delicate moment between you and the person asking about your well-being? Revealing an illness to someone may change or strain that relationship. You may risk feeling diminished in their eyes, or worse, you may be doubted and scrutinized. When you live with concealed chronic illness or pain, "How are you?" becomes one of the most complicated questions you can be asked.

For most people, revealing an illness means facing possible rejection. "I disclose pretty early," reports one woman with fibromyalgia. "One of the first questions I am usually asked is, 'What do you do for a living?' I have to reply, 'Well, I am on disability. . .and there we go." Another woman reports that she lets the people in her life know that she may need to cancel plans at the last minute. "Informing them seems to lessen some of the stress."

If one appears healthy, why would anyone believe they are not? The dilemma of disclosing often turns into the issue of control, or lack of control. Avoiding disclosure can mean maintaining distance, controlling the flow of information, and therefore preserving one's control over the entire situation. Since power and control are the very elements that diminish or are challenged when one is ill, disclosing that you are ill can further complicate the illusion of control and power. A concealed illness or condition can cause loss of endurance and function that only a discerning eye can detect. As a result of this, family, friends, and coworkers may discount the person's illness or fail to comprehend how it can possibly affect them.

Part of the success of disclosing one's illness or condition to others has to do with how comfortable you are with what is happening to your body. The more comfortable you become with your symptoms or illness, the more comfortable others will become. Strangely, that is often how it works. If it is no big deal to you, it won't be a big deal to others. Sometimes diseases such as AIDS or certain terminal forms of cancer cannot be kept secret. However, chronic illnesses such as diabetes, Crohn's disease, chronic fatigue syndrome, and lupus can often be concealed with little effort.

Becoming comfortable with what is happening within yourself is very important. Bejai Higgins offers her clients the idea of a dependency ladder. "At the top of the ladder, you are completely independent and you don't need any help from anyone. But as you go down the rungs of the ladder, you need more and more assistance from other people and it becomes obvious that there is something wrong with you. By the time you get to the bottom of the ladder, you're having to be fed and bathed and are back to a totally dependent stage, and our culture doesn't like people who are dependent. I mean, I have never been to a Dependence Day parade! Dependence is considered a failure. Therefore, I have to help people understand that dependence is a cultural value, not a basic truth. We must learn how to ask for help and how to tell people about an unseen health condition in a way that does not rob us of our individuality or our sense of control."

Higgins recommends disclosure of illnesses to workplace supervisors. To give one example of the benefits of discussing a chronic health condition with an employer, let us examine the case of someone with ulcerative colitis, a chronic illness that involves inflammation of the colon. This illness affects many young people and can be extremely disruptive to their work life and career. "Let's say in the middle of a meeting, you have to run to the bathroom," says Higgins. "This behavior has been noticed for awhile, and you are edgy and evasive. If you go out to eat with others in the office, you don't eat or aren't able to eat with them. If that weren't you, what would you think is wrong with that person? Drugs? Probably. Therefore, what is truly wrong is often not as bad as what people think is wrong."

How do you go about revealing your chronic physical condition to your supervisor without risking the security of your job or your position in the company? One suggestion that Higgins offers is to go in and say, "'You may or may not be aware that I have some physical problems. I'll make sure that they don't become your problems. Just allow me to do my job.' That's what a manager wants to hear. That you have a problem, you are getting it treated, and that you will make sure it does not affect your job or become a problem for your manager. This is a very in-control way of saying that you have health difficulties, but that you won't let them impact your job."

What if you choose to keep your condition secret, but you have to miss work here and there because of the symptoms? When there are frequent absences, management tends to think that the person is just not committed to the job. Under those circumstances, Higgins encourages her clients with ulcerative colitis, for instance, to go to their supervisors and say, "I have a condition which results in unpredictable gastric distress that is usually only troublesome for a day or two, so know that if I am not here, it is not because I'm out playing at Disneyland, it is because I'm sick." Higgins warns, "If you don't do that, you may find yourself marginalized as far as promotions are concerned. It may be assumed that you are simply playing hooky from work."

"We are always entitled to stand up for and get help regarding our legal rights. However, it is not always necessary to play hardball," states psychologist Michael Wrobel.[3] "If possible, express understanding of your boss' position and then do some problem solving. One can still do worthwhile productive work in an appropriate capacity. If you have to miss work, you can always make up the time. You may be able to prepare certain reports and correspondence from a home computer. By the way, once everything is appropriately discussed and addressed, disabled people are often found to be more productive than average workers."

Developing a plan for disclosure is a valuable project. This helps you determine how and what information will be revealed. The decision to disclose or not disclose is a very personal decision. Either way involves some risk. Will you lose your boss' respect if you tell him or her about the status of your health? The other side of the coin is that you may be granted more reasonable hours and assistance with your workload. Will you be able to take more breaks, or will you lose out on promotions or special projects? Disclosure can be a double-edged sword; there are arguments that can easily be made for revealing, or not revealing, a disability.

Learning not to define yourself as your illness is essential. "I am not my disease and I do not describe myself by this disease," reports one person with Crohn's disease. "When I do impart the news of my illness to others, I usually refer to it as the-disease-with-the-stupid-name." When people with the illness look upon their illnesses as something they have, rather than something they are, it can help lighten the dark cloud of disclosure. Another person explained: "I am bipolar, but that is simply something I live with and have to be aware of. It does not define the human being that I am at my core. It is simply a chemical imbalance and an illness that I must contend with." Another individual with a concealed illness described the situation by saying "I will forever have this disease, but as long as I can help it with an overdose of humor and good friends, it will not have me."

Have a Good Day Anyway

How do we change our priorities and perceptions about life and learn to redefine our self-image, our productivity, and our worth? How do we live a full life despite chronic illness or pain? We need to learn to redefine the meaning of a good day. Those of us who live with a concealed chronic illness or condition may have to relearn how to have a good day. We may have to teach ourselves how to be at peace and to redefine what feeling well or feeling fine truly means. We may need to challenge our previous notions of what faith and spirituality are and the roles they can play in our new lives. We may need to learn how to laugh again.

In many ways, individuals with concealed chronic illness or pain are given a chance for a new and different life. We have to learn to take care of ourselves with a gentle touch and modify activities so that they are more reasonable and realistic. Roles in our family may shift and wiggle about. Some family members and friends may initially resist new roles and responsibilities because they liked things just the way they were. We look the same, so why can't everything remain the way it used to be?

We may appear the same as we used to when we did not struggle with chronic symptoms; however, priorities may have to be adjusted and limitations must be taken into consideration. For example, if you cannot be as active outdoors as you once were, why not keep your mind active by using a computer? Write about your feelings, or start a novel. Express yourself through art. Pick up those felt pens or watercolor paints you once dabbled with in school, and attack the paper with whatever energy you do have. Many people, because of their illnesses, discover the gift of hidden talents.

Change is difficult but often opens new doors. Sometimes, it can help you explore old passions, hobbies, and talents that have been lying dormant for some time. This could very well be a new season of your life. Rediscovering some of your buried talents or latent interests allows you to rekindle new ways of getting involved with them once again. "The talent might be art, or music, making jewelry, or even personalized scrapbooks," says psychologist Geneé Jackson. "Even if you only spend fifteen minutes at a time reconnecting to these old hobbies that once gave you pleasure, it can help enormously. Maybe the person who used to play an instrument well but does not feel that he or she has the energy to do so now can still find great enjoyment in listening to the kind of music they used to play." Get in touch with other aspects of yourself—those areas that you can feel good about but are easy to forget because they are drowned out by the fatigue and pain of chronic illness.

"Many of us are overly identified with our work-world personas," adds Jackson. "We have learned to value ourselves in a doing mode. We define ourselves by what we do, have done, or will do in the future. We have to find a way to appreciate our being, as opposed to our doing."[4]

One woman felt her life had derailed in many significant ways when she began experiencing the symptoms of chronic fatigue syndrome. Panic can quickly seep in when the familiar patterns and tasks of everyday life become impossible to maintain. "I had to leave my job, school, exercise classes, and refuse some interesting career opportunities. I couldn't have a social life or travel. I lost friends and became isolated. I couldn't care for our family the way I used to or take care of the usual errands and chores. I could not buy tickets for entertainment activities, because I would most likely be too ill to attend the event. Our financial situation eroded. I don't know when, or if, I'll be able to resume a career and get my life back."

The Trauma of Travel

Diane M. has a young daughter and a husband to care for at home. She used to be a career woman with energy and goals. Now her goals are uncomplicated ones and are closer to home. She used to travel a great deal with her family, but as many people with chronic illness and pain quickly learn, traveling away from home is not always easy. There are the worries about feeling well enough while on the road, getting enough rest, eating the proper diet, and coping with the stress of change that sometimes unravels even the best laid vacation or business plans.

Diane and her family used to love to travel together. Now, having a good time on trips away from the comforts of home is very challenging, if not impossible, because of her symptoms. "I want to travel and not even think about the problems I'll encounter. If we stay in hotels when on vacation, I have to have a room in a very quiet area of the hotel—top floor, end of a hallway, etc. These special requests are hard on my husband. I can't sleep if there is any noise in the hotel and I often lie awake most of the night waiting for the first door to slam at 6:00 A.M. I'm usually exhausted from not sleeping on these vacations. I cannot fly anywhere in the morning. I can't take a long trip or even fly to see my elderly mother in Chicago."

"Try to focus on what you *can* do," suggests Marie Zadravec, a registered nurse. "Develop alternative activities that you are able to accomplish within your limitations." Hollie Ketman agrees fully with Zadravec's suggestion. Ketman works with patients on a daily basis who appear healthy but are dealing with a host of painful and chronic symptoms. "I try to have my patients focus on what they are able to do, such as walking half a block or warm water exercise," says Ketman. "They need to focus on the benefits of these seemingly mild activities. I urge them to start off slowly, work up to a goal, and try not to make the goal too high or too unrealistic." If a person is new to chronic symptoms and pain, and they used to travel all over the world, they may want to try short trips that are closer to home. Sometimes, just a minor change of scenery can do the mind, body, and spirit a world of good.

"We plan on going on a driving vacation, caravan style," explains Sahar A. "Of course, I will need to stop for the bathroom at every junction—especially if I try to eat like a normal person." Sahar has to watch her diet, the frequency of meals, and the types of foods she eats. "I will have a hard time with these diet restrictions. I also have to consider that I will need to rest when my family will want to play. How do I call it quits on a vacation? Am I allowed to get tired? What if I am in the middle of a relapse? What should I do? Keep popping steroids? Painkillers? Antispasmodics? What if, God forbid, I don't make it to the bathroom in time? That's my worst nightmare."

Field trips, family trips, and even family gatherings can be challenging at times. "I have to consider many personal factors into anything I agree to become involved in," says Sahar. "Once I give my word to do something, I will not back out, despite how I feel. I do not like staying or sleeping over at another person's home when we travel. I feel more comfortable with privacy. I require it, especially in light of this illness and the symptoms that are not the sort you want to share. I do not enjoy going out to eat very often. If there is something I want to eat, I would rather order take-out and enjoy the food at home without having to consider all of the other fear factors."

The list of things that people with chronic illness or pain are no longer able to do can certainly be a lengthy one. "I can no longer exercise at all without becoming dizzy," says Diane M. "When I became ill, I had been participating in an aerobics class three to six days per week. I was also beginning to teach aerobics while taking a post-master's class in exercise physiology at a local university. I had choreographed my own routine, and I was slated to be trained to teach classes at two different upscale health clubs. In addition to just keeping me in shape, I really miss the exuberance that exercise gave me. I miss the camaraderie of the people in the classes. As far as being able to mobilize myself to get places, absolutely everything in my life has to be close to home, or I can't do it. That includes doctors, dentists, counselors, my child's school, chiropractors, stores, friends, etc. Any kind of drive is out of the question, because I am too weak or dizzy to drive long distances. When I first became ill, I often prayed that I wouldn't faint while driving, and occasionally I still have that thought. All my plans are tentative. I usually have to confirm the day of an activity to make certain I feel up to it.

"I have been in leadership and helping positions all of my professional life," says Diane. She finds this new sick role very difficult. "Is it related to ego and self-esteem?" she asks. "Even though I feel comfortable with it myself, I guess that sharing this information with others puts your limitations out there in the public arena and suddenly others can comment or make judgments about you that you have no control over."

The Good, The Bad, and The Intrusive

Nancy G. loves children and always envisioned having a family. After her car accident, debilitating symptoms of fibromyalgia became her constant companions. "It changed my desire to have children because I can barely take care of myself now, let alone a child." Nancy now lives on disability insurance because of the pain of fibromyalgia. "I used to go dancing a lot, and gave that up, too, because of pain and increased sleep problems after such activities."

"My life didn't really get derailed so much as it changed course," reports Marilyn M., who lives with the chronic pain of migraine headaches and fibromyalgia. "Instead of doing a lot of physical activities, most of my activities and interests are now mental rather than physical, such as studying genealogy, computer work, and reading. I have not been able to work at a job that I would really like to have because I can't handle it physically. I cannot participate in physical activities with my kids, so I only observe. I just do the best I can and find other ways of exploring and experiencing the things that I still am able to do."

Many people with chronic symptoms and pain find pleasures in the simple things in life, the sorts of tasks and interests that got lost in the shuffle of a frantic day when they were just trying to hold their head above water. In the slower pace that comes from a managed life, the birds outside are singing a more noticeable song; the rain is falling in patterns that were missed in the hustle and bustle of the days that came before; sitting to sip some tea is a soothing respite for a body that is hurting and a mind that is trying desperately to cope. A new pair of eyes is beginning to awaken to see a fresh way of operating in this very different "country."

A chronic physical condition can lead us back to this simplicity and the enjoyment of life's little pleasures. Laurie E. discovered this after she came home from the hospital. "I spent a lot of time this summer planting flowers and working in the garden while I was recovering from my surgery. I felt better taking care of other things. It gave me a focus to have this to do, and to have something to think about other than my illness."

Kathleen H.'s life is now focused on coming to terms with the repetitive injury to her arm and the changes to a career that she loved. "I have worked very hard on not seeing myself as a victim. I am very proactive about what happens to me. This condition has been challenging and humbling at times, to say the least, but I have to find a positive in this negative situation."

"I have slowed down and enjoy whatever I do much more," says Trish G. "I have more time to develop spiritually and pursue my interests instead of being active, active, active all the time. I am much more sympathetic to other people and their problems, whatever they might be. Some things cannot be surmounted by sheer will, but must be adjusted to. This is an important lesson."

Marilyn M. echoes some similar thoughts on the challenge of living with a concealed chronic illness. "I always tell myself it could be a lot worse. I have learned to accept this new lifestyle. I grieved for my old life, and then put it away. Very few people have a perfect lifestyle; some are better than mine, and some are worse. I always try to keep that at the forefront of my mind."

Part Two

Meandering Through
the Medical Maze

Four

Waiting and Wading—
Patience and Possibilities

When you live with a chronic disorder, learning to play the waiting game is a necessity: waiting on the phone to make medical appointments, waiting for the bureaucratic wheels to turn so that you can receive disability benefits, waiting in doctors' offices with out-dated magazines sprawled across your lap; waiting for phone calls on test results, waiting at the end of examination tables in flimsy paper gowns while listening ever so carefully for the doorknob to turn, waiting in lines at pharmacies for prescriptions that may or may not help your symptoms. Most of this waiting is often done alone because your spouse or friends are at work. Then, of course, there is the waiting to awaken from the daunting dream that has become your new life.

How to be a Patient Patient

People who live with persistent symptoms try to be good patients. They try to do the correct thing for their bodies and for the people around them. The problem with the medical care system is that as symptoms worsen, patients in weakened conditions become more reliant on the healthcare system. And because their symptoms usually include pronounced fatigue, it is difficult to be proactive with a medical care machine that constantly asks them to sit, wait, stand in line, and try new treatments.

Sometimes, those in chronic pain or living with chronic fatigue do not have the energy to seek the help they need from medical or mental health professionals. They hibernate at home and isolate themselves from the outside world. Unfortunately, they focus more on what they cannot do than on what they can, and often lose faith in the medical system when there are no clear-cut tests or treatments for what ails them.

Many people experience a wide array of overlapping symptoms and syndromes. They are not merely dealing with one annoying malfunction in the body, but with an assortment of them. Those who live with fibromyalgia or chronic fatigue syndrome often experience bowel and bladder problems as well as debilitating fatigue or migraine headaches. Their memory malfunctions. Often, they cannot achieve restorative sleep. They have a higher sensitivity to noise, smell, and temperature. Those with lupus often contend with skin rashes and kidney problems. Crohn's patients not only cope with unrelenting diarrhea and fatigue, but often experience joint pain, eye issues, and a constellation of other medical woes. As symptoms present, any number of specialists become involved. What follows? More phone calls, more waiting rooms, more out-dated magazines, more frustration and despair.

Ken L. appears perfectly healthy but lives with chronic pain. His frustration lies primarily with the medical profession. Physicians initially told him that they could help him but eventually became frustrated and told him his problems were imagined. "Each doctor offers his own diagnosis but then cannot seem to help me. That's when the fear and frustration spring up inside of me. I cannot help but worry that I will always be this way. Doctors will often suggest it is all psychological once they run out of tricks from their medical bag."

"No one can possibly understand what it is like to live this way every day," reports Ethel Z., an energetic senior citizen who lives with ulcerative colitis. This is a new diagnosis for Ethel, who has never had a problem with her digestive system. She is now trying to come to terms with the limitations the disease imposes on her active life, and she has difficulty talking to her friends about the illness. "You are not allowed to speak up about your symptoms, and that is what is so hard. The medical professionals tell you to talk about your condition, because that will help you deal with it, but most of the world does not want to hear about these sorts of things."

Not only must we contend with a highly imperfect medical system, but we deal with physicians who are, after all, mere mortals with wildly varying personalities. Patients are individuals, as well; each enters the examination room with a unique set of experiences, expectations, and opinions. Both the patient and the doctor have the responsibility to seek a good doctor-patient relationship where both parties listen and truly hear one another. The patient must remember that doctors are not gods blessed with instant healing power; rather, they are human beings with their own perspectives, approaches, and personalities. Coping with chronic disorders is a challenge and a frustration for healthcare professionals as well.

Jill D. is a young woman with soft brunette curls framing her youthful face. Her outer demeanor and gentle smile never reveal the havoc and toll that her concealed illness has taken on her life. She feels that physicians must learn to communicate better and emphasize to the patient that the disorder is not their fault. "The physician cannot always tell by looking at a person, or even by the lab tests, what the problem or condition is," she says, speaking from her own experience. "The patient and the health provider are a team. The patient needs to be taken seriously and listened to closely. The doctor needs to work with the patient and really listen to what they are saying about their symptoms."

Kathleen H. who has suffered from the endless cycle of chronic pain has a message for the medical community. "Please listen, really listen to your patients, because when you lose your patience and become frustrated, or if you begin to lose interest in a particular case, it can be devastating to that person. Patients want to be educated about their condition. In the absence of information, they cannot make good choices. Those decisions should be made by the doctor and the patient. Share the information on relevant research and treatments with them and work together on the best approach and treatment for the disorder."

"The one thing I would urge of family, friends, and most of all, health practitioners, is to listen," says Marsha S. "Do not dismiss those of us who look well as slackers simply because we appear pain- or symptom-free. We didn't choose to be ill. I certainly didn't choose hepatitis. It chose me. We are doing the best we can. Believe us when we say that."

Mary M. wishes doctors would try to remember that their patients need understanding as part of their care. "We come to you for both help and hope. After our visits are over and your work is done, we have to live with our symptoms. We know that you cannot cure us, but we still want to be cured. We want to be good patients, but we also want to be normal."

The doctor's perspective and frustrations in treating chronic illness and pain often are not taken into account by the patient. Dr. Margaret Elizondo sees patients who have concealed chronic illnesses such as lupus, ulcerative colitis, and fibromyalgia. They often come to her office with high expectations of being fixed or cured and fervently believe this is possible if they can just find the right medication, herb, diet, or health care provider. "Unfortunately," says Dr. Elizondo, "there are no easy fixes for many of these conditions."[1]

Sadly, many doctors whose patients have hidden symptoms that are not easily explained by medical tests conclude that these individuals are malingering or are beset with serious psychological problems. "Patients with chronic disorders are actually not hard to treat in almost all instances," reports Dr. Robinson, "if you take their symptoms at face value, remain firmly committed to their care, and are perceived by them to be empathetic with their condition."[2]

Do most physicians and nurses prefer that the patient bring in a laundry list of symptoms and complaints, or should they only present the most profound and immediate concerns? The answers to this question were varied. Most physicians and nurses I interviewed stated that they would prefer a comprehensive list of symptoms in order of severity. Most indicated that they derived the most valuable insight by reading the most troubling symptoms with corresponding date of onset first. Often, reviewing such a list gives the practitioner a clearer picture of what might be going on. "It's mandatory to know the whole story," Dr. Malcolm Robinson urges. "Some things that seem trivial to a patient could be a clue to a critical diagnosis or treatment."

Dr. Douglas A. Drossman is a professor of medicine and psychiatry at the University of North Carolina-Chapel Hill. He generally likes to screen for all of the complaints and then prioritizes. "I will ask my patients to indicate all symptoms, but prioritize them from most difficult to least difficult to deal with.[3] I will speak to more general issues such as coping with the symptoms, without feeling compelled to address each one individually. In fact, it is important to remember that for most chronic conditions, there are often no immediate treatments that can be offered. The most important issues for the physician to address are coping and adaptation."

Not all physicians welcome a list of every symptom. Dr. Elizondo's schedule is often so uncomfortably tight that she does not have time to deal with a long list of complaints from each patient. "My biggest problem," says Elizondo, "is when patients don't prioritize their concerns. This can waste time on those symptoms that may not be an indicator of a serious situation."

Marie Zadravec is a registered nurse who was recently diagnosed with lupus and multiple sclerosis.[4] Her work and home life were radically disrupted by the onset of her symptoms and her inability to continue working. Prior to the onset of her illnesses, Marie was employed in a job that she loved. Her perspective on patient care is unique and valuable as she has been on both ends of the medical care system, as both caregiver and patient. "When I was working as a nurse, I always preferred to see a patient list their current symptoms placed in order of severity with the most troubling symptoms listed first. Additionally, it is useful for physicians and nurses to see a list of dates attached to the onset of various symptoms. Listing the treatments the patient has already had, including diagnostic testing and other physicians seen for the problem, is also a good idea."

Heading to your doctor's office with specific goals is useful. Do you need a new prescription because the medication you have is not effective? Do you require a referral to a specialist? Do you need forms completed for work disability or insurance, or do you need a diagnosis for new symptoms? If the patient weeds out the irrelevant details and instead identifies and prioritizes issues and goals prior to appointments, the visit's outcome will be more productive and less stressful.

When Zadravec was asked what the biggest challenge was in the treatment of individuals who appear healthy, but who live with chronic conditions and illness, her response was: "It is difficult to remember that the person involved has a chronic illness that is affecting them because it is not evident in their outward appearance. Sometimes, knowing when to limit activities is very difficult. The patient with a concealed illness often is very good at crossing over the threshold of tiring themselves by performing an activity to the point of pain. The person may not always pace him or herself very effectively or honor their limitations. This is part of the complicated picture of being in denial." Zadravec continues, "most patients want to believe they are not as disabled as they are, and they wish to keep pace and continue to function normally for as long as possible."

The most common symptoms that people with any form of chronic condition or illness may experience are fatigue, depression related to loss of function, and pain. Dr. Sidney Cassell, a rheumatologist with a busy private practice in Oregon, often sees fatigue, insomnia, general malaise, and depression as the most common side dishes to chronic illness.

Zadravec says that antidepressants can be useful in many cases of chronic illness or pain, as they can also help manage pain levels. "In many cases," says Zadravec, "pain levels often need to be adequately controlled in order to combat depression."[5] Even so, many of the physicians interviewed for this book stated that they had a great deal of trouble urging patients who needed help with their depression to follow up with auxiliary professionals such as social workers or mental health experts. "Often, patients do not accept referrals," reports Dr. Cassell, "so I don't often refer any longer."[6] Dr. Robinson has also found that most patients do not accept mental health management by psychiatrists or psychologists. "It's unfortunate," says Robinson, "even though such treatment can be immensely helpful in some cases."[7]

Depression is a common feature of most chronic illnesses or painful conditions. According to Dr. Drossman, depressive moods can occur "because inflammatory conditions can lead to cytokine activation, which leads to secondary fatigue, anorexia, and depression." There may also be psychosocial factors in the person's life that turn up the volume on the signals the brain receives from the body. Drossman says, "I don't usually need to refer patients to pain clinics or specialists, because that is the work that I do. However, I do use a psychologist, who is part of our medical team, to do supportive cognitive behavioral work and stress management/relaxation. Very often, I will use antidepressants and will present this to the patient as central analgesics since many patients are sensitive to being stigmatized with a psychiatric condition. This is particularly true for patients with concealed chronic conditions, since others will attribute their complaints (which they cannot see evidence of) as psychological in nature."[8]

People who live with chronic pain or other intractable symptoms might want to resolve to get past the stigma associated with psychological counseling and consider this sort of assistance as part of their treatment. Feeling chronically ill can take a toll on the healthiest mind. Sometimes assistance with shifting thoughts and feelings surrounding the illness and learning to live with the chronic nature of the symptoms can be enormously beneficial. Such assistence can lead to a more peaceful coexistence with the disorder.

Complementary Medicine and Self-Healing

In a perfect world, each person with a chronic illness or condition would go to medical professionals and find solutions that successfully ease every symptom. Unfortunately, there are no ideal treatments or medications for some disorders, which is why people frequently seek alternative or nontraditional practices. Many with chronic symptoms simply do not find answers or relief from symptoms and pain through traditional medical approaches and are often willing to try anything and everything to blunt the agony and reduce the unpredictability. People want to feel better. The goal is simple, but the journey can be extraordinarily complex.

Another reason people seek alternative care, complementary healing options, or self-care methodologies is because many of these treatments have only upside potential. For instance, some offer fewer toxic side effects, and patients report that they feel in better control of their treatment.

At times, people trudging down the road of chronic illness and pain collide with a variety of obstacles. They want to benefit from their medications, yet they can't seem to live with the side effects. They may find that traditional treatments do not offer enough relief from their pain or other symptoms. Western medicine, for all its knowledge and new discoveries, has its limitations. In the course of looking healthy, but feeling quite ill, people may begin to explore other avenues in their quest for healing and relief. While many are staunch and steadfast followers of strict traditional medical protocols, others attempt to obtain relief on alternative paths.

East Meets West

We find ourselves in a new and changing era, where traditional practitioners sometimes are the ones to suggest complementary treatments or alternative care to their patients. Why is this so? For one thing, chronic illness and persistent symptoms are difficult to treat. This is not only frustrating for the patient, but for the physician as well.

In addition to traditionally trained medical doctors who refer patients to alternative practitioners or particular complementary treatments, a growing number of traditionally trained medical practitioners boast practices that combine Western medicine with complementary or alternative treatments.

Dr. Roopa Chari is a traditionally trained internist who draws on her unique training as well as her experience with alternative medicine when treating patients. Although she was certified by the American Board of Internal Medicine after her internship and residency at McGaw Medical Center of Northwestern University, she also learned a great deal about natural healing methods and became certified in hypnosis, neuro-linguistic programming, Pranic Healing, and Yuen Energetics. Dr. Chari's ultimate goal is to help her patients by teaching them to heal themselves using natural remedies. "Conventional medicine is becoming more accepting of complementary treatments than it was in the recent past," says Dr. Chari.[9] "The new generation of trained physicians is often more open and accepting of natural remedies. They see the public's demand for such healing techniques and are aware of the public's heightened awareness about these matters. Also, traditional physicians are starting to use natural remedies themselves and experiencing the benefits of these remedies firsthand. They are also seeing and appreciating the scientific documentation of some natural supplements and treatments."

The main disorders Dr. Chari sees in her practice are chronic fatigue, high blood pressure and cholesterol, fibromyalgia, candida, allergies, and arthritis. She offers her patients tailor-made treatments based on their unique needs and requirements. This includes nutritional counseling, herbal remedies for strengthening the immune system, hormonal balancing, and detoxification. (Detoxification programs use herbal remedies and/or diet changes to cleanse the colon, liver, kidney, skin, and lungs.) "I have had a good success rate in treating chronic conditions due to the fact that I address the physical concerns and the emotional needs of each individual client. As a result, many of the underlying causes of their conditions can be addressed."

Most of Chari's patients seek her assistance out of frustration with the side effects of conventional medications and their inability to obtain more time with physicians. "They feel that no one takes the time to listen to what they have to say. They are also overwhelmed and confused with the wide array and potential dangers of some of the natural treatments available for their specific condition. Most of my patients mention that they seek my assistance because I have a traditional medical background as a medical doctor, and at the same time, I am familiar with natural remedies. I am able to guide them in the best of both worlds. I also spend quality time with each client to ensure their concerns are addressed." Dr. Chari tapers the patient's medications accordingly and recommends nutritional supplements based on individual needs and comfort levels.

Dr. Jill Van Meter is a licensed acupuncturist with a master of arts degree in Traditional Chinese medicine. She, too, feels that conventional medicine is much more accepting of complementary treatments now. "Medical doctors are witnessing more and more of their patients having good results with the various complementary therapies available. Many conventional medical physicians appreciate the limitations of Western medicine and are starting to understand the enormous benefits of blending the two approaches."[10] Van Meter sees many patients with digestive disorders and chronic pain. She utilizes a combination of acupuncture, breath work, visualization, and herbal therapy in her practice. "Patients come to see me when they are not getting better with traditional health care. They have heard how effective Chinese medicine can be and are ready to try it. They also crave more user-friendly services and greater attention to their physical challenges."

Van Meter has had varying degrees of success with her patients who suffer from chronic illness or conditions. "So much depends on active participation and desire for real change on the part of the patient. Chronic fatigue and fibromyalgia require permanent lifestyle and diet changes. Many patients are not willing to commit to this." It also requires a substantial investment of time to observe positive results. Many people become frustrated and quit too early; for others, the financial cost of long-term treatment is too draining. "Patients who are able to comply show the greatest improvement with Chinese medicine," says Van Meter. "For instance, I have worked very successfully with patients who have rheumatoid arthritis and have been able to help alleviate their pain. I have also had great success with treating digestive disorders such as irritable bowel syndrome and Crohn's disease. Cancer patients respond well to acupuncture and herbs for pain management, nausea, or lack of appetite. Acupuncture is not used for treatment of cancer in my office. However, it is a means of obtaining symptomatic relief."

Someone who successfully combines the advantages of Western medicine and alternative therapies is Hope M. "For the past fifteen years, I have used a variety of alternative therapies, not to cure my condition, but to ease the pain of my condition." Hope lives with painful structural challenges in her body that have plagued her since birth. Although she has utilized such techniques as chiropractic, acupuncture, massage, cranio-sacral massage, qigong, tai chi, and movement therapy, she may need to consider back surgery in the near future to fully relieve the pain. "I have successfully combined both Western and alternative medicine as they both have their benefits. Why not utilize them both if you are looking for the greatest results to your physical challenges?" Hope originally had difficulty with Western medicine's approach because it seemed to treat the symptoms and not the cause of the problem. "I feel the alternative practitioners were able to help me feel as though some change and progress could take place, even if it was subtle. I also seek out alternative medicine for preventative measures to help me care for my overall health, but when and if I need surgery, I will not hesitate to call on modern Western medicine. Nothing else can compare to the miracle it provides when people are facing a life-threatening illness."

Cheri Reeder is a public health nurse who was employed for many years in traditional medical settings such as surgery centers, cancer centers, chemical dependency units, and psychiatric and rehabilitation facilities. She eventually took a 125-hour course in reflexology, became nationally certified, and has been a practitioner for over a decade. Reeder is also a certified hypnotherapist and yoga teacher and has received certificates for her study and practice using essential oils to promote health and vitality. "People seek my attention for physical symptoms and soon gain insight and awareness into their own disease process. They come to realize the importance of balancing the physical body with their mental thoughts and patterns. Conventional medical schools still teach allopathic medicine, so even the new graduates are not taught the science behind holistic medicine." Reeder says the good news is that many doctors now study beyond what they were taught in school. They are learning from their patients that there is a great deal of validity to complementary treatments. "I am hopeful that America will continue to be a melting pot, and we will all become much wiser about healing."[11]

Although Reeder has studied many conventional approaches to medical science along with holistic methods, she does not refer to her services as treatments because she is not a medical doctor. Instead of using that term, she refers to her approach as assistance in the healing process. "I have been able to assist hundreds of people. One person came to me with chronic tinnitus (ear ringing), and it was gone within one session. Another man's recurring migraines vanished after my assistance. He did not need to take his migraine medication again. I am here to assist the body in balancing itself so that it can heal itself, and in this process, awareness is key. The person needs to become aware of their thought patterns, emotional judgments, and spiritual alignment. This awareness, along with a few lifestyle adjustments, can set anyone on the path to improved health."

Several renowned medical teaching hospitals and nursing schools began offering courses or full programs in alternative medical therapies in the early 1990s. Many pain clinics throughout the country combine conventional medicine with alternative treatments. In fact, a significant number of medical facilities and respected hospitals throughout the nation now offer patients an integrative medicine department so that they will have a raft of options for better health and faster healing. Treatments offered may include the following: mindfulness meditation, biofeedback, massage therapy, healing touch therapy, guided imagery, yoga, watsu water massage, herbal, and vitamin consultations. "This sets the stage for furthering more systematic research effort," says Dr. Geneé Jackson.[12] "The biggest challenge is attempting to apply conventional research methods to study systems that come out of a completely different paradigm, such as that of Chinese medicine. If nothing else, it will increase our understanding of the strengths and limitations of Western medical practices. There are numerous privately run professional clinics around the country structured out of an integrated model of treatment with varying combinations of specialized alternative and traditional caregivers." Patients whose symptoms have been resistant to traditional medications or palliative remedies are rushing to these centers in hopes of benefiting from an integrative approach to care.

"Chronic problems are, by nature, systemic, impacting several organs and systems, as well as mental and emotional well-being," says Jackson. "The complexity of these illnesses lies in the interplay between the medical, physical, emotional, social and, for some, spiritual issues heightened by long-term pain, suffering, and degeneration."

Dr. Artemio G. Pagdan is a board certified neurologist who received his training from the University of Louisville Hospital in Kentucky, Northwestern University Medical Center in Chicago, and the University of Michigan Medical Center. He is also trained in acupuncture. When Dr. Pagdan started applying acupuncture in his practice several years ago, he met with snickers and silent contempt by his Western medicine colleagues. "Now, some of these same physicians are referring to me their patients with pain who do not respond to conventional treatment. Physicians practicing Western medicine are gradually coming around to accepting acupuncture."[13]

Most patients who seek Dr. Pagdan's help are those with migraines or chronic pain that has not been alleviated by conventional pain medications. "The model and pathology of chronic or ongoing pain is different from that of acute pain," says Pagdan. "Hence, the pain medications that are effective for acute pain do not work well with chronic pain. For example, I use the novel antiepileptic drugs and tricyclic antidepressants to treat chronic pain due to nerve injury. Not all physicians know how to use these medications effectively." Dr. Pagdan also notes that chronic pain due to muscle overload or spasm does not respond to conventional pain medication. "I use neuroacupuncture, which is my own technique for treating myofascial pain. It is extremely effective. I have also used Botox alone or in combination with neuroacupuncture to treat chronic pain conditions."

Some alternative or holistic treatments involve mental or spiritual efforts. Meditation, relaxation, guided imagery, and hypnosis are but a few of these approaches. Scientists believe that the brain's ability to change physiologically through natural, self-produced chemicals is extraordinary. Historically, the existence of mind/body interactions was considered nonsensical by many traditional physicians who exclusively practiced Western medicine. However, there is a growing recognition that unconventional treatments work well for a certain percentage of patients who participate in medical studies but are given drugs with no medicinal value. This reaction, known as the placebo response, is thought to be a result of the power of suggestion, which can result in actual physiological changes. Ironically, the very scientific methods utilized by conventional Western medicine in the testing of medications have provided the best scientific support for the existence and power of the mind/body connection. Given the proper environment, the mind itself is powerful medicine, able and willing to connect to and heal the body despite the absence of traditional medical treatments.

Alternative or complementary treatments can include combinations of mental and physical activities such as yoga, tai chi, and qigong. These treatments can loosen chronically tight muscles and tendons, and the slow, controlled breathing techniques can induce relaxation which alone can improve or even restore general physical well-being.

Physical manipulations such as massage, reiki, and acupuncture are other forms of complementary treatments. Many practitioners believe that these treatments can relax tense muscles and tissues and release the body's own healing ability. For instance, the acupuncturist does not administer medicine through the acupuncture needles. The medicine or healing capacity resides within the patient. Needles provide a little help; they simply open those areas that are blocked and thereby allow the body to heal itself. The tiny needle pricks inform the body that it is time to release its healing potential.

More and more, patients opt for complementary treatments as an adjunct to conventional medical care. The relaxation of tension and the sense of empowerment patients gain by contributing in a positive way to their own healing can be extremely beneficial. If symptoms can be decreased through pain management, quality of life is improved, even if the underlying disorder remains. Traditional Western practitioners are becoming more receptive to and supportive of these trends as they, too, realize the important role of the human spirit in the healing process.

Understandably, many practitioners in the field of alternative medicine do not like the term "alternative" since many of these treatments are, and have been for centuries, considered conventional in much of the world. For instance, Western medicine is a more recent form of healing than acupuncture. In Africa, ancient America, Australia, Europe, China, and India, self-healing and self-care existed long before written history.[14]

Today, many physicians and researchers trained in Western medicine use alternative forms of care in addition to, or in lieu of, traditional treatments. The bookstore shelves are lined with works by doctors who are trained in Western medicine but also employ some complementary approaches. They represent the work of a growing number of doctors who educate and assist patients with treatments that include vitamins and herbal supplements, ancient Indian healing practices, and breathing exercises. The list of Western medical practitioners utilizing complementary or alternative medicine in their practices is a lengthy one. An article in a 1996 issue of *Life* magazine reported that "a recent survey of family physicians found that more than half regularly prescribe alternative therapy or have tried it themselves."[15] Additionally, many insurance companies recognize the value of alternative therapies and reimburse for treatments such as chiropractic and acupuncture. In fact, many costly marketing campaigns promise clients alternative treatment coverage in order to attract new clients and increase membership. "The federal government has been steadily increasing the budget earmarked to investigate alternative and complementary treatments," says Dr. Geneé Jackson.[16] "This is most likely because of the demand for integrative approaches from consumers. As in the private health industry, the government recognizes the growing market demand from this group of consumers. Future direction of this effort will undoubtedly involve establishing more credentialing agencies and accrediting bodies that offer reliable research-based information on the various treatment modalities."

William Osler, M.D. once said that "the person who takes medicine must recover twice: once from the disease and once from the medicine." Drugs can sometimes increase and complicate a patient's condition or symptoms. Many people with autoimmune disorders cannot easily tolerate medications' side effects. Their bodies are simply too depleted or sensitive to contend with a laundry list of adverse reactions. Thus, patients seek physicians who are willing to combine holistic with conventional Western medicine to help them live with challenging symptoms. A person with lupus may find a physician who suggests homeopathy. A particular rheumatologist may encourage fibromyalgia patients to take nutritional supplements such as magnesium and malic acid.

Gastroenterologists are beginning to see the value of nutritional supplements such as L-Glutamine for their gastro-challenged patients, according to Vijaya Pratha, M.D.[17] There is new medical research suggesting that high-potency probiotics can sometimes help Crohn's disease, ulcerative colitis, irritable bowel syndrome, and pouchitis. Although probiotics are not marketed as a medication, they are being used as one treatment option for these difficult to manage disorders.

The next chapter includes a partial survey of complementary care options.

Five
Medicinal Medley

Acupuncture

One-quarter of the world's population uses Chinese medicine, which is the oldest professional, continually practiced medicine in the world. This approach to healing treats a full range of chronic and acute conditions. It works by reestablishing harmony and balance within the body. Using a combination of tongue diagnosis, pulse diagnosis, and other diagnostic tools, the practitioner can determine the pattern of disharmony which requires rebalancing. This rebalancing often involves the use of Chinese herbal medicine and acupuncture.

Acupuncture seeks to regulate the flow of energy and blood within the body by inserting fine, sterile needles at certain acupoints. Chinese medical practitioners also use styles of Chinese massage such as tui na or amma, or they may prescribe corrective or preventive exercises such as qigong or dao yin. Practitioners typically counsel their patients on lifestyle and diet issues in accordance with the theories of Chinese medicine.[1]

Dr. Richard Gold serves on the faculty and Board of Directors of California's Pacific College of Oriental Medicine and is the author of a book on Thai massage. For over twenty years, Dr. Gold has studied, practiced, and taught oriental medicine. He has participated in advanced studies in Shanghai, China and has studied shiatsu in Osaka, Japan. Dr. Gold also holds a doctorate in psychology. "Many people today are suffering with autoimmune disorders such as multiple sclerosis, lupus, Sjogren's, and colitis. These disorders are particularly insidious because the very aspect of our being, which is designed to protect us, turns against us and attacks us. I also treat people suffering from chronic pain such as migraine headaches, sciatica, lumbago, and chronic neck pain. My clinical work employs such techniques as acupuncture, cupping, massage therapy, herbal medicine, nutritional counseling, and emotional/spiritual counseling."[2]

People seek Dr. Gold's assistance for chronic ailments that have not improved with conventional therapies. They also come to his office for preventative care because Chinese medicine supports immunity and enhances deep relaxation. "My patients prefer a more natural approach to healthcare. Over the years, more individuals have come to utilize my services as primary care, and not just after they have become dissatisfied with conventional care."

In many instances, Dr. Gold's patients have been able to cut back or simply eliminate drug usage. In his twenty years of practice, he has witnessed a dramatic cultural shift in awareness and acceptance of what was once considered alternative medicine. "For the past eight years, I have lectured to medical students and received direct referrals from medical doctors. It would be difficult to overemphasize the scope of change in America in reference to Chinese medicine in particular, and alternative approaches to healthcare in general."

"More doctors are allowing for the possibility of effectiveness from acupuncture treatments," states Julie T. Chang, a licensed acupuncturist with a background in microbiology and molecular genetics. "This is due to the increasing number of acceptable rigorous studies, and the growing empirical evidence that acupuncture works. As studies reveal acupuncture's mechanism of action, doctors are more accepting of the validity of acupuncture." Unlike Western herbal supplements which use single herbs, Chinese herbal medicine uses herbal formulas. Since studying formulas is more difficult than studying individual herbs, there is not as much acceptance or research in this area.

"Success rate," says Chang, "depends on the severity and duration of the condition, the general health of the patient, and the patient's commitment to treatment." Most of Chang's patients do not seek her assistance until they have exhausted all of their options with Western medicine. "I'm often their last resort."

Chiropractic

With her spine out of alignment and her sacrum locked, Hope M. found relief from her back pain with chiropractic adjustments. Laurie E. carried a lot of tension in her neck due to chronic migraine headaches, so she used a chiropractor to adjust her neck. "There was a period of time when I lost my ability to balance due to an existing health challenge in my ear," says Laurie. "If I caught my foot on something or stepped wrong, I would lose the ability to catch myself. As a result, I had a number of bad falls, and these falls created a great deal of pain throughout my body. My chiropractor discovered that most of my body was out of alignment. The pain in my shoulder and ankles stopped after just one treatment. I'm not sure how quickly my body would have been able to heal on its own with so many joint problems and pain. It took an amazing chiropractor to help me get back on my feet. No pun intended."

Many chiropractic offices today offer additional services such as massage, nutritional counseling, and muscle testing. Dr. Daniel Kalish is a chiropractor who has successfully treated more than 5,000 patients in the past decade. The chiropractic techniques he uses include Sacro-Occipital Technique, applied kinesiology, visceral manipulation of the internal organs, deep tissue muscle therapy, and cranio-sacral therapy. "SOT was originally created by an osteopath and chiropractor in the 1930s," says Kalish.[3] It offers a distinctive and clinically effective model for detecting and correcting musculoskeletal conditions such as headaches, neck pain, back pain, sciatica, jaw pain, and many other disorders. In applied kinesiology, there is a primary focus on the correction of nutritional balance, emotional balance, and structural balance—a health triad.

Over the last ten years, Dr. Kalish has seen a clear pattern in the reasons why people seek him. "There are two groups of patients. The first makes up about 10% of my practice; they have just recently suffered an overwhelming setback in their overall health, such as a recent car accident, fall, or back injury. The majority of patients, however, come in because of some chronic health condition that doesn't seem to want to leave. These patients have invariably been to many Western medical doctors and have either received little relief or gotten worse with time. They are desperate and find themselves forced into the world of alternative medicine."

Dr. Kalish also notes that after many years of suffering and being disregarded by their health team, these chronically ill patients begin to doubt themselves and their own condition. They wonder if they are imagining their symptoms or are just depressed. They speculate if it's "all in the head," as their doctors imply. "In the face of chronic illness or pain," says Kalish, "medical doctors will often run a series of lab tests and pronounce the person fine when nothing glaring shows up. They will usually recommend antidepressants or some type of pain reliever and close their books on the case."

If there is any doubt that chiropractors are in high demand, many practitioners like Kalish gather patients by word-of-mouth only; they do little, if any, advertising. "I accept no insurance, only cash, and I have had a full schedule of twenty to thirty patients per day for the past seven years." Prior to becoming a chiropractor, he trained as a teacher of the Alexander Technique. "This is a three-year program taken five days a week. The technique is based on teaching a person the alignment and organization for movement that will relieve chronic musculoskeletal pain patterns. I use the technique on every chiropractic patient, teaching them how to maintain their adjustments with changes in their movement patterns." The wonderful thing about the Alexander Technique is that people can learn self-implementing protocols so that they do not become overly dependent on practitioners. "The Alexander Technique allows the person to maintain and benefit long-term from chiropractic care."

The symptoms of fibromyalgia are often treated in the chiropractic office of Dr. H. Ginakes at the Integrated Medical Center. "We believe that the majority of our patients seek our assistance out of frustration, after going from one physician to the next in search of relief. Often each practitioner—the primary care physician, the internist, and the rheumatologist—all have a different focus on care based on their own individual specialty. As a result, treatment options and approaches are different from doctor to doctor. Some may recommend medications, exercise, physical therapy, or diet and nutritional changes."

Although these treatments may address some, or most of, the patient's complaints and symptoms, they often do not address them all. "In our office, we look at each patient as an individual who requires customized care and options from both a traditional and nontraditional standpoint. This allows for a more complete treatment plan blending Western medicine with physical therapy, diet, massage, exercise, and chiropractic adjustments."[4]

In this medical office of integrated approaches to healing, a medical physician is available to meet with the patient, assess the initial complaint, and track the progress of the accompanying chiropractic treatment. In this way, the patient feels that all of the bases are covered and feels free to raise questions about medication or chiropractic treatment with a medical physician as well as a chiropractor. Dr. Ginakes' patients experience pain reduction as well as increased functionality. "Once treatment has ended in our office, it is critically important to have the patient maintain a prescribed exercise and/or diet program on a regular basis. This is quite possibly the most important component to care. Often we see patients returning to our office for additional care because they felt better and stopped doing the things that we prescribed."

People who have fibromyalgia and other chronic pain conditions are often wary of going to a chiropractor as they feel it will be too harsh on their body. However, many chiropractors offer gentle adjustments so that those with delicate and painful conditions can be adjusted with little or no trauma. Ménière's disease, chronic migraines, asthma, chronic fatigue syndrome, fibromyalgia, and arthritis are just some of the conditions Dr. Cynthia Leeder successfully treats in her chiropractic care facility. "I always look at the spine, but I also do muscle-response testing to determine what type of treatment is needed. I also offer cranial work to balance the cranial bones which helps a great deal with Ménière's disease and migraines."[5]

Compared to most of her colleagues, Dr. Leeder became a chiropractor rather late in life. She has studied herbs, homeopathy (the use of tiny doses of natural substances from plants and minerals to stimulate a person's immune system), acupuncture, nutrition, applied kinesiology, cranial work, and other special areas of healing. Most patients see her because they are dissatisfied with current modes of treatment. "Drugs aren't making the problem go away, and many times traditional chiropractors are not able to locate the real source of the problem. Sometimes, they come to see me simply because they are desperate and tired of hurting. I don't advertise, so the clients I see are normally those who are referred by other patients or relatives. Some of my patients complain about the large amount of pharmaceuticals and NSAIDS (nonsteroidal anti-inflammatory drugs) they have to take that offer little to no relief. Others find the drugs are helping the original problem, but are causing other problems in conjunction, such as stomach pain, bloating, rashes, constipation or diarrhea. My patients are constantly expressing their frustration and desperation about their efforts to obtain more significant, long-term relief."

Dr. Leeder provides her patients with a carefully designed diet and supplementation program. "Conventional medicine is becoming more accepting of complementary treatments. For instance, ten years ago a radiology group told me that they could not x-ray my patient because I was a chiropractor. Now they are soliciting my business and the business of other chiropractors. I have also had a few neurologists and orthopedists tell their patients to continue being treated by me because of the positive response they are getting. I believe the body is not just a physical entity, but a combination of spiritual, emotional, mental, and physical bodies. For the most part, traditional medicine addresses only the physical component."

Dr. Susan Cameron is another chiropractor who has spent many years on an intensive search for methods of self-healing and integrating body, mind, and spirit. Conditions she treats in her office include migraines, chronic fatigue syndrome, asthma, hypertension, and chronic pain. Through the use of cranial-sacral and trigger-point therapy, she offers assistance to those who seek a more natural approach to healing and to those who have not received good results with medications or traditional medical treatments. "Those in traditional Western medicine have come to see that more people are seeking alternative, natural approaches that are gentle and more holistic, as opposed to symptomatic, compartmentalized curing."[6] Dr. Cameron feels that traditional medical doctors should educate people about healthier lifestyles that prevent illness and disease. Exercise, healthy diet habits, meditation, and prayer reduce stress, which she feels will prevent or alleviate many chronic conditions.

Meditation

Steven Hickman is a psychologist at the University of California, San Diego. His individual and group work with patients revolves around meditation and the cultivation of mindfulness-based stress reduction (MBSR). "Mindfulness, at its simplest and most basic level, is moment-to-moment, nonjudgmental awareness," says Dr. Hickman. "It has its roots in Eastern traditions of Buddhism, although its application is universal and not tied to any spiritual context."[7]

The practice of mindfulness is cultivated through meditation, gentle yoga, and other techniques devoted to settling the mind, keeping attention on the present moment, and recognizing the mind's tendency to create worrisome moments and imagined scenarios, or relive previous experiences. Mindfulness can be taught on an individual basis, but Dr. Hickman prefers to utilize the MBSR eight-week group model. "This is an intensive training in mindfulness meditation and stress reduction wherein participants attend eight two and one-half hour group sessions (in groups varying in size from four to forty people) and then are expected to practice the learned techniques for forty-five minutes per day." This is an often daunting challenge, but the group format allows for a great deal of support, problem-solving, brain-storming, and education. "An added bonus of this program" says Hickman, "is that many of these individuals lead very socially isolated lives, and the interpersonal interaction provided by such a format is often valuable. The groups become quite cohesive and supportive."

Many attend mindfulness workshops, which are held all over the country, because they either recognize that they have a problem with depression or anxiety (that may or may not be related to their pain or illness), or they are looking for an alternative to medications and their side effects, or they are trying to avoid invasive treatments and traditional allopathic views. "I like to joke that the job of practitioners like myself is partially dedicated to undoing the work of Descartes, whose position was that the mind and body were completely separate entities with no relationship to one another. Modern Western allopathic medicine has adopted that approach and we (in the West) are only now recognizing the limitations and fallacy in that theory."

In his MBSR groups, Dr. Hickman is absolutely amazed to see patients transform during the eight-week course in terms of their fundamental relationship with their pain, their bodies, and the world in general. "I teach them that we are thinking outside the box by learning to look deeply at what is present in each moment, without letting it take us to all the places it could take us. Rather than distracting from the pain with guided imagery (e.g., picture yourself on a beach), or self-hypnosis, or breathing exercises, I am directing them to stop and look directly at the pain or illness or depression or anxiety and examine it closely. Often, what they find is that it has a much different, more manageable quality when they separate it from their beliefs, worries, fears, guilt, and associations about it. There is a fundamental change that seems to occur for many patients with respect to their relationship with their own bodies."

Many of Hickman's patients would prefer not to be in their bodies at all, which of course sets up the ultimate tragic paradox, because there is literally no other place they could be. "Rather than constantly struggling to be somewhere other than in their bodies, my patients begin to gain an acceptance that this is where they are in this moment, and that any struggle to be elsewhere only uses up valuable resources that could be better used to live their lives (as opposed to just existing). These people learn to gain back some of the trust that they used to have in their bodies, or to develop a new trust where none existed."

The work that patients do with Hickman is intended to serve as an adjunct, not a replacement, for their particular medical treatment. Hickman finds that when people can accept that this intervention of mindfulness is not a cure but simply a way of changing their relationship with life and with illness, the quality of their lives increases dramatically. "My work is not in treating or curing bodily illness per se, but in altering its impact on people's lives and renewing or revitalizing their own natural tendencies to heal and gain satisfaction from life, no matter what they face on a daily basis. In many cases, people rate the intensity of their pain sensations or other physical symptoms about the same after completing the MBSR course or individual therapy with me, but their psychological symptoms (depression, anxiety, anger, grief, fear, etc.) are greatly reduced and their quality of life is enhanced immeasurably."

Evidence of the benefits of meditation is mounting. For example, one study shows that "women who meditate and use guided imagery have higher levels of the immune cells known to combat tumors in the breast. This comes after many studies established that meditation can significantly reduce blood pressure."[8] Additionally, new research using the most sophisticated imaging techniques shows how meditation can train the mind and reshape the brain.

Many physicians trained in modern Western medicine refer their patients to meditation programs. They are doing this not because it is the fashionable thing to do, but because scientific studies are showing that it works. "I have a great deal of contact with medical students and interns and residents," says Hickman. "They are reaching out to complementary therapies, Eastern and other approaches, and the whole idea of integrative medicine as part of their training. These individuals will form the heart of medicine in this country in another generation. They can see the genuine benefits and potential break-throughs inherent in having an open-minded, inquisitive and inclusive approach to all forms of medical intervention. Often, these students and trainees insist that their schools and training programs incorporate aspects of complementary therapies into their training."

Yoga

Yoga is especially beneficial for chronic conditions including fibromyalgia and arthritis. The gentle stretching assists with these and other chronic pain disorders. Diane Roberts, in an attempt to heal her own serious back injury, began practicing yoga and alternative therapies twenty years ago and then began teaching others to do the same. She studied with chiropractors, yoga instructors, cranio-sacral therapists, massage therapists, acupuncturists and medical doctors. Then she created a hatha yoga system that allows all body types and physical conditions to safely heal and strengthen. "I most often treat people who have acute and chronic musculoskeletal pain caused by traumatic accidents, structural imbalances, or chronic illness," says Roberts.[9] Most of her clients live with debilitating conditions such as fibromyalgia, digestive disorders, neck and shoulder pain, chronic fatigue syndrome, breast cancer, sciatica, and degenerative disk disease.

"I have a student who suffered from constant sciatic pain for four and a half years. He tried everything from acupuncture and chiropractic treatment to injections, pain pills, muscle relaxants, and physical therapy. By his second class with me, his sciatica was gone and has never returned. Another student suffered from severe fibromyalgia. She received tremendous relief from attending yoga classes and having an occasional yoga therapy session. She is now able to be productive and function in her life again."

Roberts encourages her students to work at their own pace and modify each pose to suit their needs. She encourages them to rest when they feel tired, back off when they feel stress or pain, and listen to their bodies for feedback. "I teach each person to respect the body's limitations, get to know the places that are ready to be strengthened, and to be patient with the places where they discover resistance."

Most people seek Roberts' classes because they are looking for an alternative to back surgery, have not had their complaints of pain taken seriously by the medical community, have been told there is nothing that can be done for them by their medical doctor, do not want to take muscle relaxants or pain killers, or have tried their doctor's recommendations which have not proved successful. Most recently, however, Roberts has been seeing people who have been referred to her by their own medical doctors, chiropractors, or massage therapists. "Yoga is becoming more accepted as a viable treatment for a whole host of what ails people." The number of clients who have been referred to Roberts by medical doctors has tripled in the last three years. Additionally, her students now include orthopedic surgeons, physical therapists, and internists. "There seems to be a greater shift toward understanding the contribution yoga can make to physical health and comfort."

An astounding number of people with chronic health disorders (even those with long-term, chronic symptoms), experience relief from their symptoms and a general sense of renewal with the regular use of yoga. For those who live with chronic pain, yoga is often the only form of exercise or movement that is feasible. Lori Baker suffered with sciatica and lower back pain from the age of eighteen. She began to experience pain and stiffness in her hips as well. Although good holistic health care was available and Lori believed strongly in it, her budget would not cover it. Instead, she decided to start practicing yoga. "Although I had a bit of a rough start, I kept going and found that if I practiced every day (even a little yoga is effective if it is accompanied by a good attitude) my pain seemed to dissipate."[10] Lori is not only pain-free, her joints remain flexible and she feels happy again.

The benefit of yoga is that you do not need a lot of fancy equipment or even special clothing. You can take it wherever you go and use it anywhere at any time, because the essence of the practice is breathing and body awareness. "I practice in the car, at the grocery store, on my bike, and at the bank," says Baker. "Yoga is not a fitness regime or sport, as it is noncompetitive. It is a tool to be used as a way of life." Lori is now a yoga instructor and helps others benefit the way she did. "I instruct others so that they may also integrate wellness (yoga, meditation, and nutrition) into their own life." The only time Lori's back bothers her now is if she overworks it without paying attention. "I can easily rectify my situation within one day by practicing yoga." Lori also meditates. As she explains, "Meditation is a practice of stillness with awareness. Yoga is a practice of movement with awareness. I am completely free of pain as long as I am consistent with my practice. Even when I stray from my path, as soon as I'm back on track, I am okay. I find that exercise, nutrition, and relaxation are the most effective ways to stay healthy."

Reflexology

According to Christine Issel, a nationally board-certified reflexologist with over thirty years of experience, reflexology is the systematic, manual stimulation of the reflex maps of the feet, hands, and outer ears. The application of pressure to these areas results in stress reduction and relaxation, which in turn can produce other physiological changes within the body. "Reflexology is known and used throughout the world. Not only can a person apply reflexology to others, it can be applied to oneself," says Issel.[11]

Issel's clients usually report reduction, if not elimination, of their pain and gain more mobility and flexibility along with a more positive outlook on life. Used with such conventional treatments as chemotherapy, Issel's clients report relief from pain and nausea as they go through the treatment cycle. While reflexology may not be a cure, its use adds quality to life. Reflexology can also give family members who learn this practice a sense of empowerment because they can help a loved one who might be going through an illness or unpleasant medical treatment. "Feelings of isolation can be replaced with a feeling of still being loved," says Issel, "and no one will argue that feeling loved is pretty strong medicine."

According to Issel, the acceptance of complementary therapies has always been consumer driven. "The positive White House Report in 2002 on complementary medicine has opened the door to more dialogue between complementary and conventional medicine at the governmental and educational levels. In addition, the probable study under consideration by the Department of Health and Human Services utilizing an alternative system of medical insurance billing codes may provide the public with greater access to practitioners in the near future."

Massage

Many people in chronic pain seek massage therapists for relief or an improved sense of well-being. "Massage allows me to be more present in my body," says Hope M., who lives with a chronic and painful back disorder. "It also helps me relax and gain compassion for myself and my body as it fully surrenders."

The key to any bodywork such as massage, reflexology or cranial-sacral therapy is locating a therapist who welcomes feedback regarding the degree of pressure used and the body's general response. Debra Peterson is a full-time certified massage technician. "Fibromyalgia, arthritis, multiple sclerosis, migraines, and other forms of chronic pain respond well to a gentler therapeutic touch including, but not limited to, acupressure, Swedish massage, or Zen Shiatsu (a gentler style of Shiatsu that works the meridians with the heel of the hand, not with the fingertips). For clients with muscle fatigue or chronic back pain, a deeper style might be used such as sports massage or deep tissue work. Quite often, integrated styles create a unique session geared toward each individual's needs." Peterson says that every attempt is made to ensure that clients are comfortable expressing their needs with regard to their tolerance to pressure. "Most people who seek my assistance are looking for an alternative, natural means of relief from symptoms. Some clients seek massage as a complement to their traditional medical regime. I find that each patient or client knows inherently what is best for them. They are tired of taking muscle relaxants and pain medication without seeing actual progress. Or, they realize that the use of pain medication does not eliminate the cause of the pain; it only eliminates the sensation of pain. Sometimes that's enough and sometimes it's not. There are those who are looking for a more hands-on approach, literally and figuratively. They want a massage professional to help them facilitate their own healing process."[12]

In the 1970s, massage was sought for relaxation only. Since that decade, we have come a long way in our understanding of the value of therapeutic touch. Hospitals commonly use volunteers for their long-term infant patients. The simple act of holding and touching is a gentle way of encouraging premature infants to thrive when they might otherwise become ill or fail to gain weight. They respond to human touch, and adults are no different. "We have learned to disconnect from those basic responses and needs, but when we are hurting and in need of caring contact, we respond to human touch again and truly feel its ability to heal." Peterson maintains that both traditional Western medicine and alternative methods of healing have their place. "Striking a balance between the two approaches is often the shortest pathway to actual healing and long-lasting relief from chronic symptoms."

"Massage is simply a treat that I give to myself," reports Rob H., who suffers from chronic pain. "Some people enjoy chocolate. Others indulge in ice cream. For me, it's regular massage. There are few things that feel better than lying still for an hour while someone tenderizes my muscles that are knotted. Massage is very holistic and grounding and is even covered by some medical insurance plans. I can't say enough about how this simple pleasure helps me in my pain management routine."

Karen Jolley is a practitioner of cranial-sacral therapy, a form of massage therapy. "Cranial work is based on the spinal fluid pumping into the head," says Jolley.[13] "As this fluid pumps up into the cranial cavity, the bones of the head are supposed to expand to allow the fluid to fill. If the bones are not expanding, then a complete flow of fluid is hindered and optimum health is prevented." Cranial-sacral practitioners are trained to slowly and very gently (five grams of force—the weight of a nickel) release the cranial bones from their fixed positions. "The results of freeing the bones are usually quite varied," says Jolley. "Sometimes it doesn't fix what the person came in for but does alleviate some other malady."

"You can never know what symptoms will be helped," Jolley continues, "but very few clients do not obtain some results. I recommend to clients who get no relief from their first treatment of cranial work to seek another type of treatment, as the problem does not seem to be in the bones of the head. Further treatments will most likely not produce the desired result." One of the things Jolley likes best about cranial-sacral therapy is that while it helps many, it does not build false hopes or exhaust funds that would be better spent on another therapeutic modality.

When Laurie E. first started treatments of cranial-sacral therapy for her chronic head pain, she was told by the practitioner that her head felt like cement. "He couldn't feel any movement in my cranial bones at all due to the severity of my pain and previous surgeries. The doctor needed a lot of time and patience to get some movement in the cranial bones. Over time, he began to feel the natural movement of the bones and my body began to heal." Hope M. has found that cranial-sacral massage is a useful therapy for treating trauma to the body. "This therapy has helped me throughout the past five years. I've been able to work through some of the pain from a very core place inside of my body."

Chiropractic offices often house not only chiropractic doctors; some offer massage services and traditional medical care. Kevin Klatt, a Holistic Health Practitioner, works at such a facility. He has offered massage in a chiropractic office for several years and works side-by-side with chiropractors, physical therapists, and physicians. This particular office treats a large number of fibromyalgia patients as well as those with repetitive stress injuries. "Chiropractors perform adjustments and do trigger-point therapy," says Klatt, "while our physical therapists assist in active and passive stretching combined with exercises that promote strength and endurance in the problem areas. We also offer traction to some of our patients, which helps stretch the musculature of the neck and promotes the c-shape curve in the cervical spine."[14]

If needed, the medical physicians in Klatt's office have the ability to write prescriptions for the patients as well as prescribe massage if there is a medical necessity. The majority of Klatt's clients prefer a more natural approach to healing, but he believes a combination of the two forms of medical care, Western and alternative, is extremely beneficial. "It is the best of both worlds for our patients, because every patient's situation is different and each person reacts differently to medication, massage, stretching, nutritional supplements, and exercise." Klatt combines relaxing Swedish massage with the rigorous movements of Hawaiian massage to assist his clients. Each person requires a different amount of pressure, so Klatt makes a determination in the first visit as to the type of massage approach that is best. "Some people with fibromyalgia or other chronic pain conditions require a very gentle touch and others like a deeper massage. I talk to my clients and assess their particular needs. We work together to make the massage time most beneficial to them." Klatt believes that the medical community is beginning to realize the benefits of alternative medicine.

Six

Case Studies and Combining Forces

Complementary Care—Up Close and Personal

Laurie E. has used various forms of alternative medicine since the beginning of her health challenges. "I truly believe that I would not be here without the assistance of alternative healthcare. I also would not be here without Western medicine. For me, the marriage of Western and alternative healing helped me cope with my conditions which include mastoiditis, chronic ear and lung infections, and frequent and severe migraines. I needed a traditional surgical procedure for my ear problems. I needed alternative medicine to deal with the headaches and migraines that traditional medicine could not help. Traditional pain medications simply did not work for me, so I had to search for other methods of relief to help ease the pain."

One of the things that Laurie has incorporated into her daily routine is nutritional supplementation. "I do a lot of research on the supplements that are appropriate for me, and I consult with alternative practitioners for their guidance. Since my immune system is constantly challenged, I have relied heavily on herbal and nutritional supplements to keep my body as healthy as possible. Through the combined contributions of Western medicine and alternative healing, I have been able to deal with my illness and pain. Being a participant in my healing process is important to me, and I am able to do this through natural medicine and the support of some amazing traditional medical doctors."

Nancy G. has suffered from fibromyalgia for many years. She uses traditional antidepressant therapy to assist with the sleep disorder component; she combines this with chiropractic care and regular yoga practice to help ease her complex array of symptoms. Nancy also treats herself to regular therapeutic massages to help her ease the frequent muscle pain that accompanies fibromyalgia. "I learned to combine conventional Western medical treatments with diet changes and alternative therapies. Prior to my car accident, my health practice was almost exclusively alternative medicine. Initially, alternative care did not cure my symptoms, so I resorted to traditional medicine and medications. So, for the past eleven years I have fluctuated between alternative approaches and conventional medicine. I prefer alternative approaches, especially after I experienced more and more side effects with the medications. I really dislike the toxicity of medicine, especially with long term use." Nancy found that the most useful approach to her symptoms was the detoxification of her body with wheat grass, raw foods, juice fasts, colonics, and regularly scheduled swim sessions. "Biofeedback was initially helpful for overcoming my pain from the car accident. Gentle yoga is always effective, though I need the structure of a class to do it consistently. Sometimes my symptoms interfere with attending class and I lose ground. Meditation is helpful, but very hard to do if I have not slept well. Swimming regularly affords great benefits, especially for my emotional sense of well-being and productivity. Psychotherapy has been helpful in adjusting to the changes in my life and my new limitations. My spirituality is what sustains me above all else."

Lynda P. has lived with a chronically inflamed colon for over a decade. She sees her physician on a regular basis but has also switched to a macrobiotic diet which has helped increase her endurance and quiet her gastrointestinal symptoms. She also incorporated Transcendental Meditation, qigong (a movement practice similar to tai chi), and the Alexander Technique (a type of bodywork that releases painful muscle tension) into her daily regimen. Her symptoms have decreased with this successful combination of treatments. Transcendental Meditation is recognized as a viable way to lower blood pressure, alleviate insomnia, and reduce chronic pain.

"I turned to alternative medicine because of Western medicine's slow pace in diagnosing and treating my chronic illness," says Lynda. "I was at a crisis level with my fissures, extreme weight loss, and severe abdominal pain. In desperation, I went to an acupuncturist which was a first for me. This acupuncturist made an immediate and accurate diagnosis. He told me it might take ten to twelve treatments to control the ghastly pain, but within three treatments, my comfort level had improved significantly." Lynda's acupuncturist also prescribed herbs and eventually recommended dietary changes. Lynda remains on this diet and is able to control her symptoms without the use of medicines, herbs, or invasive treatments. "Eventually, I located an M.D. who diagnosed my disorder by utilizing invasive tests, as opposed to the acupuncturist's noninvasive diagnostic methods."

Lynda recently began a serious study of qigong (some call it Chinese yoga), which is moving meditation. "I incorporate it with my practice of Transcendental Meditation that I first began thirty years ago." She believes the combination of qigong, meditation, acupuncture, and an altered diet have led her to a state of wellness that she otherwise would not have reached. "A wise M.D. whose opinion I highly value once told me, 'you're a well person with an illness.' That made a lot of sense and offered a great deal of comfort to me."

Hope M., who lives with a chronic back disorder, also experiences great benefits with the practice of qigong. "This is a wonderful holistic method of exercise that has been a form of moving meditation for me. It offers a way to harmonize my body and mind while fostering an inner quietness."

Anita M., who lives with the chronic pain of endometriosis and fibromyalgia, attends a support group for pain. The participants in this group are offered useful and relaxing breathing techniques to help them deal with chronic symptoms. "This type of exercise is very calming for me. I look forward to these meetings because it is gratifying to have a painless technique work so easily." Many years ago, Anita started using homeopathic medicines because she often had adverse reactions to prescribed medications and was eager to try something new.

Medications can generate a cavalcade of adverse side effects that are sometimes worse than the condition or symptoms they are trying to bring under control. "Acupuncture treatments were also successful for me," says Anita. "Acupuncture is a powerful healing method that is not painful and truly allows me to relax. I walk away from my treatments with a euphoric feeling and a great attitude."

Nancy T. found that acupuncture helped her Crohn's disease symptoms. "The night sweats and fatigue from the blood loss went away after my treatments. I really enjoyed the entire experience." Amma therapy is a needle-free form of acupuncture that stimulates acupuncture points through massage. It is another treatment Nancy has used to help calm her symptoms.

Jill V. has suffered with severe symptoms of chronic fatigue syndrome for the past three years. Although she uses many alternative treatments and takes nutritional supplements, she also uses prescription medication to help her manage her symptoms and get through the day with greater success. This combination of conventional and alternative treatments sometimes works best for people with chronic symptoms.

Sahar A. is a domestic violence counselor and holds bachelor's and master's degrees. Crohn's disease never stopped her from reaching her educational goals although it did slow down her progress at times. She finally decided to complete an accredited degree through the mail so that she didn't have to worry about fatigue and hunt for restrooms between classes. "Prior to formally being diagnosed with Crohn's disease, I wasn't quite sure what ailed me. The symptoms worsened over the years, and I knew I was at odds with my own body. Frustrated, physically weak, and feeling rather disgusted, I turned to the only source of comfort that held any consistent usefulness, which was, and still is, prayer—and a good sense of humor. Prayer has allowed me to keep everything in perspective and not become self-destructive. It prevents me from indulging in a personal pity party. That's not to say that I stopped using certain herbs and vitamins, but I believe it is the combination of all of these things that was successful in my case. I use peppermint tea to help with spasms in the intestine. I also drink tea for the sheer comfort it gives me. There is something about the warmth of tea that helps sooth the pain and cramping. When body aches make sleeping difficult, I drink Valerian tea. To treat my stomach cramps, I heat up an herbal bag and place it on my stomach."

Joanne Mason is a registered nurse as well as a licensed therapist. As a nurse, she worked in the pain clinic of a major hospital. She now works as a therapist who treats many people with fibromyalgia. "Prior to my private practice, I treated a variety of pain problems running the gamut of migraines, carpal tunnel syndrome, chronic back, neck, shoulder pain, and osteoporosis.

I currently offer stress management with relaxation techniques, guided imagery, mindfulness meditation, and what I call learned hopefulness." Mason's therapy is always in conjunction with medical care, but since many pain conditions are chronic, there are at times, treatment hiatuses. "My clients generally use my services to deal with their feelings of grief, anger, and depression due to pain problems and insomnia. Conventional medical professionals are generally pleased to have assistance with their chronic pain patients, as they too feel the frustration of treating these conditions." The good news is that clients are more aware these days of the various methods and treatments available outside of conventional medicine. "The patients are the ones seeking out these other forms of treatments on their own."

When Mason worked in hospital pain clinics, most physicians referred their patients to her, assuming that the pain clinic performed conventional treatments. "Most were unaware that we offered meditation, acupressure, yoga, bodywork, jin shin and jitsu, Feldenkrais (a movement therapy), guided imagery, and biofeedback."[1] Biofeedback is used to treat a variety of chronic pain conditions that include Raynaud's disease, irritable bowel syndrome, and many others. It is a way of learning to change the body's responses in a manner that improves health.

When she was in her forties, Marilyn M. started using biofeedback for her own benefit. "It was a positive experience for me. I found it to be calming and portable, with none of the complexities of pills and their side effects. Once you learn the technique, you can take it with you anywhere you go." Marilyn became very good at lowering her stress level in a short period of time. She was given relaxation tapes to listen to, and she reached a point of conditioning where she could fall asleep about halfway through the tape. "It provides relief from my inability to fall asleep. An added bonus is that it lowers my blood pressure."

Bridging the Gaps

With increasing frequency, physicians and nurses are advising patients to explore areas of alternative medicine but caution the patient to discuss possible treatments with them first. Some nurses and physicians may not believe that all forms of alternative medicine are valuable.

Hollie Ketman, a nurse who works in the field of rheumatology, approaches her patients with a few words of caution. "We welcome patients who want to try alternative treatments but tell them to bear in mind the extra cost and to beware of herbs that have not been formally tested."[2] As long as an alternative treatment is within reason and offers hope and relief, many physicians are open to considering these options for their patients.

Dr. Drossman does not normally discount alternative or nontraditional treatments, "since it is well recognized that patient belief systems are pivotal on how well or poorly people do from a health outcome standpoint. It is less important to me whether these treatments are effective as much as how strongly the patient believes in them. If they are planning to use alternative treatments,

I would want to be fully apprised of the nature of these treatments. I will generally allow them concurrently with the treatments I prescribe. I am also very careful to monitor these treatments and will let patients know if I think that there may be health risks. For example, one patient was taking megavitamins including large dosages of vitamins A and D and was a moderate alcohol drinker. I informed her that the fat-soluble vitamins such as vitamin A can cause liver toxicity. Since she was at high risk for liver disorders, she needed to stop taking the fat-soluble vitamins."[3] Dr. Drossman also tries to stay current on the side-effect profiles of various herbal supplements so that he can advise his patients on the latest findings.

Dr. Margaret Elizondo sees many people who mention a variety of alternative treatments during office visits. "As long as the treatments do not seem dangerous," she says, "I encourage people to explore avenues of treatments that they feel will be helpful. However, I cannot specifically recommend most of them, as safety issues are always a concern."[4]

There are some physicians who firmly discourage their patients from trying alternative treatments of any sort. They are simply not comfortable with alternative medicine, especially herbs. "Most are poorly documented or not scientifically studied in terms of either safety or efficacy," says researcher and gastroenterologist, Dr. Malcolm Robinson.[5] He urges his patients to be wary—and to watch their wallets. At the same time, he understands the lure of these treatments. "For suffering patients, it may be almost irresistible. However, the major problems with natural supplements are as follows: no standardization of such products, poor-to-totally-absent meaningful scientific data on their efficacy, unknown interactions with conventional medications, and uncontrolled hype regarding their benefits. Nevertheless, patients widely use alternative medicines despite physician disapproval, and it seems likely that some of these products could actually be beneficial in selected patients. It is very important for patients to tell their doctors about any complementary medicine utilization, although they virtually never do so. Doctors should ask, but almost always don't."

"I am generally supportive of alternative medicine or Integrative medicine as it is known today," says Dr. Bill McCarberg, physician and director of the pain clinic at a large hospital.[6] "However, patients with chronic disease are sometimes vulnerable to treatments that may be of no value, or even dangerous, such as some herbal preparations. There are not enough studies or good information available on many of these nontraditional treatments for doctors to give reasoned and clear recommendations. St. John's Wort, for example, is used widely in the United States to treat depression yet interferes with common medications taken by many patients. St. John's Wort may even interfere with the effectiveness of birth control pills."

Dr. McCarberg's general advice to his own patients who want to use some of these alternative forms of treatment is threefold. "Let me research the treatment to see if there is anything about known dangers. I also ask the patient what they believe about the treatment. If a patient is firmly convinced that the alternative treatment will help, then it probably will. Western medicine tries to understand, in a biomechanical way, why treatments are effective. We often understand the process, but sometimes we do not. For instance, we are not sure how acetaminophen actually relieves pain, but we recommend it all the time." Dr. McCarberg also examines whether a particular alternative treatment will require frequent visits (for instance, chiropractic twice weekly for a year) and/or a large financial expenditure. "If yes, then I am more hesitant. Patients with chronic illness are often desperate and willing to try anything. I do not want my patients going bankrupt on untested therapies." Most conventional practitioners of Western medicine caution their patients to beware of products or services advertised as miracle cures. Though desperate in their search for relief and good care, those with chronic disorders often fall prey to peddlers of quick-fix treatments or promises of fast and easy relief.

A wide variety of health challenges find their way into the acupuncture office of Dr. Elissa Blesch. She sees people with asthma, migraines, chronic pain, digestive disorders, chronic fatigue, fibromyalgia, environmental sensitivities, and more. The people who seek her care share a common goal: they want a better quality of life and haven't been able to find the answers they need. Some are dissatisfied with their doctors while others are tired of their prescribed medications. "These drugs are costly, sometimes ineffective, and produce side effects," says Blesch.[7] "Patients want input about what is happening in their own bodies, and they feel that their medical team is not really listening to them." Others want the best of both worlds. They want to try various forms of complementary care in conjunction with their traditional medical team.

In the past few years, Blesch and other alternative practitioners have seen Western medicine and alternative medicine pull together in ways that they could not even imagine a decade ago. "Medical doctors are opening their eyes and minds to alternative healing modalities because they can no longer deny its existence," says Blesch. "More and more of their patients are seeking acupuncturists, chiropractors, massage therapists, and naturopathic physicians." Unfortunately, quite a few of Blesch's clients do not inform their M.D.s that they are seeing her or other alternative practitioners for fear of being chastised. Even so, more and more multidisciplinary clinics and medical facilities are springing up nationwide. Acupuncturists and other alternative medical practitioners are included on staff. "No one healing modality is going to cure all chronic illnesses," says Blesch. "There needs to be a group effort with a variety of healthcare practitioners working towards the same goal: healing the patient."

"Integrated clinical settings across the country are seeing increasing numbers of patients with fibromyalgia and related chronic problems, primarily because they need a multileveled comprehensive assessment at the point-of-service to determine the specific areas of intervention needed," says Dr. Geneé Jackson. It is extremely important for practitioners, in all forms of healing, to work with the patient as a group effort. A potential for danger is if, for instance, an acupuncturist, biofeedback specialist, psychologist, and medical doctor, all work with the same patient to address pain management, yet do not communicate with one another about their respective treatment programs. "Any one treatment could interfere with, or even neutralize, the effect of another," says Jackson, "which can undo many of the benefits."[8]

Dr. Jackson works in a collaborative referral network of independent practitioners that includes traditional medical doctors, nutritionists, acupuncturists, chiropractors, and integrative psychotherapists. The network was formed in response to patients who were seeking a wide array of alternative treatments with the supervision of traditional medical practitioners. Some of Jackson's patients are direct referrals from medical doctors who recognize the need to treat patients at multiple levels. "In my work with patients, I ask them to consciously decide how far they want to go. Some want symptom relief; some want to get functional (be able to return to work, take care of children, have energy to socialize); others say they want to seek vibrant health and well-being beyond what they have known." Jackson encourages her patients to raise their own bar as high as possible.

People who have little hope of a cure (chronic pain, chronic illness, HIV, etc.) are acutely aware of the limitations of current medical treatments available. These individuals welcome the role of complementary therapies and nontraditional adjunctive treatments as a means of providing relief and improving quality of life. Coverage of complementary therapies appears with increasing frequency in magazines, on the Internet, and in traditional medical journals. Patients often come into the examining room with a list of potential treatments or promising therapies that they have gleaned from other sources not typically available to patients only a decade ago.

Whether the mystery lies in medication or in our own cells, everyone must find his or her own personal path to healing. If an individual ventures into alternative medicine, or stays on the path of Western medicine, or perhaps tries to manage a balancing act between both approaches, they must ultimately become their own best judge of what protocol works best for their body and situation.

Part Three

Interactions and Reactions

Seven
Family, Friends, Foes, and Fumbles

Doubting Thomases and Other Foes

Some would like to believe that their illnesses are not real. In many ways, doubting and/or denial can be comforting. Others find it very difficult that those around them doubt the seriousness of the illness and its symptoms. Since family or friends cannot see the illness, how can it exist? And how can someone believe that the illness is real if everyone around them doubts or scrutinizes it?

Many must contend with such scrutiny. No one can see the illness or condition. The disbelief and doubt witnessed in the words and faces of co-workers, family, friends, insurance companies, and even medical professionals can be discouraging and disheartening. "When I reveal my illness, my surgeries, and my pain, I can see the wheels spinning around in their minds as they give me the once over," says Laurie E. "They look as if they are trying to see my pain, and the pain must be seen to be real."

People with lupus, Crohn's disease, fibromyalgia, or any number of chronic but concealed illnesses often appear perfectly healthy and vital. They seem to be free of physical challenges as they participate in family outings and activities. They show up at work and perform well, but no one sees the fatigue, pain, and other symptoms lurking just beneath the surface. The pain is real, the symptoms are real, and the suffering is real. Even so, family and friends fail to see the symptoms, let alone the anxiety and weariness, by-products derived from hiding difficult challenges and symptoms on a daily basis.

There are some emotional reactions to diagnosis that are universal: fear, pain, anger, and powerlessness. "If it is a visible and well-known illness," says Bejai Higgins, "you can be sure of receiving concern from family and friends, a caring medical team, general understanding, and offered support (as opposed to the kind you have to ask for)." However, if you have a little known illness or condition, and if the symptoms are not visibly apparent, the reactions you receive can change dramatically. "Those with hidden illnesses are often treated with disbelief and thought to be hypochondriacs, whiners, malingerers, or difficult patients," says Higgins. They can sometimes receive dismissive medical treatment. These discounting reactions from health professionals, and sometimes the patient's family and friends, can begin to generate self-doubt. Self-doubt, left unchecked, can lead to depression and isolation.

"Well-meaning family members think my symptoms are all in my mind," sighs Leslie W., who lives with lupus. "According to them, if I think healthy, then I'll be healthy. If I don't think about my depression, it will go away. They believe that this illness is all in my mind. I feel as though I'm on this long, difficult journey all alone."

The disadvantage of a concealed illness or condition is that people do not give you the support they would otherwise extend. There is also the problem of having to explain a very misunderstood and complicated disorder that many people think is psychosomatic or hypochondriacal in nature. Lynn E. lives with the debilitating pain and weariness of chronic fatigue syndrome and fibromyalgia. She feels that it is not what people say, "but their silences and how they gaze at you. You can almost smell their doubt and scrutiny." Nancy G. often sees the disbelief in the eyes of other people as they discount her symptoms and pain with their scrutinizing stares. ". . . what they can't see, they don't believe."

People have questioned the existence of Shawna F.'s illness more than she cares to remember. Many people, including some physicians, all have scratched their heads at her concealed, but chronic symptoms. "I have heard the word hypochondriac whispered behind my back. Even though that was years ago, I still sometimes feel I have a chip on my shoulder, as if I have something to prove. I feel as though I lead a double life at times. My world feels safer when I go to great lengths to hide my physical pain."

"This is a very slippery slope," reports psychologist Dr. Geneé Jackson, "since maintaining a healthy sense of reality can become difficult. Our self-image is mainly formed through the eyes of others who mirror to us what they see. If others see us as being well, and we know we are really not well, we are left with an inaccurate or incongruent mirror. What is needed is to be able to fill in the known but hidden aspect of your health picture for yourself, and then reinterpret others' impressions with that in mind. This requires a great deal of reflection and attention at first and can be confusing and exhausting."[1]

Self-trust is an important piece of the puzzle for this process to work smoothly and successfully. "Over time," adds Dr. Jackson, "trusting yourself to know what is and is not true about your experience becomes easier—what does and does not define who you are—and that your suffering is truly valid. To the extent that this belief is held by you, the one who lives with the illness or pain, the message of how real your illness is tends to get clearer over time to those who interact with you on a regular basis."[1]

People in pain and discomfort will often seek others who are suffering with similar symptoms in order to validate their own. Validation and support can often be found in support groups or by simply connecting with one other person who lives with similar chronic symptoms. One man says "many people, like my parents for instance, cannot accept an illness that they cannot see. One of the ways that I have coped with this is to make friends with people who truly understand the challenges I'm dealing with."

One woman's husband constantly makes excuses for her when she lacks the stamina to attend an activity. In addition, he goes alone when she is physically unable. She feels guilty about this as do so many others with chronic disorders, but there seems to be no alternative. She finds herself wondering if others think she is not with her husband because she doesn't want to attend, or because she is just using the illness as an excuse to stay home. Since she appears perfectly healthy, why would she not accompany her husband?

"Others don't seem to understand my illness at all," explains a petite energetic woman who appears to be the picture of health. "If they have heard of it, they consider it the 'disease du jour' and do not take it seriously. Since I have so many different things wrong with me, and because there are so many different symptoms, they think I am a hypochondriac." She also speaks about the difficulty her husband has in understanding that she has a real illness. "I asked him to accompany me to a support group meeting where a respected physician was speaking. After hearing about the disorder from group members and from the doctor, he believes me a bit more. It was quite exasperating to not even have my own husband believe or understand what I was going through."

The additional challenge of an invisible illness or condition is that many people doubt the validity of the debilitating symptoms it generates. "I would like people to not judge me and to believe me when I say I physically cannot do something," says one frustrated woman. "I wish they would not make sarcastic remarks. If I had a disorder that put me in a wheelchair, no one would say, Get up and walk! Right?"

Dr. Drossman feels "the biggest challenge for patients with concealed illnesses and hidden conditions is that their family, friends, coworkers, and at times, even their physicians do not believe that the symptoms are as severe as they describe. Thus, they may not report how severely they feel them, and therefore, they suffer alone. When they do report their symptoms, they feel that they run the risk of being stigmatized as hypochondriacal."[2] Dr. Drossman adds that support groups can often be a great benefit in these situations where the illness experience is shared among persons with similar symptoms and challenges. Psychotherapist Jan Yaffe agrees. "Support groups are wonderful. People feel connected to a world of others who are going through similar situations. There is nothing more validating."

For a variety of reasons, people with chronic disorders often feel hesitant to routinely discuss their symptoms or fears with their spouse. Friends may not understand what they are going through. The person with the chronic condition does not want to become what they perceive as a burden to family, friends, and coworkers. A good alternative is to join a room of kindred spirits, a support group. Not only can the group provide strength, compassion, and empathy, it also spawns some great ideas, coping strategies, and humor. These people have already been through, or are currently facing, similar challenges and identical obstacles. Support groups are good places to learn where to turn for particular types of help, or they can be places to vent or ask questions.

Marilyn M., who suffers with fibromyalgia pain, found group therapy and support groups helpful. "Talking with people who understand what you are going through has a positive effect. You obtain tools to work with so you can think about your own health situation more clearly and with much less anxiety. There is a social component to belonging to such a group that is quite healing. The group helped me cope with my depression when I was feeling isolated from the rest of the non-hurting world."

The value of support groups and Internet news-groups that offer resources and camaraderie is profound. However, it is important to stay on the lookout for groups that may put the majority of their focus on expressing anger and negativity; ideally, support groups productively uplift their members' emotions and outlook. Some people like to carry on about the terrible hand life has dealt them. They can't see positive attributes in any part of their existence and focus exclusively on negativity and fear. If you find the group dynamics in a particular support group dragging you down, find a different group. Complaints and tears serve as a release, but the perennial focus on a half-empty glass is counterproductive.

Dr. McCarberg finds that patients in his pain clinic who appear well yet suffer from chronic illness and chronic pain such as fibromyalgia, irritable bowel syndrome, or chronic fatigue syndrome, often blame themselves for not improving on their own. "They feel that the illness is their fault, and this is often a belief that is confirmed by others. Even their doctors can sometimes not locate a reason for their pain or discomfort or the array of symptoms they are experiencing. And sadly, sometimes, their spouses do not and cannot understand the illness."[3]

Dr. McCarberg assures his patients that illness or pain is not their fault. He also tries to help his patients focus on ways to achieve an enhanced quality of life. "My job is to provide expert, competent medical care and to diagnose and treat injury or illness. However, when medicine fails to understand a condition adequately, then I must empower the patient. This means to help them accept their new place in life, which may include continued symptoms and pain. I treat the symptoms. I trust the patient's complaints. Yet, only patients can move on. Only they can live in a new physical reality and make the most of it. My responsibility is to help patients see this new reality and not dread it."

What if you make plans with friends and at the last minute are not able to join them because you are not feeling well? This is a common dilemma for many who live with chronic and unpredictable symptoms. Sometimes after awhile, doubt arises among family members, friends, or work supervisors about whether you are reliable; they frequently assume that you are just making excuses to not do certain things.

"I am not able to be the reliable, responsible person I used to be," reports Cindy V. "I constantly have to rearrange my plans because my physical condition changes throughout the day. Sometimes, I can only commit to something within a few hours. I don't take classes or volunteer as much as I would like to, because I cannot rely on myself to be functional or to be able to follow through."

Bejai Higgins often encourages her clients to give their friends and family members this warning: "I have every intention of being there, but sometimes things happen on short notice, and I end up in trouble and can't really get out. It is not about you, it is about me."[4] Higgins maintains that if you make this clear early on, and the event comes and you find you can't go, you can call your friend and say, "Remember when I told you that this might happen? Well, it is happening now."

Higgins learned to do this herself because of her own physical challenges and disorders. She became disabled in 1984 and lost her primary career. That was a devastating time as she had loved her job and her old life. Higgins went back to school and got another bachelor's degree and a master's degree in counseling. Was it difficult? "Absolutely!" exclaims Higgins. Since she did not appear disabled, she had to tell people that she may or may not be able to do what she had committed to do, but she found that if she told them up front, people were very understanding. "When I take on a new patient, I inform them that there may be times when I will have to change appointments at the last minute. That reality needs to be okay with them. It takes the entire sting out if I let them know up front that this is the way it is for me. This is the heart of my practice; how to stay in your world as much as possible, and make room for a disease or condition that is not going to go away."

Higgins sees many clients with hidden disabilities. Early in the sessions, she asks her clients to research and learn about the newly-diagnosed disease or condition. She then asks them if their symptoms ring true and if they sound familiar and fit their experiences. "It's his or her own body. The rest of us are guessing. If after research and reading about the symptoms, the diagnosis feels correct, then patients need to get active and get treated. If it doesn't feel right, they need to continue the diagnostic and discovery phase, because maybe the first diagnosis isn't correct. Maybe they finally have a diagnosis, and it is the wrong one! That happens." One of Higgins' patients reported that she and her mother had spent hours of their time searching for information and people to help her with her diagnosis. "Between the two of us," the patient stated with a gleam in her eye, "my mother and I have become great researchers."

People have to own their illnesses. If they do not, they cannot make the necessary changes to live with them. "If they are unsure and are not accepting of their own diagnosis, I always ask them to go for a second opinion," adds Higgins. "If they have a painful condition or illness that I am not familiar with, I tell them that I am going to research it and they are going to research it, and the following week, we are going to talk about it in the session."

Dr. Wrobel urges his clients to develop "healthy boundaries between themselves and the truth, and what others might say. If you have too many people doubting your illness, you may start to question the validity of it yourself. Don't." Instead of doubting your illness or condition, Wrobel suggests trying to ignore and doubt the Doubting Thomases around you and to assertively express the truth as you know it. Learn to recognize and respect the truth in your own body, not in the words and erroneous conclusions of others. To give power to other people's words when they have not walked a mile in your moccasins makes what you are going through seem invalid, and that is not your truth.[5]

"Surround yourself, whenever possible, with people who are compassionate and sensitive," suggests psychotherapist Jan Yaffe. "Learn the art of detachment when you are with family members or others who are critical. So much depends on how we perceive and receive other people's judgments. We can and should make conscious choices about this."[6]

Carol C. is a woman in her mid-thirties who has endured her share of health challenges. She was once a model but now lives with her husband and several Siamese cats in their rambling ranch-style home. She has hepatitis C and had to undergo a liver transplant at an early age. She also has ulcerative colitis. This dual diagnosis would shake up any young life. "I felt as if I had been hit with a double whammy because three years after the transplant when I had rebounded and was disease free, I suddenly discovered I had another disease to contend with. After getting through my first illness, it still wasn't over. I live with a compromised immune system and getting people to understand that is very hard because I appear perfectly healthy. I've had some people actually say to me that I let myself get this way by letting the illness enter my body. They say to me, 'If you tell yourself you are well, then you will be well. If you tell yourself you are sick, you'll be sick.' This makes me feel inferior, as if I am not strong enough to ward off illness." On the other hand, Carol feels as though she has been given a new set of eyes to see with even though her liver, not her vision, was impaired. "I feel as though I have a second chance at life, even if living is on borrowed time. I have the precious gift of life. I feel so fortunate. Someone else had to die and donate their liver so that I could live on."

Disability Insurance: the Discouraging Labyrinth

Many people face a series of daunting obstacles, either from their employer or from the government, when attempting to obtain disability benefits. If an application for Social Security disability insurance or work-related disability is rejected upon the initial request for benefits, some people begin to doubt the diagnosis. Sometimes an illness or condition is not recognized as a "reasonable disability" by the state or a private insurance company. This often results when there is no definitive diagnostic medical test. The inability to diagnose does not mean that no malady exists; it simply means that no accurate test is currently available.

"I had a cancer patient who was unable to work and was terminally ill," reported Bejai Higgins.[7] "When this person applied for Social Security disability benefits, the request was denied. She was dying, and she was denied. So when people get turned down, I say to them, 'You know what? Just about everyone gets turned down the first or second time. It's automatic. So, don't let this process impact your own belief about what is happening to you.' They don't know what you are going through and what happens to you on a daily basis. I always encourage people to go after whatever benefits they are trying to obtain—Social Security disability insurance or disability benefits through work—and to ignore the process. If you looked at these matters thirty or forty years ago, no one would have diagnosed bipolar or lupus as a disability, so it's just a matter of timing. Some people are discounted by a lot of these insurance organizations, but they cannot afford to discount themselves or question their own credibility. That's the danger. If they do, then everything can start to slide out of control."

Cindy V. had a job that she very much enjoyed. She got along wonderfully with her boss and coworkers and wanted to maintain employment, but her flare-ups were too severe at that time. She was forced to take too many sick days from her job, and she knew she couldn't continue to maintain employment and good health. "I really wanted to keep working, but my illness was just too severe at that time. I had tried applying for disability benefits, but was rejected. I appealed time after time, and it eventually came to the point where I was to appear in court before a judge. I did not really feel I needed a lawyer but hired one anyway, since I thought he might be somewhat helpful to my case. My lawyer did not think I had a very good chance of getting disability because I looked too healthy." Cindy did obtain disability status, but it took extraordinary perseverance on her part.

Don K. lives with rheumatoid arthritis, a painful and progressive illness he has had since he was a youth. The thought of not working is devastating to him, not because he identifies himself with his job, but because he wants to project a positive work ethic to his two sons. "I was told several years ago I could take a disability retirement, but how can I teach my sons to be proud workers, strong men, and leaders if their father doesn't work?"

When the cognitive and stamina difficulties that often accompany chronic illness or pain seem significant, nurse Marie Zadravec approaches the issue with the patient by discussing some sort of modification of work habits or encourages them to apply for disability insurance. "Most patients resist this initially but come to accept it if they have a supportive health care team pointing out their limitations and the long-term effects of the disease process."[8]

Before recommending that his patients apply for Social Security or other disability programs, Dr. Douglas Drossman likes to get further information about what they can and cannot do. "Often patients feel unable to work, yet they can do similar physical activity outside of work. Therefore, I try to determine whether they have a physical or cognitive impairment or one that is situation-specific. For example, if someone is having more stress at work or feels stigmatized by coworkers, they may feel less energy or ability to perform that work. Assuming that there are situation-specific measures, I will try to address these issues directly. If there is general impairment in functioning, I will often try to determine what they feel good doing and not doing and try to redirect much of their energies into gratifying activities, perhaps with less physical challenge."[9]

The impact of listening to others about an illness, condition, or pain being all in your head is damaging in a number of ways. By living in a state of denial, the person is not in a position to make optimal self-care decisions. This belief system also precludes loved ones and coworkers from being able to clearly understand and appreciate the problem and provide effective support. Cognitive behavior therapy is often helpful in these situations where the person can learn to recognize and disregard irrational or skewed thoughts. "Examining irrational thoughts can be a useful way to assess your level of denial and how it negatively impacts your life and the lives of those around you," says Dr. Geneé Jackson.[10] "Until the denial is penetrated, the emotional and spiritual integration necessary for healing cannot occur."

"When you change one component (yourself), other components in the system (everyone else) have to change as well, by default," continues Jackson. "Knowing this, I focus primarily on helping people convince themselves of the validity of their illness. If their own belief is firm and they are clear about what their condition really means for them and for the others who share their lives, the rest seems to flow fairly easily. They are now able to educate and convince others. Sufferers who are around someone who holds strong negative biases toward illness and who cannot be supportive, have a larger, perhaps more long-term issue of moving away from that person's sphere of influence. However, they must do this for the sake of their own healing."

Whether moving through the state insurance system, or facing scrutiny from family members or physicians, it is easy to get sidetracked or forget that the person who lives with the symptoms is the only one who truly feels the impact. The effects are day-to-day, week-to-week. Those who are ill are the ones who ultimately must cope with the obstacles and limitations. They are to be believed, not ignored.

It is sometimes necessary to enlist an advocate, a person who is planted firmly in the corner of the person with the health disorder who can be that person's mouthpiece and strength. Advocates can help with the disability paperwork, or simply accompany them to doctor visits, or talk to the nurses at the hospital on their behalf. Since those who are in pain or are dealing with chronic symptoms are often not in the best position to be proactive, they should utilize their advocate—a friend, family member, or professional— who can be their voice when they do not have the stamina to do battle. Advocates can help fight the battles with persistence and justice as their weapons; they can win the war for you, and with you.

"Don't be afraid to speak to your doctors," insists nurse Zadravec, "or have your advocate speak for you. Tell them what you need. Tell them what you would like to try, and if they are not responsive, get another doctor. There are caring understanding doctors out there who will help you. Do not waste time on a doctor who tells you it is all in your head."[11]

Grappling with the Green-eyed Monster

"I envy other people's view of a long life unfettered by medical issues," reports Cari D., a young woman in her twenties. "Most of my friends are in their late twenties and simply do not have to deal with what I do, such as frequent fevers, having blood tests every couple of weeks, rectifying insurance problems, colonoscopies and x-rays, medications that may cause cancer in the future. The list is endless and quite scary at times. I envy those who do not have to face these things until they are in their eighties!"

Many people who live with concealed but debilitating symptoms often envy those around them who seem to be living carefree, pain-free lives. They see others working effortlessly and playing with great gusto and boundless energy. These feelings of envy or resentment, however, can make a person feel even more isolated. When asked if they envied friends' and family members' physical stamina, monetary accomplishments, mobility, and freedom of movement, many people with concealed disabilities answered yes. Unfortunately, envy minimizes a person's own sense of accomplishment. Everyone must recognize their accomplishments, no matter how small or insignificant they may seem.

"I would love to be able to go anywhere at anytime. The thought of that makes me feel very jealous," says Sahar A. "I envy every person I see running or playing sports. I love to play and have fun, but since my diagnosis, the only running I've been doing is downhill."

"I feel envy for my friends' good health, but I am happy that they don't have what I have," says Marsha S., a mother of two sons, two stepsons, and one stepdaughter. Marsha lives with the chronic pain and symptoms of fibromyalgia.

Shawna F. has endometriosis, a painful condition of the reproductive system that causes the uterine lining to grow outside its boundaries. She often feels envious of the good health and pain-free existence of those around her. Shawna's competitive nature rears its head when she starts to wish she could slip back into her former self—the one who did not have to live with chronic pain and symptoms. "I see Olympic softball players with just as much talent as I had, and they're doing what I want to be doing—what I could be doing if things had somehow gone differently."

Trish G. is a teacher who finds that her energy has lessened significantly since her diagnosis of ulcerative colitis. "I frequently envy well people who, through no effort at all, lead such comparatively simple lives with no doctor appointments, medications to keep track of, symptoms to monitor, or explanations to make to family and friends. They don't seem to appreciate how fortunate they are to be free of all of those worries."

"Hearing about everyone else's great life is very difficult for me," says Linda N. "I wonder why I have to deal with my illness while they are out having fun and working."

Laurie E. is a lanky young woman with long blond hair and a supermodel smile. Few people would detect that she has suffered for years with daily migraines and an ear disorder that leaves her dizzy, disoriented, and hard of hearing much of the time. "As each year passes, I am still dealing with my illness and pain. I do envy healthy people. I feel that many people are not completely thankful that they are healthy. They take their good health for granted. I have noticed that I have become very sensitive to others who abuse their bodies and treat them in a variety of harmful ways, as if that is no big deal. I don't understand how someone can pay money to damage themselves physically through smoking, drinking alcohol, or drug abuse. I want people to understand how important their health is and to treat their bodies with the utmost grace. I get irritated if I hear someone complain about their health when they have been abusing it. I do not want to give someone sympathy who complains to me about their hangover. I think of how hard I struggle to feel well. My illness did not come about because of my careless behavior or damaging lifestyle habits. Each day I do everything possible to live the healthiest life I can so that I can feel the best that I can. I envy those people who never have to give their health a single thought."

Although difficult, a most worthy goal is to reduce the resentment of others who seem to be trouble-free and pain-free. It is important to learn to take the focus off what you can no longer do, and place your focus on what you can do, and more importantly, on who you still are. Focusing on what you can do each day, even if the accomplishments seem small in scale, will chip away at the envy and self-pity and alleviate some of the stress and unhappiness that can accompany concealed chronic illness and pain.

All in the Family

Having a concealed disorder can affect family members in a multitude of ways. Some of the people interviewed for this book mentioned that the dissolution of a marriage or a job loss occurred shortly after their diagnosis. In the majority of instances, however, this was not the case. Chronic but concealed illness becomes a family condition; it stretches well beyond the boundaries of one life into the lives of others. This shift can result in a radical redefinition of illness and can even influence the course of the illness. Learning to gracefully accept a chronic condition is essential.

Those who live with and around the person with chronic illness have had their world and roles altered, too. Friends, family, and coworkers become detectives of sorts; they look for signs of discomfort or pain in their loved ones. Sometimes this new role of scrutinizer or detective is not a welcome one. At other times it comes quite naturally. This requires an adjustment, large or small, on the part of the loved one.

The willingness or reluctance of friends, family members, and associates to embrace the individual with a concealed illness can throw another monkey wrench into an already complex melange of feelings and fears. The individual with the chronic disorder may wonder: What if my partner does not love me anymore? What if I'm not fun to be with? What if I cannot be productive? What will be my worth in the eyes of others? Some of those in the vicinity of the ill person can remain supportive and even help the patient feel part of life again, while other family members and friends have difficulties with new and unexpected roles. They may distance themselves and become uninterested and uncommitted. Their eyes may dart around the room in search of a quick escape route.

"My boyfriend has been very supportive," reports one woman. Even so, she feels that his new role scares him a bit. "He initially met and dated a very strong, healthy, successful woman. He fell in love with that girl. And for over a long time, it remained that way. That's what he was accustomed to. We both realize that life never stays the same, but this has been a long journey, and many changes and adjustments have been made. I now have physical limitations and have suffered financially from my inability to work at this time. The most significant change, however, has been my emotional state. I push him away at times, but I do try to explain why I'm doing it. Sometimes I don't even know why I'm doing what I'm doing or why I'm thinking what I'm thinking. Overall, it's been very challenging, but his faith in me and his patience, support, and love have kept us together."

A young mother feels that her hidden disease has hit her son the hardest. "He constantly fears for me and has bad dreams about my dying. I'm not sure why. He's very close to me, but I wish he could accept this situation better. His anxiety wears me out, and I'm already dealing with all of the other emotional baggage that comes with having a chronic illness."

Another man sees that his health challenges affect his family members in a variety of ways. "My wife seems to have the most difficulty accepting my condition. I feel that if I could truly accept the condition myself, she would be able to do so as well. She seems very sympathetic to my problem, and I am sure she is, but there is a lot of tension at times. Primarily, I think this is due to my symptoms and how they vary from day to day, or even from hour to hour. This wears on me. From her perspective, I seem to be ignoring her, but that's not the case. I can also see the worry in her eyes as she watches someone she has always thought of as a strong and invincible man change before her eyes. I need to learn to communicate to my family that I am having a severe attack and not just feeling grouchy. I can't expect them to just know. I try to face each day with new hope that I am getting better. However, on days when I am experiencing symptoms, I can become depressed, which sometimes has a negative impact on my family. They tell me, 'Just don't worry about it,' which is easy to say when you are not the one suffering from the condition. Outwardly, I try to portray the strong, independent person I had always been prior to this illness. I think this behavior confuses my family very much. They had always pictured me that way, which makes accepting that I have sometimes significant limitations very hard for them."

Marie Z. is now on disability income because of lupus. She shares some of these same feelings about a role change. "I have always been on my own and able to handle life. Now I feel vulnerable, as if I am not able to take care of myself financially."

"The person who understands my hidden illness the least is my husband," reports another woman. "I feel that I have finally come to accept this illness, and I wish he could, too. I finally had to put my foot down and say, 'no more vacations that bring on my symptoms.' They are not one bit enjoyable for me, and I cannot do these sorts of trips anymore just to make him happy. There had to be some compromise, and we had to find a vacation we both could enjoy. After some time, we have managed to do just that. Every now and again, however, he will bring up some place we used to go, and I have to remind him that I cannot take advantage or enjoy that sort of setting any longer. He still does not seem to understand my limitations."

Many people feel that their family and friends walk on eggshells around them, because they don't want to do or say the wrong thing about the illness or condition. One man feels that his wife and kids are too cautious around him. His other relatives protect him from bad news for fear that his illness might worsen. "This has always had a reverse effect, because I become angry when I am left out of the information flow. I hate not being told about things."

Then there is the man with diabetes who has to adhere to dietary restrictions. He doesn't like others to suggest which food items are allowable. He doesn't like to be told what he should or should not order in a restaurant. "I hate when people ask me, 'How are your sugars?' I know they mean well and are concerned, but I hate hearing it." He also doesn't like people to ask, 'Can you have this?' in reference to a particular food item. Those with Crohn's disease or ulcerative colitis, two serious digestive diseases, also voice this sentiment. Are you sure you can have that? Maybe you shouldn't order this. Is that dessert allowed? Won't you become sick? Although most people mean well, there is a loss of control and dignity to the person with the illness when others question their judgment or fuss over them.

One woman says that her husband does not know whether to touch her or leave her alone if she is in the midst of a flare-up. "If I am having a bad day, the last thing I want to do is become intimate, despite the fact that I am madly in love with my husband. I wonder if he is getting to the point where he thinks I just don't want to be with him. This disease is debilitating on so many levels. It has made me question my womanhood like nothing else ever has done."

Another woman suffers from an illness of the reproductive organs that can cause great pain with sexual intercourse. For this reason, she has had to make significant adjustments in her intimate life. "I used to take extra pain medicine before I would have sex with my husband. This left me feeling like a bad wife. Now, I've learned to communicate much better. If sex is painful, we stop. When there is too much pain to even try, we don't."

Telling a spouse or partner when you're having a bad day is very important. But how does a loved one learn to help their partner, child, or parent cope with the pain that they cannot see? Therapist Bejai Higgins suggests using a number system instead of adjectives. For instance, when you come home from work, ask the person with the invisible illness or condition how they would rate their pain on a scale of one to ten, instead of asking for a narrative description. "One would be no pain, whereas ten would be at the other end of the spectrum—barely tolerable pain. This tells you immediately where they are in their pain spectrum."[12]

"Make a list of the things that help you cope with or soothe the pain even if they offer minor relief," suggests Higgins. "Be sure you have already discussed at what number on the one–ten scale you will need your spouse or friend to step in and help you. For instance, if you suffer back pain, at what number would a massage or other source of comfort from your list of useful coping mechanisms benefit you? What point on the scale would be best to simply have your loved one go away and not try to help you? Have this information sorted out before the pain strikes so that you both have a workable formula for figuring out what can be done, or not done, at various points in the spectrum of pain."

What if the pain or the nature of your condition prevents you from being able to experience physical intimacy with your partner? Some people who live with ulcerative colitis or Crohn's disease feel as though they want or need to keep their partner at arm's length if they are having pain or experiencing too many trips to the bathroom. A woman with endometriosis may associate sex with pain because of her condition. Those with arthritis or fibromyalgia may not want to be touched as the sensation can cause more discomfort than pleasure. Perhaps someone with chronic fatigue syndrome simply does not have the energy or interest to participate in sexual relations. Or someone with major depression might not be able to muster up an interest in physical intimacy.

"I was single when I was first diagnosed with diabetes," said Steve B. "At that early state, I was still sexually active and there was no impact on my performance whatsoever. After marrying and having two kids, I was and still am concerned about passing diabetes on to my children. Often, antidepressants and other medications can result in male impotence. There is a disproportionate amount of guilt for not being able to provide your spouse with a fulfilling sex life, especially when you're in your forties or fifties. It is always in the back of your mind that it shouldn't be that way."

A young married woman with ulcerative colitis expressed a lack of sexual feeling and the accompanying guilt. "I feel guilty because I don't feel as sexual as I'd like to." She adores her husband, but sometimes the wear and tear of the illness and pain on the body affect the libido. Even though trying to enlighten a sexual partner about this lack of interest is very difficult, she still tries to communicate her feelings to her husband. They also attend support group sessions where he is able to hear about other people with similar challenges.

Intimacy is not only sex, even though sex can certainly be a part of intimacy. Higgins breaks intimacy between partners into four important components. Each component is a tool for self-esteem that does not involve sexual activity: 1) sharing thoughts, 2) sharing dreams, 3) sharing feelings, and 4) sharing bodies. Higgins also adds that you should use "I" statements such as

I am feeling ———, I am experiencing ———, when communicating with your partner. This conveys your feelings in an effective, non-blaming manner as well as explains how you feel and what you think. However, do not expect the other person to understand exactly what you are going through and what you are experiencing. "If they comprehend 50% of what you are saying, you are at a good starting point. Attempt to have several small conversations about this issue, not one big one. Don't forget to communicate good news as well as bad. And if you have a good day, don't forget to say so."[13]

Diane M.'s family continues to help accommodate her illness. She says they have been doing this for so long that "adjustments are second nature and part of how we live now. Despite my normal appearance and my attempts to attend holiday events with family, they understand that my stamina is low and are not offended when I have to leave early, or eat something if dinner is running late, or if I have to lie down."

One woman, who has lived with a chronic illness for thirty years, appreciates collateral reassurance and hearing important reminders from her support community, such as "I know how awful this is right now, but if possible, try to remember that you've experienced the remission/relapse cycle countless times. You will certainly improve. It's simply a matter of when."

Perhaps your loved one feels helpless and does not know how to assist you when you are in pain, or you have a friend or family member who lives with a chronic condition and you don't know how to help them. The best advice is to simply be there for the other person, and listen. That's all. Don't reassure them. If you are the one with the concealed symptoms, do not ask for reassurance. Instead, ask for presence. Presence is the best present one can give someone who is in pain. There is something very powerful, calming, and magical about the expression, "sitting up with a sick friend." That is simply the best you can do for someone you care for. If they are in bed, lie down beside them. Don't stand over them talking. Get down to their level, and just be with them. The presence of another person during a time of need or pain is one of the most powerful healing tools available (and doesn't require a prescription)!

Friendship: Strains and Gains

One of the things that seems unfair to those who live with chronic disorders is the effect on friendships and potential friendships. Many people have difficulty making new friends when they have an unseen chronic illness or a condition that keeps them from being more active and socially involved. Since the disability is invisible, there is fear of skepticism and distrust even before the first hello. "I usually do not say much to anyone about my illness until I get to know them fairly well or an occasion arises where I have to explain my illness," reports Marsha S. who lives with hepatitis C and fibromyalgia. There are some activities she simply cannot do, as they aggravate one condition or the other. How do you explain the inability to be in the sun or do something physical when you look completely fit and in good health—when you look just fine? "My fibromyalgia limits me from taking trips with friends and going out at night," sighs Marsha. "The sun allergy keeps me from doing any outdoor activities."

"Making new friends is very hard," reports Diane M. who suffers from chronic fatigue syndrome and frequent migraines. "I would love to have new friends but don't have the energy to maintain the ongoing needs of others."

Mike E. tried for years to keep up with the crowd by acting like he was okay even though he was experiencing debilitating fatigue, rectal bleeding, and the side effects of steroids. "I finally learned that blending in is not as important as staying healthy. What I did was to resist using the bathroom for long periods of time even though I had to use it very badly and urgently. This caused great discomfort and increased my symptoms. Not smart."

Jaye B. is convinced she will never be able to have more close friends in her life because of her illness and its limitations on her life. "Occasionally, an acquaintance will suggest that we get together and do something that I know I cannot possibly do. For instance, someone asked me to join a class with her. This is something I would have jumped at prior to my illness. But realistically, I knew that I could not meet the physical demands at this time because of my symptoms and fatigue. I chickened out and wasn't able to do it."

Other people find that sharing experiences strengthens the bond they already have with friends and family. Kathleen reports that she didn't lose any friends during the worst time of her health challenge. "On the other hand, I wasn't such a good friend myself. I withdrew. My friends called all the time, and I just didn't call back or respond to their e-mail. They are still there, however. Since they are good friends and know me the way they do, they all gave me the space I needed and didn't feel offended when their calls were not returned. They would send e-mails just saying: Hi, how are you? Thinking about you. Call me when you feel better. Or call if you need anything. They understood, because every single one of them had experienced their own dark periods for whatever reason. Each could understand and appreciate and respect the way I was handling my pain."

When you look perfectly healthy but cannot participate in activities such as trips, movies, or walking around the neighborhood, explaining why is difficult and tiring. "Having a hidden illness is very challenging," explains Linda N. "This illness interferes with a lot of my activities. I get tired of explaining to others why I cannot do this or that."

Carol C. feels misunderstood. "Many people expect too much from me. I feel I am letting them down in some way or another if I cannot keep up with them." Carol feels that she might spoil the day by getting ill if she goes out with them. "They think that I can do all of the things that they can do. They eventually find out that is not the case. I have lost a lot of friends because of this."

Lee T., on the other hand, feels that her friendship circle has grown since her diagnosis of Crohn's disease. Although she is no longer able to work full-time as a graphic designer, she says that she probably has more friends now because she has more time for friends. "I also have a greater need for friends now than I did before." Lee knows that she would not have met, befriended, and grown close to all of the special people in her support group had she not developed this disease.

Often, friends want to know what they can do when someone they care about is in pain or battling fatigue. Most of us reflect on the times we have been ill or when a loved one has been very sick, and we realize that discreet expressions of sympathy and compassion were always welcome.

The intense sense of isolation that may accompany illness cannot be completely alleviated, but considerate words and gestures (nothing fancy, simply heartfelt expressions by phone or letter, a living plant, a basket of personal care items, or best of all, your presence) can be very valuable to the unwilling traveler in the land of ill health. Offering to help the person who is ill with shopping or cleaning can also be a most welcome gift.

Leslie W. loves to receive little beauty gifts from a friend such as bubble bath, perfume, or dusting powder. "That is a small contribution, but it keeps giving and giving and giving." Having friends who offer to color or lighten your hair for you can help lift your spirits. This small act allows the person who is not well to feel like she has a new and fresher face to present to the world. "The nicest gifts I have received when ill or recovering from surgery are lip glosses or special hand lotions. These are the little things that pamper me and allow me to feel better and look better. These things can perk up my spirit."

Pampering yourself or a friend through a flare-up is simple yet very powerful. If you know they love coffee, how about bringing a special mug with one of those flavored coffee mixes? One woman with lupus loves to pamper herself by sitting in her backyard in a chaise lounge with her feet up, drinking a mocha cappuccino she fixes from an envelope and hot water. "I put it in a good china cup, prop my feet up, and read a good book," she says. "Sunday is a vacation from the rest of my life. This special and peaceful rest period keeps me going throughout the week."

Spending quiet time with someone who is ill and simply being there in quiet stillness with them, or watching a sunset together, or reading in the same room, can offer great comfort and peace. Being in calm camaraderie with a caring person is often the most healing gesture of all. Quiet companionship is, indeed, potent medicine.

Take responsibility for pampering yourself and seeking resources and strategies that will be helpful to you. Caring for yourself as you would a friend and pulling in the reigns when you are tempted to cross the line, whether with physical exertion or eating the wrong foods, can become a full-time job.

"Make full use of the range of pain management techniques available," suggests Dr. Geneé Jackson.[14] "Whether you use guided imagery, meditation, exercise, or a heating pad, pick and choose what you feel is best for you in that moment. Always be kind to yourself. By virtue of the illness' pattern, your path will always have its highs and lows. However, with a good measure of self-acceptance, self-love, patience, and appropriate self-care, your emotional and physical highs and lows need not be extreme. Find creative ways to keep the things you love most in your life, and live as much as possible in the present moment." If one day at a time is too difficult, try one hour or even one minute at a time. Some days that will be the best that you can do for yourself, so congratulate yourself for a job well done.

The Romance Dance

Every one of us is flawed. That is what makes us human. For some, it is psychological. For others, it is physical. That seems to be the nature of human beings: to feel we have something to hide from the world. This idea comes into play in the arena of relationships and romance. Ken L. has difficulty explaining to others that he is not able to work because of his chronic pain and epilepsy. It's not so much a problem with his male friends, but "it's a major turnoff for females to know that I'm not working. Dating is nearly impossible. I'm twenty-nine, unemployed, can only drive short distances, and I live at my mom's house. Yeah, sure, women want me."

Prior to her marriage, Cindy V. had a great deal of trouble disclosing her disease. "When I was younger and in my dating phase, I avoided telling any of my dates about my disease or the symptoms of my disease. I truly felt that no partner could accept me with this disease. I was so afraid of rejection that I would do everything I could to hide the illness. When I would start getting too close to someone, I would break off the relationship. At that time, I felt I couldn't risk anyone finding out about it. This went on for many years."

Even when Cindy was dating the man she is now married to, she did everything she could to hide her disease from him. "I would purposely not eat before our dates. Sometimes I would go five days with only water and bananas just to avoid having a problem around him. At the time, eating very little reduced my chances of having symptoms. If I was in his apartment and needed to go to the bathroom, I'd jump in the car and drive home thirty miles away, without an explanation. However, I didn't want to break off the relationship as I had with other men. It was scary, but fortunately he truly loved me too, and he ultimately accepted me, disease and all."

Those with chronic health challenges who find themselves in bad marriages are often reluctant to leave damaging relationships because they are afraid no one else will want them. After all, they are somehow "flawed." They must realize that, at times, a relationship itself can be unhealthy, much more so than the individual with an illness.

Dr. Geneé Jackson recently saw a patient whose life and marriage had been greatly impacted by her long-term illness. "Its ambiguous etiology had disfigured her life in ways that greatly challenged any of her efforts to recover physically," says Jackson. "It changed the quality of her married life, her friendships, her ability to be socially connected, and her decision to become a mother. She and her husband had been married for several years and her husband had become increasingly unsupportive. The more we talked, the more she realized that he was also depressed and feeling helpless about how to support and fix it for her. She said that he often tried to do things to help, but had difficulty helping in the ways she really needed."[15]

This patient was seeking help for a variety of problems. Her immediate goal was to relieve her physical pain. However, her more fundamental needs were to normalize her marriage and social relationships and be able to continue to work.

The impact of illness on family systems has been a subject of a great deal of theoretical and clinical research. "The family members are as affected as the challenged person in terms of caretaking demands, identity, role, and how needs are negotiated," says Jackson. The sense of normality and fitting back into a larger social network of friends and extended family is stressed and stretched to its limit. "This patient's husband was likely unaware that he was equally impacted by his wife's illness. He was simply showing a different constellation of emotional and physical symptoms."

Another woman I interviewed is still not sure how her concealed chronic illness will affect her love life and the potential partner she is now dating. "I've just renewed an old friendship from high school, and I'm delaying telling him about my illness. Eventually, my illness will have to come up, but I just don't know when. I guess I'll continue letting the relationship grow first. I'm not sure how I will explain the lupus to him. If we eventually break up, I'll always feel that my illness was the factor, when it might not be that at all."

Dating has become nonexistent for Lynn E., an attractive young woman with short blond hair and a ready smile. Lynn struggles with chronic fatigue syndrome and a sleep disorder. "My hope of finding an appropriate partner has all but completely faded because of my chronic illness. If I had the energy to pursue and develop a romantic relationship, I would have no problem attracting someone. However, once potential partners learn of my disabilities, the majority of them choose to be with someone more energetic." Lynn lives on disability insurance now after years of an active career and social life. She has had to get used to spending most of her time alone, since socializing is an effort and activities are unaffordable. "I look just fine. I believe the fact that I am still highly verbal and present myself intelligently can also be deceiving. People have a hard time believing that someone who seems so competent can be truly disabled. People who see me slowly walking my dog in the neighborhood don't have a clue. They cannot see my pain when I bend or squat. Many of my friends have been in denial the last three years, saying everything from 'try adding certain vitamins' to 'try more positive thinking.'"

"I have the dating issue come up a lot with breast cancer patients or men with testicular cancer, which is a young man's disease," says family therapist, Bejai Higgins.[16] "I encourage people to start dating and not to mention their illness or condition right away. If you get to the point where you think you may want to spend a significant amount of time with a particular person, let them know that you have something serious to discuss with them." Don't spring it on your new dating partner as they open the door. Trying to be as up-front as possible is a good idea, but it's best not to talk about having a debilitating disease or illness in the first couple of dates, or to include every detail until you know you have strong feelings about this person and want to continue the relationship. Try to share your story with confidence and matter-of-fact conversation, not pessimism and fear. "Talk to the person you care about in a place where you are going to be safe and you're going to be able to have a serious conversation," says Higgins. "Tell the person how nervous you are to talk about this so that they are not flippant in their response, then take a chance and tell them. It can be wonderful, because people are surprisingly considerate and loving when given half a chance."

Deciding whom to tell and when to tell can become an anxiety producing decision. The person with the illness may feel that if the person they are dating or are about to date will freak out when they are told about the disorder, then that person is not for them. You should have someone to talk to about your feelings surrounding your condition or illness; however, that person should be a family member, friend, coworker, physician, or therapist. To present the illness early in a new relationship does not allow the other person a chance to get to know you. It only allows them to get to know you with an illness. If you're not sure how to tell a person you care for about your condition and how it affects you, you can role-play a conversation using someone you feel close to who already knows of the illness.

Emotional support systems are often influenced and altered by the intrusion of a chronic illness or condition. Old friends may become uneasy and fade away, while new ones may emerge. Some friends may try to fix the person who is going through the roller-coaster ride of chronic illness. Others may want to rescue that individual with fervently-held religious or philosophical beliefs.

The most important thing a person with a chronic disorder can do is to become comfortable with their new self. There often needs to be a significant adjustment period for friends and family members to this new way of being together, playing together, or working together. Often, others will not feel at ease with illness unless the person with the illness is comfortable with their new situation. What may be required is time, self-examination, real patience, or perhaps even some counseling sessions to get to a point of comfort and acceptance with a new self and a new way of being. It is a lofty objective indeed, but an extraordinarily worthy goal.

Your Child with a Concealed Chronic Condition

The parents of a child who lives with an unseen illness or condition often struggle with feelings of guilt and remorse related to how their child became ill. "They often blame themselves for things they could not have controlled," notes psychologist, Dr. Geneé Jackson.[17] They should seek support to work through these issues for the sake of their child and for themselves. "In one particular case, a father was so angry about his son's illness that he projected his anger onto the child. He was also so fearful that his son might die (an irrational thought in this case based on the child's diagnosis), that he put an emotional barrier between the two of them and only interacted with him when absolutely necessary. This ultimately hurt everyone in the family."

In addition to the parents' need to educate themselves, they have to adjust to the limitations placed on their personal lives and their family's lifestyle. "The parents hold the major responsibility for helping the child accept their challenges and the ways in which they are different from other children," notes Jackson. "This is not easy because the child's needs and issues change during different developmental stages. For example, adolescents tend to have the most difficulty with medical compliance because the desire to be just like their peers is strongest at that time of life. Adolescents are also less likely to be as closely supervised as they were when younger."

Children with a chronic illness tend to miss classes and after-school activities. This impacts and often retards emotional development so much that the child is often emotionally younger than others the same age. Parents must be aware of this extra layer of developmental challenges and must adjust their own expectations accordingly.

Another often overlooked problem for these parents is how the healthy siblings of chronically ill children are affected. The needs of siblings are often misunderstood and ignored by parents, teachers, and caregivers. "They typically suffer from feeling invisible and unimportant because of the high need for attention that goes to the sick child in the family," states Jackson. Parents must help them see that they play unique, valuable roles in the family. This piece of a family's reality should be reinforced on a regular basis, or the siblings and their needs might easily fall through the cracks.

There are a multitude of challenges for parents who have children with chronic diseases and conditions. The tendency for children to internalize their frustrations, feelings of isolation, and sadness is a natural one. Not surprisingly, these same feelings can affect and overwhelm the parents. "Parents can easily feel worry, pity, and over-protectiveness for the child," suggests Jan Yaffe.[18] "A parent may feel frustration and anger that their child is sick or flawed in some way." Often, parents project their pain and fear about the condition onto the sick child. "They begin to see everything the child does or feels as a function of his or her illness and forget that the child is a person, an entity going through life stages. Letting go, letting the child fall or fail is a challenge. They need to help the child be in charge as much as possible in their life so that the child can feel empowered." The most important element to remember is that a parent's reaction to a child's illness can greatly affect the child's own adjustment to it.

Eight
Running the Race

The Hurdles and Fumbles of Work and Income

Leslie W. lives in a small, quaint, cottage-style home near a large university. When we first met to discuss her concealed illness and its effects on her life, I noticed that her front yard was spruced up with newly planted flowers and shrubs. Her small living room walls were lined with bookshelves holding hundreds of videos and DVDs. Leslie was a film reviewer for a local television station. This was the ideal job for her as she was an avid movie buff, but Leslie lived in fear of being discovered. She felt that if they learned of her illness, she would soon be dismissed–literally and figuratively. As a result, she kept pushing herself beyond her limits, even as her energy faded. She felt she had no choice but to cover her tracks. She had a young daughter to raise on her single-parent income and a mortgage to pay. She couldn't afford to let her guard down and reveal that she has lupus.

Some people feel that it is appropriate to withhold mention of their illness to an employer or a prospective employer. Many fear they will lose their jobs if they disclose their physical challenges. Other times, they fear they will lose the respect of their supervisor and coworkers. The fact of the matter is that many illnesses, including many forms of cancer, do not necessarily get worse with time. Instead, the symptoms of most of these concealed conditions ebb and flow. The fear that an employer will not accept or understand the nature of chronic illness often muzzles employees. They live with the burden of a great secret. Since their illness or pain is concealed and difficult to detect, it encourages this pattern of silence and nondisclosure. However, the act of successfully hiding a condition from supervisors, coworkers, or prospective employers does not necessarily relieve anxiety and the fear of disclosure. "I never allude to my condition during job interviews," reports Rick D., a Gulf War veteran who suffers from hearing loss, "for fear of not being hired because of it."

If you are in the process of looking for a new job and have a disability, when and how should you broach the subject with your potential employer? Too soon, and you risk being eliminated before the selection process begins. Too late, and you could damage the relationship with your new boss, if it appears you were not up-front about your illness.

There are practical as well as legal issues involved around disclosure in the workplace. Generally, companies are not supposed to inquire about disabilities before making a job offer. But if a person needs some sort of accommodation, the employer must know about any physical limitations or illness. Sometimes the candidate's best approach is to let the employer know what they are in for, especially if the disorder requires a workplace modification. Revealing one's illness or condition can provide tremendous peace of mind. They are no longer harboring a horrendous secret. On the other hand, this revelation can hinder the chances of receiving a job offer.

If someone with a disorder is not experiencing any significant symptoms when meeting with a potential employer, that individual is not required to disclose the illness during the interview. If, at some point, absences arise during flare-ups, medical tests, or treatments, that would be a good time to approach a supervisor to discuss the illness or condition and its impact. The individual must weigh the pros and cons of disclosure in each situation and determine what is most appropriate.

Many who work outside the home and experience chronic illness or pain find that jobs or careers become derailed somewhere along the line. "I don't have the stamina of my young coworkers," reported one young woman. "I tire easily and must pace myself to get through a day's work." The issue for people with concealed chronic disorders is not about getting a job, but how to perform and sustain one.

"I have had to create an entire new life," reports Lynn E., who lives with chronic fatigue syndrome. "In being unable to maintain regular employment, and being totally disabled, the biggest adjustment has been trying to survive financially. Most people in America are worried about how much they earn and if they will save enough money for retirement. Those worries now pale in comparison to the difficulty of not knowing, month-to-month, if I can survive as a single, disabled person, especially after exhausting my savings account. The forced loss of income has meant never being able to afford to take a trip out of town or go out to dinner, buy new clothes, or pay for recreation. It means the loss of dreams and aspirations."

"I don't like to be blamed for missing work when I cannot help it," says Jill D., a bright and attractive young woman who lives with inflammatory bowel disease and clinical depression. Below the surface of her cherubic face and sweet disposition sits a great deal of frustration about not being able to declare financial independence. She is angry because her illness derailed her career. Even though she is in her thirties, she has to live with her parents to help make ends meet or to live in the townhouse her parents own. She was forced to give up her dream of supporting herself and maintaining a full-time job when the fatigue and symptoms of her illness made full-time work impossible.

Cari D. had just moved into a new townhouse when we first met. Her moving boxes still lined the living room floor and kitchen area, and the new carpet on the stairs was covered in plastic. Cari appeared to be the cover girl for good health. No one would ever suspect the severity of her concealed illness and how it had thrown her for a loop just two years prior to our meeting. For the past twenty-four months she had been on and off many medications for her easy-to-conceal illness. Ironically, she was now working as a pharmaceutical representative for a major drug company. She was amused that after taking so many drugs, she was now peddling them back to physicians. Cari found her previous job had created too much pressure, so she found one that better suited her and her illness. "I quit my job as a manager with a large company and sought a job that would give me more flexibility for doctor appointments and less stress to aggravate my illness."

Harry K. wishes he could have completed schooling in telecommunications and gone into television production. "This illness changed my mind and my career." Having his own business has its positive and negative points. Self-employment and flexible hours are very helpful because he never knows when he'll experience a flare-up that will land him in the hospital. On the other hand, not having a pension to look forward to is frightening to him and his family. "I will need to work through what would otherwise be my retirement years in a semi-retired status in order to make ends meet. Having a chronic illness can definitely determine your financial security, or lack of it." Harry has met some wonderful people during his self-employment and has enjoyed his work even though his career path has little in common with his original plan. "I've met great people I wouldn't have met otherwise if I hadn't developed this disease. Many have become very good friends."

People with concealed chronic disorders that force them to quit jobs or rely on disability insurance checks are often regarded as lazy or worse–as malingerers. However, a reduced workload is often an unwelcome necessity that is profoundly difficult to accept. Marilyn M. can no longer maintain a full-time job because of her painful symptoms. "I can and do work outside the home but only at a part-time job. I physically cannot handle full-time work now. I currently work in a job that is enjoyable but one that I am way overqualified for." Laurie E., on the other hand, has been unable to work at all for the past few years. "I cannot always plan things in advance since I don't know how I'll feel on any given day. When I do plan something, I know that I may have to cancel if I am not feeling well enough. This year, I have been living on disability insurance. I hope that I improve physically so that I will be able to work again soon."

When Mike E. was working, he told his employer that he had diabetes rather than reveal the truth: he had been diagnosed with kidney disease and ulcerative colitis. Michael engaged in the deception because he felt his employer would more easily understand a relatively common disease than the ones he actually had. "Although a person with diabetes may not appear disabled either, diabetes is a familiar illness and thus would not require a lot of explanation. Also, explaining diabetes is far less embarrassing than explaining the symptoms of ulcerative colitis. In a sense, I have sometimes wished that I appeared disabled or had a more acceptable or recognizable illness."

Leslie W. would love to ask for time off from her job so that she could rest and summon the energy needed to finally get some things done at home. But "to ask for disability so that I can take a little time off would mean disclosing my illness. I don't need to add that stress to the worry that already exists. By doing my job as usual and keeping up my home, I give the impression to coworkers that I am a strong and independent person." This is the way Leslie wants it and needs it. She cannot risk losing her job. "I must have the income to pay bills and pay for my home." But pretending at work and resting on weekends in order to get up and do it all over again becomes a vicious and draining cycle.

For Leslie and many other people who live with a chronic concealed illness, balancing exhaustion with maintaining a job becomes a way of life. "I save all of my energy for work because that's my only income. Weekends are spent relaxing at home as much as possible so that I can have enough energy to go to work on Monday. My social life is almost nonexistent. My home is no longer neat and clean all of the time. My bills are sometimes overlooked. I don't exert much energy at home because I don't have much energy to exert."

Kathleen H. suffers from chronic pain from a repetitive injury, but her injury and the severity of her pain are invisible. She looks perfectly healthy, well-groomed, attractive, and presents a strong demeanor. "In dealing with an invisible condition, I find that you have to prove yourself to be honest and credible, and that's not an easy task. I just don't want to come across as a malingerer. I feel that one bonus in explaining my particular situation–and I've become somewhat of an activist on this–is to educate my supervisors that the same injury that happened to me is happening with alarming frequency to my fellow coworkers. With my own knowledge and experiences thus far, I try to inform them regarding ways to prevent some of these injuries. Hopefully, I might somehow help reduce further incidents of this condition to my fellow coworkers.

Mary M. is a woman who has lived with Crohn's disease for several years. "I always try to give the impression that I am strong and independent. The only people I give a clue to that this is not the case are my doctors and my family. These are people I simply cannot hide it from. I have become a very unsocial person. I rarely go out for fun, but I do go to support groups to learn and to support others. I don't get personal with people at work and often have to turn down offers to do lunch. Now, they don't even ask."

Nancy G. described her career as totally derailed after she tried hard to continue working with the symptoms of her illness. "I had my own business which I was forced to close when I could no longer work. My financial situation changed drastically. I was no longer in control of my income, and I was no longer able to live in the lifestyle I had before."

Having a chronic illness or living with chronic pain often means plans must change suddenly. Sahar A. had a promising career and active life before becoming ill. She has earned numerous degrees but is not well enough to use them in the workplace. "I am concerned about my professional life. For instance, do I still have one? I can do so much to help my community, but the pain and discomfort have left me wondering about where I am going with all my cumulative degrees. Studying makes me feel hopeless. I tend to get to the point where I tell myself not to bother. What is the point? What is worse, I have absolutely no control over this illness despite my best intentions, and this makes me quite angry."

What do people do when they realize that they cannot work nine to five any longer? Kathleen H. has recently been faced with the reality that she cannot return to her chosen profession as a court reporter, which she had loved and enjoyed for many years. "This has been the biggest tragedy of all. . . that I am already finished with a career that I loved. I had always told myself that if I ever became bored, or perhaps after my daughter finished college, I might try something new. I had viewed this as an option to use at my discretion. Now, due to unfortunate circumstances, the decision has been made for me. I was not even close to opting for a new career or prepared for one. I was happy where I was working and with what I was doing. I was also very content with the financial aspect of it. I felt very secure in knowing that I was accruing retirement, putting money away for my daughter's college fund, and being covered medically. I felt secure in the fact that I was preparing for my future. Security has always been a mandatory theme in my life. Now it is elusive."

Since Kathleen had no control over the decision to end her career, she was not prepared mentally or emotionally to handle the paralyzing, ever-increasing fear about her inability to work. Her mind raced out of control each day as she imagined the worst-case scenario. "I am disappointed in my body. I feel like it has let me down, and the timing couldn't have been worse. I hit a stone wall. I'm not quite sure what I can do career-wise because I still have many limitations. I'm tossing a lot of ideas around, but it's a frightening prospect. I'm not opposed to change, but why should I have to? I've been in my particular profession for over fifteen years and have been very comfortable and happy. Starting a new job or even thinking about starting a new career is a scary venture. I question whether I can reeducate myself in a way that will challenge me, and whether I will do well at it. I haven't been to school in years, and that's a completely different environment. I have many doubts, and after thirty-nine years, it's a brand new feeling for me."

Marriage and family therapist, Bejai Higgins, reminds us that having a chronic illness often means feeling powerless and out of control. "The damage is directly related to the degree of self-esteem the person with the chronic illness or pain associates with their career. The higher the association, the harder it is to be disabled."[1] When Higgins sees a client for the first time, she always asks the person, "How high up in your self-esteem is your career title or job position?" Some people are confused by this question when she first poses it. This is a very interesting inquiry that reveals how much trouble the person is going to have when they cannot work full-time, or at all, or if they have to change the way they work in order to accommodate the illness.

Jaye B. is a former registered nurse who feels that she would have continued her education if she had not become sick. Her chronic symptoms affected her ability to work at a job she loved. "I had to give up working as a nurse, even in a part-time capacity, because I couldn't get through even half the day. My energy level was too unpredictable and unreliable. Too much energy was being drained from my life by working. Luckily, I was able to quit work and still be financially secure. Now, I do volunteer work which makes me feel happy and worthwhile. Most importantly, I can choose the hours I want to contribute."

Carol C. is an English woman who currently seeks employment. She has concerns about disclosing her liver condition to potential employers, but she also knows that there is a risk in withholding the information. "If I tell my employer from the beginning that I have a debilitating disease, he will not hire me. On the other hand, not telling an employer about my illness that is not otherwise visible, will cause worry on my part. Because if he finds out later, I will get fired for having to take too much time off, or for being late, or for simply not disclosing the disease to him in the first place."

Some people, out of fear or actual experience, insist that working outside the home with set hours and the added pressures of deadlines to meet and time clocks to punch exacerbates their illness. One individual reported, "I feel that I might make my disease worse if I work outside the home because I cannot avoid stress. I can do housework, but I know when I need to take it easy, and I can do that at home." Staying aware of limitations and withdrawing from activities, a job, or intimacy because of symptoms or fear can help you cope with your restrictions. Conversely, a person must avoid using illness as an excuse to evade activities or responsibilities. One bad experience need not determine future outcomes. Fearful junctures present opportunities to challenge assumptions and evaluate whether restrictions we have imposed on ourselves are sensible or simply fear based.

David K. discovered a gift that came with his diagnosis. He made a career change he otherwise would not have. At age fifty-one, he accepted an early retirement from his government job and started a new career as a substitute teacher. "I enjoy working with the kids, have much less stress, feel much better physically, and appreciate not having a boss over me all the time. I am much happier in my new career. When I heard about several of my former coworkers who could not afford to retire and learned that they have either died or had major problems such as heart bypass surgery, I was very glad that I took the early retirement." His new life and career proved beneficial and enjoyable.

Many people feel that they have to outdo their coworkers, friends, or family members in order to be perceived as good enough despite illness. "I have had firsthand experience with discrimination in employment," reports a man who lives with chronic illness. "In my foolish attempt to be up-front and honest about my condition, I told a former prospective employer about my illness. I ended up getting the job and working there for seven years, longer than I have worked anywhere else. However, I did not get the job until I signed a waiver stating that I would not attempt to join the company's health insurance plan as I would have driven up the cost for everyone else. I lived up to that agreement and spent the next seven years proving myself to be a completely dedicated and loyal employee, demonstrating an excellent work ethic and exceptional quality of work. I felt I had something to prove. What I got in return was a lot of patronizing pats on the back telling me what a great job I was doing. But compensation was low, bonuses were nonexistent (I was the only one in the entire company who was not on some sort of bonus program), and the last straw was the withholding of my Christmas bonus. According to my employer, I got my Christmas bonuses during the year because of all the doctor appointments I had to go to, which I got paid for. The fact that I was a salaried employee and put in countless extra hours for the company was irrelevant."

Sometimes you hit your head against the wall in an effort to appear to be just like everyone else, whether at work or in social circles. Ironically that special effort and over-extension can dramatically backfire and deplete your stamina and health status. It's a risky strategy.

Kathleen H. is not able to work. She feels that the chronic nature of her condition has affected not only her beloved career but her entire life. Her diminished sense of accomplishment and ability to support herself and her daughter has been devastating. "A lot has to do with ego. I have always been strong, healthy, and independent. I am naturally athletic, from gymnastics to bowling to throwing darts. Since I have a difficult time asking for help and since I was used to doing almost anything I wanted to by myself, this pain has curbed my desire for activities that I used to love and possibly new ones that I have yet to explore. This condition has changed the balance in my household. It was a big adjustment for my daughter and myself. It has also changed the balance in my personal life. I wasn't the only one who had to make adjustments. I currently have to look for new activities and interests that won't exacerbate my condition. I have yet to find many, but I'm staying positive and still looking."

The Case to Pace

Many people who live with a chronic illness or pain cannot predict, from day-to-day, what they will be able to do. This makes planning activities a real challenge. Learning to keep pace with a body that has a new speed–slow–is a tough adjustment for most people. "I cannot make plans ahead of time," reports Marilyn M., a mother of two who lives with the constant pain of fibromyalgia and migraines. "By the time the activity comes along, I might have a bad day, and I won't have the energy to do whatever it is. I need most of the day, and sometimes two, to do the laundry for two people. I take longer to do errands or chores. That is, if I can do them at all."

Jill V. is just starting to learn the intricate rules of the pacing game and how easily she can try to play catch-up when she happens to have a good hour or day. "Sometimes I start to feel better, get excited, and feel that I should take advantage of feeling better. So I begin to get things done and end up doing too much. I crash, get scared, and panic that I'll never get better, let everything go and rest, start getting better, and the cycle begins all over again. I've only just learned that instead of trying to get a lot done while feeling well, I need to temper that phase so that I don't crash. This is so obvious and yet so hard to do, because it is so exciting to feel good. I have asked friends and family to let me know if they see me in my higher functioning phase when I am doing too much. Their feedback really helps me."

Ana H. lives in the rural countryside on the outskirts of San Diego, California. She lives with the difficult symptoms of fibromyalgia. For the past two years, her husband (and a few hardy relatives) have been building a new home on their property. They are doing much of the work with their own hands. When I went to meet Ana, I found her living in a small trailer on their mountainous property. She and her husband, along with their five dogs, three cats, and two birds somehow fit into this small space. Ana could not wait for their house to be completed. She was a delightful woman with sparkling eyes, dark curly hair, and a quick wit. She greeted me with enthusiasm, and her movements were quick and energetic as we made our way up the muddy hillside to her house-in-progress. "This condition has been terrible for me," she said, with a big grin on her face that never seemed to fade. I found myself having difficulty believing she was so ill. After all, she appeared so fit and sturdy. She walked briskly and wore such a carefree expression. Then I remembered that people said that all too often about me.

Ana was obviously a survivor and had that familiar vibrant spirit that many people with concealed chronic illness seem to possess: a tough outer skin with a glow in their expression. No wonder people have difficulty believing their stories. "I feel like I have a flu that will never go away," she stated. "I can't really let anyone know how helpless I feel most of the time. I don't like to seem old or sick because I don't want to be either," she laughed. "Many times, if you seem active and healthy, you pay for it later by overextending yourself and becoming overtired. When everyone leaves and I am finally alone, I have to sleep for days afterward in order to recover."

The struggle of pain and exhaustion is a daily concern. Fatigue is a part of many chronic conditions, and making a place for this unrelenting weariness becomes a way of life. After awhile, it becomes impossible to remember what it is like not to feel exhausted. "It is important to recognize that you may be able to perform some of your previous activities, but less frequently or for a shorter duration of time," says psychologist Sarajane Williams. "People with chronic disorders can learn to work with their bodies and to recognize their limitations, but it often takes a bit of time and some trial and error."

"I have to structure rest periods during the day," reports Trish G., a teacher who has been diagnosed with ulcerative colitis. "I do not plan full weekends like I used to. I plan one or two things so that I don't get too tired. I also avoid long excursions like the ones I used to take such as overnight camping trips. They just don't work. Bathrooms aren't close at hand, and they are too tiring for me anyway. I miss camping and backpacking a lot, but on the other hand, I may have phased those activities out of my life as I got older anyway."

Families may have to find a new way of playing and having fun together when one member of the family becomes chronically ill. Old hobbies and recreational trips may make way for new and creative replacements. Playing board games rather than camping, for instance, can keep families connected and involved in each others' lives.

Resting and recuperating as preparation for repeating the cycle–again and again–can become a new but common routine for those with chronic illness. Pacing yourself becomes a difficult but essential survival technique. "I have learned over the years," says Dave K., "that you play and pay." He had to learn to weigh each chore, trip, or task at hand, and decide if the end result was worth the effort. "Sometimes the answer is yes, sometimes no."

Maria D. contracted an incurable form of hepatitis. Before her illness tackled her to the ground with debilitating fatigue, she had been employed full-time and enjoyed a flourishing career. She is no longer able to work, and that is a difficult adjustment for her. "I have centered my entire life around my disease. When I go out with my husband, we cannot be out for the entire day. The sun really tires me out as does too much walking. I avoid most of the things I used to do. I have to clean my house in shifts, a little at a time. By the time I finish, I have to start again. Basically, everything is a challenge when you live with chronic illness or pain. Some days are a challenge just to get up in the morning. Everything is usually done at a slower pace. Some days, there are things that simply do not get done. I have learned over the years to weigh the trips and tasks at hand with the question, 'is it worth the pain and fatigue I will pay later if I do this?' That question helps me limit what I do or don't do each day. I can do housework, but on a limited basis. Some days I can do almost anything (and of course, I tend to do too much on those days and pay for a week afterwards), and other days, all I can do is get myself a meal."

The Fog of Fatigue

Steve B. lives with numerous physical impairments and sleep deprivation. The lack of deep rest and debilitating fatigue keep him in a state of exhaustion, physically and emotionally. "This impacts everything I do in life."

"Some people couldn't figure me out," smiles Gloria P. who suffers from Sjogren's syndrome, an autoimmune disease marked by inflammation and eventual destruction of the body's exocrine (moisture-producing) glands. "Some days, I would have lots of energy, then need to rest the entire next day. Walking had to be done for limited periods and in shorter distances. I could not sit very long without getting extremely tired and stiff. I had to give up playing board games, cards, and working puzzles. I used to love doing all of those things."

"Before I got this illness," reports Lynn E., who lives with chronic fatigue syndrome, "I could hop in the car after a full day of work and run two or three errands. Now, a good day is having the energy to run any errands at all. When I was well, simple things like trips to the laundry room were taken for granted. Now I must often return to bed for brief periods during and after the laundry chores. I used to work forty-five hours a week, led a relatively active social life, walked my dog in the morning and evening, regularly exercised, and made plans to see friends. Now, in spite of not working, just exercising the dog is a challenge. Because of my disabling fatigue and malaise, some days do not permit any activity whatsoever. I frequently tell people that the hardest part of all of this is not getting anything accomplished."

Weakness and exhaustion are major symptoms. "The problem with fatigue is, it doesn't look like much," says therapist, Bejai Higgins, whose client base is primarily those with chronic illness and pain. "I try to educate the family around them. I tell family members, "If you're tired and you take a nap, you will wake up feeling refreshed. On the other hand, if your ill family member feels fatigued, and they lie down and take a nap, they will still wake up feeling fatigued."[2]

Higgins gave a group of siblings, whose parent had been experiencing debilitating fatigue from chronic pain, a challenging and revealing exercise. She asked them to get into their bathing suits. "I then told them that I wanted them to go outside and run around in the pool. They came back, and they were all exhausted. I said to them, 'Okay, that's what your mother feels like when she walks through the dining room.' You have to try to figure out a way to make the people in your life see your fatigue by feeling it in their own bodies. If the people around the patient can be more understanding, life is much easier for the patient."

"If I am not working, I am resting," reported Leslie W., who experiences lengthy periods of extreme fatigue. She sometimes felt left behind at work because keeping up with her coworkers was becoming harder and harder. When we met for the first time, Leslie was struggling to maintain her secret of having lupus from her supervisor and coworkers. A year later, her illness gave rise to more challenging symptoms and fatigue than she could endure. Even though she looked perfectly healthy and just fine, she was quite ill and fatigued much of the time. Leslie was forced to request permanent disability benefits and leave her beloved job.

Jaye B. finds that she needs to take extraordinarily good care of herself as she tries to balance the highs and lows of her illness. She checks to make sure that she's not taking on more than she can realistically do. "Otherwise, I'm exhausted all the time. I don't live a normal person's life. I'm in bed by 8 P.M. and get up around 9 A.M. If I am taking high doses of steroids, then I am in bed resting for longer periods of time. I feel tired all of the time. This medication affects everyone differently. Some folks who are taking steroids can work circles around what they used to do. But for me, well, I'm at a low energy point on this medication."

Some people who live with chronic illness or pain and the associated limitations are tired of being tired. At this point, they sometimes decide to challenge their limitations or else let limitations be overridden by the sheer force of their willpower. Some people have the mental determination but lack the corresponding physical stamina. It's as if the mind and physical body vibrate at different frequencies, and race or rest at entirely different levels. "In my mind, I have all of these ideas or projects I'd like to accomplish, articles I'd like to write, jobs I'd still like to hold," says Leslie W. "I still want to run things. I am an energetic person even though my body may not be energetic."

The Pain of Exercising in Pain

"I envy other people when they are doing things that I cannot do," reports Joan R., a raven-haired woman in her mid-fifties with porcelain skin and large expressive eyes. Joan lives with the pain and fatigue of fibromyalgia. The bounce in her step and her bright eyes show no signs of illness or pain. "I love tennis. I played for years. I cannot play anymore. If I were to play, I would require cortisone shots and have tons of pain. The last time I played tennis, I literally cried because of the pain. Even for me, this pain was unbelievable. I just wish things were different."

Exercise can seem overwhelming and unrealistic to someone with chronic pain, such as those who live with fibromyalgia or rheumatoid arthritis. Pain is not the only obstacle. Fatigue can be equally debilitating in these and many other chronic conditions. It is always useful to look at exercise as multidimensional. Exercise doesn't have to mean jogging around the track or swimming laps. "It could be taking the stairs when normally the person would take the elevator or just walking more than one would normally do," says Dr. Drossman.[3] "When you are looking for a progressive rehabilitation, increasing your walking 20–30% can have positive effects over a longer period of time."

Dr. McCarberg feels that with any chronic illness, exercise is key to achieving maximum functional status. Whether the patient has fibromyalgia, chronic daily headaches, IBS, or depression, "Many patients with pain complain more about functional loss than the pain itself," says McCarberg.[4] "Exercise improves function, yet is an elusive goal. Pain or chronic illness decondition us. Exercise not only appears an insurmountable task, but when we try to exercise, we are injured or symptoms worsen. For example, exercise sometimes exacerbates fibromyalgia and chronic fatigue syndrome." McCarberg advises his patients to start very slowly under close supervision of a structured program.

"Walk half a block, or use warm water exercises," suggests Dr. Cassell to his patients with arthritis or fibromyalgia. "Start off slowly, work up to a goal, and try not to make the goal too high or unrealistic." Dr. Cassell feels that a structured program in exercise, if appropriate, is beneficial for patients with joint pain or muscle problems.[5] On the other hand, Dr. Robinson feels that exercise is fine conceptually but is often rejected by patients; at certain times, it is totally impossible. "I have no problem with patients who opt to avoid exertion and would never be pushy in that arena."[6]

Dr. McCarberg's patients often try too hard to exercise, or try to exercise too heartily. As a result, they become injured. However, with a cautious approach, a physician's vigilance, and a very low-impact program (water exercise, slow walking, low-impact aerobics, low-tension exercise bikes), a minimal time exercise program can help even those with chronic conditions slowly become more fit. "Indeed, exercise can induce endorphins, improve sleep, elevate mood, facilitate weight loss, and increase stamina," Dr. McCarberg said.[7]

Nurse Marie Zadravec advises patients to determine their exercise level by their energy level (or lack thereof). "It is always counterproductive to push past endurance levels. A person with chronic pain or fatigue will learn to know when he or she has no energy reserve left and must learn to respect that pain no matter how much he or she would like to push further. A lowering of the basic immune response as well as potential injury can result if a person does not rest at the appropriate times. I find that most patients find that small, frequent periods of activity work better than longer periods of exercise. Frequent naps also help conserve as much energy as possible. The person must always remember to get past the guilt that is sometimes associated with taking frequent rest periods or even naps during the day, as these are sometimes perceived in our society as a sign of weakness."[8]

Learning to "Be Here Now"

The person who lives with chronic symptoms must constantly play the trade-off game. What can I cut today? What has to be done, and what can be shelved for awhile? How can I save my energy? How can I reshuffle the responsibilities before me so that I can maintain my stamina?

Marsha S. suffers from fibromyalgia. She also experiences frequent and severe migraines. "I have difficulty going out in the evenings now. I am so tired that I feel as though my brain is shutting off around 5 P.M. Paying attention in a meeting or even remembering names of people or words that I am trying to say is extremely difficult. This is very embarrassing. I have heard it called "fibro-fog" and I sure know what that means. People don't understand this and think I am being a party-pooper for not going out."

People who live with these draining disorders discover that they must make trade-offs to survive. If they don't alter their lives in significant ways by juggling, pacing, and simplifying activities, they cannot live their lives very effectively or efficiently. Marsha can deal with the pain, but the fatigue just stops her cold. "I cannot seem to find anything that helps except to give in and rest. When I feel good, I go, go, go! When I don't feel good, I stop and rest a few days. When the migraines go on for days, they really depress me. I truly feel that these headaches affect the brain chemistry. As soon as they go away, I am not at all depressed."

Simplifying a life means eliminating clutter. Large and small compromises and sacrifices can help a person with a chronic hidden illness to carry on more successfully. If it is possible to hire others to cook, mow the lawn, grocery shop, or clean the house, the precious energy conserved dwells in the body's storage tank for use during the rough patches.

Delegating is a crucial survival skill that chronically ill individuals must develop. This is often difficult, especially if a patient links self-worth to tasks completed. For instance, someone with chronic back pain or arthritis may have difficulty asking the grocery store bagger to assist them to the car. Accustomed to being self-sufficient, many with pain or chronic illness may equate help with weakness and the loss of dignity. They desperately want to remain self-sufficient and are loathe to surrender to fatigue and pain. Others, however, may regard such a request as a way to reserve and restore some energy and preclude the most persistent pain.

"Be prepared for others to ask what they can do to help," cautions therapist Jan Yaffe. "Don't think of these reactions as demeaning. If they can assist in some way, they will feel less helpless."[9] Learning to accept help can actually be a favor to others. Accepting aid from friends and family may be easier if you look at it in this way: You are helping them to cope. "Give some thought to how these individuals can make your life easier. Can they drive you to doctor appointments, pick up groceries, or just visit when you feel alone? Learning to feel comfortable with this healthy dependency is time and effort well-spent. That is a lesson we all need to learn."

People who live with chronic illness or pain often simplify the demands of their day. They must examine core values, beliefs, and desires and hold onto what best reflects or supports them, then let go of all of the rest. While holding fast to the core of who they are and what they enjoy, the individual who is ill may need to take radically different approaches toward reinforcing priorities.

"I try to remind these people that simplifying often equals strength," states Dr. Michael Wrobel. "For example, resting after breaking a leg is realistic and helpful. Why should someone with a chronic illness that is affecting their health, their stamina, their mood, and their ability to do things be any different?"

Energy levels vary wildly for this population; acknowledging that is an enormous self-care tool. That said, Dr. Geneé Jackson reminds us that this process can be lengthy. "You may need a considerable amount of time to actually dismantle a current lifestyle and build something different. This includes rethinking your place of residence, type of work (if you are able to work at all), friends, family members, spending and eating habits, as well as what you do for fun and long-term financial plans."[10]

Making decisions, making changes, and dealing with the unexpected can be overwhelming to someone living with pain and illness. "Energy levels have to be assessed and respected on a regular basis," suggests Jackson. "All plans must be made with the expectation that they may need to be modified."

People who live with concealed disabilities talk in terms of good days and bad days. If the bad days overshadow the good days, self-care and activity levels wane. Performing one major task per day helps many people who are ill manage their world, if only in small bites. Deciding what is a priority and what can wait becomes a science. Pacing and juggling tasks and pleasurable activities become skills that optimize chances for a manageable life.

Along with delegating tasks, many people with a concealed illness must learn to manage their guilt about not being able to do the things they used to do. If they cannot get to the living room today to pick up all of the old magazines, they can learn to become more flexible.

Pacing is a skill that takes time to acquire. Many people who are forced to let their routines fall by the wayside on a bad day find themselves struggling to catch up during the good days. A good day can simply mean a bit more energy. What may become problematical is that many individuals who wake up to a good day find two weeks of chores and activities waiting. And thus, the vicious cycle perpetuates; it is easy to again overdo and exhaust an already depleted stamina. This frustrating and dangerous cycle confounds most people with chronic disorder.

No Pain, No Gain?

Chronic pain often accompanies chronic illness. Unfortunately for the patient as well as the physician, pain is invisible and can only be measured subjectively. Chronic pain is usually defined by pain that persists longer than six months and can manifest itself as an aching, throbbing, burning, shooting, or stabbing sensation. Frequently, chronic pain seemingly exists in a vacuum; although more than fifty million Americans live with chronic pain, many live without a concrete diagnosis or explanation.[11]

How does one live with debilitating, ongoing pain with no hope of relief on the horizon? Living with pain, day after day, can lead to severe depression, low self-image, unemployment, and financial devastation. Often the best approach is to adapt to the pain rather than to wait for recovery. A vexing challenge, this adaptation requires a great deal of courage and a fair amount of time.

Sensations that generate excruciating pain in one person might barely be noticed by someone else. This can be an enormous problem for the treating physician. Magnetic resonance imaging of the brain has confirmed that some people do, in fact, feel significantly more pain than others. Their brain scans register quite differently from those who barely feel pain. "When researchers compared the brain scans in a recent study with the pain rating of volunteers, they found parts of the brain known to be involved in experiencing pain were more active in people who said they felt more pain. In particular, they found increased activity in the primary somatosensory cortex, which deals with pain location and intensity, and the anterior cingulated cortex, which handles unpleasant feelings caused by pain."[12]

Intractable pain was once seen as an inevitable consequence of some underlying injury or illness. However, pain is now becoming recognized as a separate condition. It is best served by pain specialists and clinics for both assessment and solutions. Pain management has become a huge industry, with specialty clinics and pain treatment centers now affiliated with hospitals throughout the nation. Treatment can include medication (and medication adjustment) or nonmedication-based management such as biofeedback, counseling, and physical therapy. Sometimes, despite the best efforts of the physician and modern medicine, relief remains elusive.

People who live with chronic pain frequently believe that they alone live with such physical distress. This perception can, in turn, engender a sense of hopelessness and isolation–even from friends and family. Others who live with chronic pain believe that their value is measured by the number of tasks and activities they accomplish. By not being able to participate or achieve what they used to, people with chronic pain can be left with feelings of guilt, insignificance, or loneliness. They can become angry, not only at the community of medical professionals who cannot seem to cure them or ease their pain, but also at themselves for being in pain in the first place.

Peggy S. is a lively and talkative woman, but she lives with the daily pain of fibromyalgia and feels as though she always has the flu. "I used to be able to do absolutely every sport and activity, but now I suffer for it afterwards. I still participate at times but often realize it is just not worth it. I went with my husband to hit a bucket of golf balls. I hit two of them and thought I'd have to go to the emergency room later that evening!"

There are four major sources of chronic pain: muscle, nerve, bone (joint), and blood vessel (such as with migraines). The source of the pain will often dictate the best treatment method. Some people respond well to medications. Others find relief by incorporating relaxation techniques such as yoga or meditation into their daily lives. Dietary and biomechanical adjustments can also improve quality of life. The best way to manage chronic pain is different for every individual. Unfortunately, in this one-size-doesn't-fit-all universe, some will never find complete relief. Getting better is sometimes not an option. Some people will have to learn to cope as best they can and adopt a new attitude and way of life that is challenging but still fulfilling.

Raelene Paulus is a registered nurse at a large veterans hospital in Southern California. She finds that during certain periods, especially when there is moderate to severe pain that lasts for days, the use of some noninvasive techniques along with medications may be the most effective way to relieve pain. "Teaching the patient about new strategies to help relieve pain, such as acupuncture and biofeedback, increases the number of pain-relief options available."[13]

But what is chronic pain really like to live with? If you have not experienced it, it is difficult to wrap your mind around such a steadfast companion. Chronic pain goes on and on with no end in sight. One woman reports that chronic pain is different from having a baby where there are breaks in-between contractions and epidural anesthesia to ease the worst pain. You can only take unrelenting pain for so long. Women endure labor pains because they understand that their pain is finite and they'll be rewarded richly for their efforts. When you are in chronic pain, however, there is no end in sight.

"It starts to grate at your nerves," explains Diane M. "Sometimes I think that I'm holding my breath waiting for a break in the pain. If the pain lasts for extended periods, I don't want to be anywhere that is noisy or in a social setting where I have to act happy and pleasant. There were many times that my daughter wanted to invite friends over for a sleep-over, and I had to say no. I knew I could not handle it. And then there were times when I felt guilty as a mom and did say yes to her requests and regretted it later. Now I try to be honest about what I can and cannot handle."

Kathleen H. told me that she has tried everything to ameliorate her chronic pain. "I'm still open to suggestion, but I bought a magnet pillow. It didn't work. I've changed mattresses thinking it might be my bed. It didn't help. I've bought every product with wheels on it. I lived for a year slathered in creams. It didn't help. I've been on anti-inflammatories, muscle relaxants, and painkillers, but they offered me only a very subtle and temporary respite. I've had physical therapy, hand therapy, neck therapy, and trigger-point injections. I put two tennis balls in an old ski sock to reach and massage my shoulder blades. It feels great but doesn't help the pain. I've been to a work conditioning rehabilitation program. That was a joke. They had me strap on a heart monitor, get on the treadmill, and measure my heart rate. Then I did leg stretches. I was supposed to do that three to four days a week for four weeks. That one pushed me to the edge. I kept asking, 'How does this help my right arm, shoulder, and neck problem?' I've had acupuncture. I have had every kind of wrist and arm brace you can imagine. I've tried a massaging heating pad. I've tried ice. I'm still searching the web looking for any new treatments. In the end, I have come to accept my condition and learn to trust my own instincts and make healthy decisions for myself. I am now trying to move forward."

"Just last night, I had a flare-up and could not go to a much anticipated baseball game," says Steve G. who lives with ulcerative colitis. "So, not only was I in pain, but I was missing out on something I wanted to do. When I have my pain, or discomfort, I just want to be left alone. There is nothing anyone can do and my friends and family can't understand what I'm going though. My wife does a good job of knowing what I need and if I want to be left alone. She will check in on me every hour or so. I feel angry toward my body and this whole situation. When I experience pain, I cannot seem to identify what causes it to come on."

"Chronic pain is a real struggle of character," states Bejai Higgins.[14] She teaches her clients non-drug relief techniques for all forms of chronic pain. "Anything that works for more than five minutes goes on a list because it's a useful tool no matter what it is. I ask my clients to go through the list and try everything. Drugs are on it, but often drugs take away your mental acuity and lessen your feeling of being in the world. I teach my clients practical relaxation, guided imagery, and self massage techniques. I teach children how to massage the palms of their parent's hands if the parent has chronic pain, cramping, etc. A pleasurable sensation in the hand will block some of the pain messages. I do this exercise with them so that they can do something useful and generous for their parent and something that will help both of them feel better. It helps the child of a parent with chronic pain feel worthwhile."

Higgins does pain work with almost all of her clients who live with a concealed disability. "I ask them to come up with a log and record their pain for a week and then bring in the log. Okay, the pain is worse in the morning. That means you have a window of opportunity in the middle of the afternoon where you can schedule all of your social events because you're likely to feel better. This gives people who live with chronic pain a feeling of control again." Higgins also asks clients to identify what they are going to do each day. "They should identify one of the tasks on their daily to-do list as a flat tire task, so that if they have a flat tire kind of day, they have one thing on their list that they do not have to do. There should also be something on the list that is purely pleasurable, purely for them, and that they are not allowed to drop. Getting out of bed in the morning is often painful, and if all you have scheduled for the day is shoulds and musts, you might not make it. We have to guarantee ourselves that we are going to be able to do that pleasurable thing, no matter what. I do this exercise for myself every single day. I make sure that I have something each day to look forward to that is just for me, and I never allow myself to drop this item from my list."

"The basic question," adds Yaffe, "is not what do I have to do, or who do I have to please, but rather, will this activity or person add something to my life right now? If not, I know it is not essential and I can let it go."[15]

Activity and pain logs are helpful. See what you are able to do on a daily basis without overextending yourself. Also, examine what time of the day you are able to function best. Stop chasing the things that you are not up to doing, and start maximizing the time and energy that you do have.

You have to be realistic about how many functioning hours you have in a day. If you set yourself up for six hours a day and can realistically function for only four, then you have to ask yourself, What am I doing? By trying to exceed your physical limits, you are encouraging everyone else to assume that you can do more than is comfortable. "You have to be more realistic with your own expectations," explains Higgins. "There is a reasonably good life with a disability, but you have to give it the room it's going to take. You cannot constantly move beyond your physical limitations, or your life is going to be full of little failures."

As the head of a prominent pain clinic, Dr. Bill McCarberg always validates his patients' symptoms and lets them know that what they are experiencing is real. "It is not made up or just in their heads. I also make sure that all diagnostic procedures have been explored and all treatments have been appropriate. I survey patients about the impact of their pain and the illness on their lives."[16] McCarberg asks his patients what their expectations are of him. He administers antidepressants, anticonvulsants, muscle relaxants, opiates, and other medications as necessary. He also enrolls patients in a six-hour cognitive behavior program designed to empower the patient with new skills that will help them deal with their chronic symptoms.

"Most patients with chronic illness," says McCarberg, "will present with particular predominant symptoms to their disease. For irritable bowel syndrome, there is usually bloating, diarrhea, or constipation. For fibromyalgia, there is global pain, fatigue, and poor sleep. For interstitial cystitis, there is urinary frequency, urgency, and pelvic pain. In addition, most patients have stress about their symptoms which results in depression, poor sleep, poor life adjustment, and social withdrawal."

The American Pain Foundation recommends that a patient discuss their pain when they see a doctor. They must let the doctor know where the pain is located and describe it on a scale of zero to ten, where zero means no pain at all and ten means intolerable pain.[17] Describe anything that makes the pain feel better or makes it worse. Is it always there? Does it move around? Do other things (diet, activity, fatigue) make it feel better or worse? What type of pain is it? Use specific words like sharp, stabbing, dull, aching, burning, throbbing, or deep pressing.

How does the pain affect your daily life? Does it interfere with sleep, with work, with exercise? Does it inhibit your ability to participate in social activates or keep you from concentrating? How does it affect your mood? Tell your physician or nurse about previous attempts to alleviate your pain. Have you taken medication or had surgery? Have you tried massage or meditation? Does the application of heat or cold help? Explain what works and, most importantly, what does not.

You have a right to have your report of pain taken seriously by physicians and nurses and to be treated with dignity. As one person with chronic fatigue syndrome sadly pointed out, "One time, I went to a physician who told me I didn't have chronic fatigue syndrome because I appeared to have too much energy."

You have the right to have your pain thoroughly assessed and promptly treated. A physician will discuss what could be causing the pain, possible treatments, and the benefits, risks, and costs of each. You have the right to participate actively in the decisions about your pain management and to be referred to a pain specialist if your pain persists. You also have the right to clear and prompt answers to your questions, time to make decisions, and the right to refuse a particular type of treatment if you so choose.

When discussing pain that occurs with a chronic illness or condition, we often overlook the accompanying psychological pain. "People do not see the emotional pain," reports Linda F., a diabetic. "I have no children because I am diabetic. I'm so tired of hearing about other people's children and grandchildren. Everyone just assumes that since I am diabetic, not having a family should be normal. It hurts. People can be insensitive about the painful emotions surrounding the disease."

Isolation and Chronic Illness
We all do our fair share of mind reading. It seems to be an ineluctable facet of human nature. But this becomes particularly damning with respect to the presumptions we make–despite a dearth of information–about how others per-

ceive those who are ill. This is especially true of those who live with concealed chronic illness or pain. This group of very ill individuals spends an inordinate amount of time fearing what people will think, how they will react, and what they will say. Assumptions are made even before the facts are disclosed. A diligent, concerted effort to overcome the tendency to mind read is an imperative first step toward combating isolation. Chronically ill people retreat and often isolate before they give others an opportunity to understand and empathize. They isolate in order to protect themselves against their worst fears.

"I tend to hole up when my symptoms flare-up," reports Trish G. "This is not entirely helpful as I get lonely and scared. But I tend to curtail activities, simplify my diet, and increase my rest when I start to feel poorly. I started putting aside one or two hours every afternoon to watch a video. Now I nap every day. That seems to suit my body rhythms pretty well since I have low energy in the afternoon. After a nap, I am able to enjoy my evenings without having to feel as though I'm waiting to crawl into bed and go to sleep."

"Most people will understand if you tell them of your limitations," reports psychologist Michael Wrobel. "Find a way to increase predictability and control. Information and knowledge bring relief for the majority of us in the long run." For instance, if you have irritable bowel syndrome or inflammatory bowel disease, find out where the bathrooms are before you go somewhere. Do some research so that you feel more relaxed about where everything is located and how long you need to get there. This knowledge can save you hours of anxiety and may just allow you to venture to places where you otherwise wouldn't dare go. "Realize that you may not be able to predict and control everything," Wrobel reminds us. "Empathy toward yourself and a good dose of humor go a long way. Sometimes the unpredictable can be fun–and funny–often making for some interesting stories later. We are normal and special people who happen to have a chronic illness with concealed symptoms. The illness doesn't define us, but becomes integrated into who we are and what we do."[18]

People who have a lot of downtime because of their illness often feel guilty about being less productive and social. Others make peace with the necessity to rest more often and accept this as part of their survival plan.

Kim H. maintains that she sets aside every Sunday to rest. She never makes plans to see friends, go shopping, or drive on that particular day. Kim knows that if she doesn't take this weekly time-out, she may run out of steam during the week. "My husband and I just make it our lazy, rainy day to stay inside, even if it is sunny and ninety degrees in the shade. We lie in bed, read the Sunday paper, chat about the week's activities, and watch old movies on the television. I turn it into my vacation-from-the-world day, so it feels like a treat rather than a forced rest."

Part Four

The Challenge to Change

Nine

Lessons Learned

The Losses and Gains

To say I'm glad that I developed my own illnesses because they taught me more about myself, about human nature, and about learning to appreciate the good, is quite a rationalization. To be elated about the worst circumstances in our lives doesn't necessarily make them joyous occasions worth celebrating. Let's put away the balloons and confetti. However, more often than not, I have seen such struggles beget tremendous happiness and insight. People discover what they are made of, what they are capable of, what they can endure, and most importantly, their self-worth. This knowledge has the potential to radically enrich lives.

Leslie W.'s lupus has been an exceptional teacher. She's learned to slow down, which allows her to appreciate life much more fully. "I write to friends much more frequently now. I quilt. I read. I plant flowers. My house looks like a fairy tale cottage. If I were not ill, I would never have taken the time to explore these more sedentary activities and creative interests."

Trish G.'s illness has helped her stop and smell the roses. "I have more time to develop spiritually and pursue my inner interests instead of being active all of the time. I find I am much more sympathetic to other people and their problems, whatever they might be. I have learned that some problems in life cannot be surmounted by sheer will, but must be adjusted to. This is an important lesson."

Dave K. was first diagnosed with psychosomatic illness—one with physical manifestations but without any known or identifiable physical cause. He later learned that his disorder was not all in his head, but rather in his intestines. He had Crohn's disease. However, he acquired an invaluable skill prior to receiving the correct diagnosis. "When my problem was supposedly psychosomatic, I learned self-hypnosis. The hypnosis helped me to relax, control my pain, and challenge my thoughts. To this day, I still use the self-hypnosis technique I learned years ago."

Lee T. clearly sees the value of the lessons her illness has taught her. "In the long run, this has forced me to look at my life more philosophically and less as a superficial series of achievements. It has enhanced my appreciation of the beauty in the world and the joy of friends and family."

Danny M.'s religious beliefs are deeply rooted in Judaism. He works in a company that manufactures exercise equipment. Danny suggested that he be photographed surrounded by the various workout machines in his company's showroom. It is equipment that he will probably never again use, but he is happy because he is still working in a job he enjoys and maintains a productive life. In addition to living with Crohn's disease, Danny had recently undergone a liver transplant—an experience that left him with a deep appreciation of each new day. "This is what life has given me. I look around and find so many people worse off than I am. If I dwell on my medical condition, that sort of focus may make everything feel worse than it really is. That kind of attention creates anxiety, at least for me." Danny spoke of the joy and strength he received from his faith. He felt a great appreciation for what he had gained through his illness; he refused to focus on what he had lost.

"I wouldn't wish this on anybody," laughs Kathleen H. "Even so, I firmly believe there is much to be learned from this trying experience. Our initial reaction to a negative or scary situation like this, is just that—negative and scary! Not all good things enter our lives wrapped in pretty packages. We just don't realize this fact of life at the time of diagnosis. I have gained more empathy for others in many different types of challenging situations. I've learned that it's okay to question the system and rely on your instinct, because you know yourself and your body better than anyone else. I believe that how you survive such an ordeal makes you a stronger person. I had to let down my guard and be vulnerable. I felt totally raw and exposed, but I survived. And my friends and family were still there, not thinking any less of me. We are all human and we have our frailties. It is not only okay, but it is healthy to share these shortcomings with one another. I believe there is a reason for everything. I rarely receive the answer to my questions on demand. But, inevitably, somewhere down the road, I get this feeling: Oh, now I get it. I always know the answer will be sent, but I just don't know when I'll receive it. I just keep the faith."

Having a concealed chronic illness or experiencing chronic pain can often force a person to review life patterns; it can eventually bring new meaning into life. For example, examining your job history or career may lead you to conclude that working so hard is a way of avoiding true intimacy with loved ones. "The illness, by default, stops you in your tracks and forces you to face-off with yourself," says Dr. Geneé Jackson. "You see who in your life is emotionally available and supportive to you and who is not. In a sense, you are forced to become more vulnerable with these special people in your life in ways that you would never have had an opportunity to do before."[1]

Jill V. found that living with chronic fatigue syndrome brought her periods of great learning and deep personal transformation. They have also brought to her "the hardest, scariest, darkest, and yet most illuminating times of my life. I know that there are great lessons and meaning in this illness as long as I am willing to see them."

The Spiritual Connection
Many people coping with physical or mental pain or other challenging symptoms seek to locate meaning in their suffering. This is where spirituality plays

such a critical role. It is the relationship with a greater force—God, a Higher Power, a Higher Self, Buddha Nature, Krishna, Christ Consciousness, Cosmic Intelligence, Spirit, etc.—that provides comfort. This belief and connection give meaning and purpose to our lives despite physical or mental anguish.

Illness is a potent life event that causes most people to ask grand and probing questions: Why am I here? or Why did this challenging event come into my life? Suffering and illness usually ride in tandem. However, some conclude that there is no divine purpose or meaning whatsoever to the suffering induced by any disorder. Regardless, once illness strikes, people can grow by using what is learned to better themselves and others who are facing similar circumstances and challenges.

People who live with chronic pain or illness may experience feelings that they are being punished in some way. Maria D., who suffers from hepatitis, said that she prays all of the time for the illness to be gone and to "just have my energy back. Sometimes I feel like God is punishing me for my past."

"I have definitely toyed with those feelings of punishment," reports Kathleen H., who lives with chronic pain. "What I do when I feel this way is to make room in my mind for a clear spot and take away all the other junk that is clouding my judgment. Then I ask myself, 'Kathleen, is that how you truly feel?' Well, the answer is usually, 'No, I don't.' I allow myself that safe place in my mind. I take the time to really think it through and reinforce to myself that I am okay, not inferior, or defective, or being punished in any way. I also tell myself that I am not a victim, and I don't want to start thinking like one."

For many, spirituality is what sustains them through life's most difficult days. Many who have found themselves in the clutches of severe pain or other intractable symptoms have searched for healing and comfort. They need to make sense of their circumstances and move to a place of wisdom that offers a tangible perspective of the big picture. They often discover a new path, a novel way of looking at the world that sustains them through the worst of times and feeds their joy of living during the best periods.

"I believe in the mind, body, and spirit connection when it comes to health," says Rob H. who suffers from chronic pain. "Regardless of the pain or condition one is dealing with, having some type of spiritual practice that allows you to recognize how your life fits into the world is vital."

Rob relies on the practice of Nichiren Buddhism as an important part of his life and to help him deal with chronic pain. "Through this practice, I become more aware of the law of cause and effect. That for every action there is a reaction. When it comes to my back pain, I know that if I don't continue my stretching, weight training, and medical practices, my pain will quickly return." Buddhism helps followers see that the key to happiness, despite illness or pain, is up to them.

There are many people searching spiritually to try to understand more about life and illness. A stroll down this path has led Kim H. to the one thing that has made the biggest difference. "In 2002, I traveled to Northern California. I was needed to be part of a support system for a close friend who was undergoing leukemia treatment at a Bay Area hospital. At the same time, my own health was not doing too well. I was rundown from the stress of travel and worry about my friend and was suffering some flare-ups of my disease. My friend, a practicing Buddhist who was concerned about my fragile health during this stressful time, started chanting for my health to improve. She introduced me to Buddhism and taught me to chant the phrase *Nam-myoho-renge-kyo* while I was driving into the city each day to visit my ill friend in the hospital. I noticed a change in my health almost at once. This practice teaches happiness and taking control of one's own life. As I practiced, I noticed my energy increasing, weight increasing (which is good for me), and my overall symptoms starting to become more normal. It was incredible, especially for a skeptic like me." Kim has been practicing Buddhist chanting for over a year and continues to experience greatly improved health. She is quick to remind others that this is not magic. "This practice promotes living responsibly. I take my medication and follow my diet along with chanting to improve my health. I have faith in the balance I am creating between myself and the energy in the universe. This balance leads to my improved health and happiness. I feel like I have much more control over my life, and my health naturally improves in this condition."

Kim's Buddhism practice reminds her that we have a connection to everything in our world. "By following this belief system, my life force has become stronger," says Kim. "I feel more connected to the world and my health has improved. When you can get outside of yourself and work for a greater cause (helping others), there is a direct benefit to your life."

Being diagnosed and living with a chronic illness or chronic pain often forces people to reevaluate their religion, philosophy, or beliefs about life. Some who live with a concealed chronic illness or chronic pain derive great strength and coping mechanisms from faith and spirituality. Sahar A., a Muslim woman, found her beliefs reinforced through her many difficult years of health challenges. "Allah (God) promises not to place a burden on anyone that they cannot handle, so obviously Allah thinks that this struggle, is within my reach. I am not being punished. This illness has helped build my character. When I reach a point where I feel deeply depressed, I pray. I cry to my Creator and make *dua* (request to Allah) for strength and guidance."

Diane M. relies on her Christian faith to help make sense of her circumstances and put her illness in perspective. Her belief in an afterlife helps her cope with her pain and challenges. "Even though I am suffering desperately now, I will be in no distress and be happy forever at a later time. I have a great faith even though I can get very angry and frustrated with not understanding why this is happening to me."

Diane's ardent beliefs, along with the support of family and friends, has helped her stay afloat during the most difficult days with chronic fatigue syndrome. "I picture my spirit as a garden. When I'm feeling my worst, the garden may be down to one rose, wilted at that, but it is always alive. When I start to feel better, that one rose lifts its head and becomes strong. On the best days, I have a whole garden of flowers, vibrant in the sun. Having this image cheers me and keeps me grounded and hopeful. When I feel my worst, however, I desperately beg God for good health. Unfortunately, my spirituality seems to go to the back burner when I feel better and am having a good day. I want to remember to remain spiritual all the time regardless of my health status."

Even the most devout concede that religious fervor can wane when the body agonizes. All too frequently, bad days eclipse good ones, and one's faith takes a beating. "I sometimes get angry at my body and God for this sickness," says Pete M. "I have found my faith in a god to ebb and flow over the years, as my illness flares up or goes into a remission."

Sallee S. is a woman in her mid-twenties who suffers from a chronic bladder condition. She prays nearly every day, not to make her illness disappear, but for the strength and trust to deal with its most painful symptoms. For her, prayer is a stabilizer; it strengthens her resolve and gently paves the way toward acceptance. "Talking about my condition and the feelings surrounding it helps me a great deal. In prayer, I can talk about exactly how I feel without leaving out any of the grim details."

Diane J. has survived brain cancer—not once, but twice. Her faith has sustained her through difficult surgeries, long periods of rehabilitation, and overwhelming fears. "I know it is hard to believe, but having had cancer has been a gift and continuing blessing for me. I am a successful human being because I have accomplished so much with my strong resolve and a determined step, literally and figuratively, although sometimes my gait is a bit unsteady! I am the one who has faced seemingly impossible odds. My doctors think I am a miracle. I have always had peace because of my faith in God, which continues to grow every day. The battle is His and not mine. I just turn all of my burdens over to Him."

Judy R. has had a difficult time maintaining her faith through the darkest days of her illness. She comes from a Catholic background and has a strong belief in God, but her faith has been tested repeatedly through each hospitalization and its aftermath. Recently, Judy was rushed to the emergency room with a life-threatening abdominal infection that had migrated into her blood stream. This is not the first time Judy has had a brush with death. "They performed emergency surgery the next morning, and I have to have another surgery in a couple of weeks. I spent two weeks in a hazy recovery. I now look forward with no great glee to the next surgery. They are going to try to put Humpty Dumpty back together again."

At one point, Judy had enrolled in a technical school for job training. "I had to keep putting off the start date because of the flare-ups and treatments for my Crohn's disease. Then this emergency surgery happened. All my plans fell to the wayside again. By the time I regained consciousness, I had lost all expectations of ever having a life beyond this disease. I had not lost my faith, but I'd definitely lost hope."

Judy was left weak, depressed, and scared by her ordeal. Her faith was tested, and she found it difficult to call upon her own spiritual strength when she felt, as she described it, kicked to the curb. Like so many others, Judy's deep faith and unflagging courage remained intact during the relatively easy periods. Her religious beliefs seemed to sustain her, even if there was an occasional bump and fall. But when death drew close, when plans to rebuild her life with schooling and training had been crushed, she became distrustful and defeated. Judy felt adrift, overwhelmed, and could not imagine recapturing the sense of confidence we all need to move forward. As she and I sat and discussed her most recent ordeal with this disease, she mentioned the phrase "God doesn't give us more than we can handle." With tears glistening in the corners of her eyes, Judy looked up at the ceiling, forced a laughed and said, "God, I think you must be on a coffee break because I don't know how much more of this I can handle." Her laughter was loud but half-hearted. What was unmistakable was the profound sadness and fear behind those forced giggles. She was a woman reaching for her faith, but the tools and beliefs she had come to rely on had fallen just out of reach—at least on this difficult day.

Faith can be an exceptional coping mechanism. During painful periods, however, people with chronic pain or illness often surrender a dearly held belief system. Lee T. has utilized meditation and other spiritual studies for many years to help her deal with the symptoms and stress surrounding her illness. "I have to admit," Lee confesses, "that at the depth of my misery, I had trouble focusing on spiritually uplifting concepts or continuing to have faith in anything." We frequently lose the tools that help us maintain strength, faith, and hope along the way. Often, we recapture them once the worst of the storm has passed.

At times, chronic symptoms can test your stamina, your faith, and your will to move forward. When you are at your worst, when you have hit the bottom of the ocean, seeing or remembering the sun shining above the dark water is very difficult. When people have been dragged down too far for too long, they often cannot recall better and brighter times. It is easy for them to forget that people care about them and their well-being. Being ill or in pain for too long induces amnesia. Some forget about life's pleasures, lose a little faith, and temporarily misplace their seemingly distracted God.

The Fickle Nature of Flares

One of the realities about chronic illness or pain is that there are good days and bad days. This is the nature of the beast—its course is unpredictable, and flare-ups will happen when you least expect them (and least want them to happen). You may be diligently pacing yourself, getting enough rest at night, staying away from problem food, meditating to take the edge off stress, and still the flare-ups come to call. Sometimes you can see a link between a particular activity and a flare-up, but at other times, there seems to be neither rhyme nor reason for your discomfort. During these volatile stretches, when symptoms unexpectedly ebb and flow, the only certainty is the difficulty associated with social events, travel plans, work, or school responsibilities.

Remission is sometimes a gift, but never a given.

"Some days I feel normal, and I think to myself, maybe I am better," says Rick D., who suffers with fluctuating hearing loss. "Sometimes I have several days or weeks without a flare-up and that always gives me hope that maybe this is going away. Then a flare-up happens, and I become pretty depressed. I always feel so good when I can suddenly hear normally in both ears. The feeling is hard to describe, but all of a sudden, my mood is much brighter. Having this hearing condition is very difficult. I never know when I go to bed if I will be able to hear when I awaken in the morning. I have lost a lot of sleep worrying about this. I especially worry about going to sleep and waking with a problem in the morning when I have an important meeting the following day or have to travel for business. I find myself waking up several times during the night to test my hearing. If my ear is plugged, I tend to have a minor panic attack. I sometimes lie awake for hours until the alarm sounds, just worrying about a flare-up. I think that the lack of peaceful sleep is one of the most upsetting aspects of this condition, and this leads to my becoming very moody and depressed during a major flare-up. I know this is hard on my family. I have been working to accept my condition and just get on with life. The intermittent nature of this condition leads to an endless cycle of hope and then despair."

Health issues can easily define the structure and pace of daily life. "I am always monitoring my level of vitality and my reserves," says Marc H., an attorney who lives with chronic fatigue syndrome. "I cannot let myself become run-down, or I will become sick later. It is just a part of my life, just as someone on oxygen is always monitoring the level in their tank."

Living with chronic illness or a chronic condition requires coping with uncertainty. Some people have an easier time going with the flow than others. People who are used to feeling in control have a more difficult adjustment to their new way of being in the world. Will they be able to take care of their children today? Will they be able to go to work tomorrow? Will they have to contend with unbearable symptoms when they go out tonight? The list of adjustments and new rules with family and friends, jobs and careers, child care, and vacations, can grow quite long very quickly. "Sacrifices must be made on many levels," Dr. Elizondo reminds her patients with chronic illness, "and you have no choice but to cope in some manner."

Crystal F. still finds herself frustrated by a severe chronic illness. She lives in a pleasant cookie-cutter suburban paradise with her children and husband. When we first met, we spoke about her illness and about how self-conscious she felt about having her picture taken. Crystal's face was still swollen from the steroids she took to control her disease. Even though the puffiness of her cheeks was not that noticeable to those around her, it concerned her and made her a bit shy. She rested her head in her hands and let her fingers surround her cheeks, hoping to camouflage what was so obvious to her but not to those around her—that this illness had dealt a devastating blow to her life as a young wife and mother. Crystal's pets and kids were running around the house as we made our way to the family room. As we sat on the couch, she spoke about the feelings surrounding her illness and discussed the intensity with which her chronic symptoms had impacted her family life. "I had difficulty accepting that I was no longer healthy," she started. "What a horrible roller-coaster ride! When the illness is in remission, you begin to live again, but then a flare-up happens, and all of your optimism goes out the window, and you start all over again. The worst part is the impact on my family. The guilt sets in when I have to cancel family plans."

"I don't adjust very well to flare-ups," reports one woman who lives with the chronic pain of fibromyalgia. "I tend to do more than I am capable of and ignore my pain. Then I suffer later, especially with disturbed and unrestorative sleep. On the other hand, if I accepted my physical state and limited myself too often, I would never get out of bed."

Laurie E. has chronic migraines and chronic ear/balance problems. "I have been dealing with my illness since 1994. I have good days and bad days and everything in-between. Slowly, and over time, I have had to give up most of my activities and the things I enjoy doing. I can't always plan things in advance since I don't know how I'll feel on any given day. When I do plan something, I accept the reality that I may be forced to cancel if I am not feeling well enough."

Some people learn to pamper themselves when a difficult flare-up comes to call. "I get into bed with a book, a cup of tea, and a heated bag of herbs on my stomach," reports a young mother of six children who lives with the unpredictable flare-ups of her intestinal disease. "The warmth of the bag feels good and helps with cramping and spasms. I wish I had better painkillers though. If I were out of pain, this disease wouldn't be so unbearable. I would just ignore it. Actually, with six children, I spend little time in bed anyway. When I hurt, I sit in one of my comfortable chairs and continue to spend time with the children and home-school them."

Jaye. B. tries her best to ride out the waves of symptoms she has lived with for decades. During our interview, she insisted that her disease was not who she was but rather what she had. "The disease is a large part of the way I am and the way I act but is certainly not my soul. As a result of the illness, the pieces of the puzzle of who I am do not fit together like they should at times. I don't care what others think of me. My illness is not something I tend to wear on my sleeve." Jaye B. has held onto her sense of humor through a very challenging illness. "I tried to make friends with my diseased ileum (the lower part of the small intestine) by naming her Isabelle, thinking that if I put a name to her, she would cooperate. Isabelle definitely lets me know she is there and that she is a powerful force in my life. I vacillate between loving her and hating her. If someone wrote a book about my life, it would be called *The Ileum and the Odyssey*."

The most important thing to remember during a flare-up is that you may not be able to control the timing or severity, but you can work on your reaction to future episodes. Some people beat themselves up during a flare-up.

What did I do to cause it? Why can't I be like other people? What's wrong with me? Why am I so weak? We must all see ourselves as human during these times. Would the ill person berate someone who is sick in the same way they berate themselves? Probably not. Their flare-up is real and their body has limits. Working on honoring your own limitations is a worthy goal.

Some people who experience frequent flare-ups try to accept rather than fight them. Flare-ups do not become best friends, but they are part of the body process and need not be the enemy. There is only so much anyone can do when their body is not behaving itself. People who live with chronic disorders must give themselves credit for doing the best they can with a difficult situation. Engaging in alternative activities certifies the ability to accomplish; it is an exceedingly pragmatic approach to dealing with chronic symptoms. If you are bedridden but can sit in bed, asking someone to bring in a large sheet of paper or writing pad and some felt pens is a good start. It is especially helpful to experiment creatively and set aside the judgment that often thwarts our attempts at creative endeavors. Leslie W. says that the good news about lupus is that she has a lot of time to rest. So she returned to sewing, a hobby she had long ago abandoned. "I had forgotten the simple pleasure of quilting."

Pragmatic planning is always beneficial and often precludes the last minute distress of having to alter plans. Resting before a big and eagerly anticipated event is a time-tested strategy. Although difficult to accept, sometimes the best approach is to earn a good day by modifying the days preceding an activity. Do not plan anything that cannot be rescheduled. For instance, make certain the tickets to the play can be changed to another date if needed. A planned escape hatch is a guaranteed safeguard that will eliminate the anxiety and pressure surrounding an outing.

Perseverance is a critically important tool for those who seek the best care. Shawna F.'s stubbornness and tenacity have pulled her through the rough times. "I just can't take things lying down and give up the fight. No matter how many times I have heard, 'There is nothing more that we can do for you; you have exhausted all treatment options.' I feel that is just not good enough. I have empowered myself with education and knowledge and have made my life's goal to find the answers that I need, that we all need, to heal ourselves. Whether I become an M.D. or a physician's assistant who practices medicine in a clinical setting, or if I get my Ph.D. in immunology and do research for the rest of my life, I will find out how to help myself and other women who suffer in the same way I do. Whenever I get to the point where I feel sorry for myself and want to give up, I think about what I have survived so far and all of the people whose lives I can eventually make better, even if only in some small way."

How to Hope, How to Cope

Contending with a chronic disorder is challenging if you have family responsibilities, but what about the countless single men and women who must fend for themselves and care for their own needs—shopping, driving to and from medical appointments, cleaning their home, cooking their meals—even when fatigued and plagued with pain, depression and other symptoms?

Many people photographed for this book spoke with great affection about pets who, during the most difficult days, had provided support and steadfast companionship. Those who lived alone and could no longer work or participate in social activities found comfort in the quiet company of their dogs or cats. A number of individuals who were photographed and interviewed for this book insisted that their portraits be taken with their four-footed companions in order to celebrate the animals' capacity to love and heal.

"My beautiful companion, Chelsea, a five-year-old golden retriever, has been of indescribable consolation," says Lynn E. "She is there for me at every moment whether I am frustrated, joyful, angry, or exhausted. She sleeps next to me whenever I feel the need to rest. She licks my tears when I cry from the pain. She is always willing to give me unconditional love. Just looking at her reminds me that there is still something important to live for, despite this illness. We are compassionate souls who found one another."

"I do not believe that suffering is necessarily a bad thing," explains Cari D. "Oh sure, I have had my share of pity parties and have had times of great depression and feelings of being all alone with my illness, but the reality is that bad things happen—disease happens—and you and I have no control over it. The only thing we have control over is our reaction to it." Cari copes with her illness by taking one day at a time. "A better treatment could be just around the corner for me. I am very hopeful and very thankful that I live in a time of great strides in modern medicine. I also cope by remembering that there is always someone better off than I am, but there is also always someone worse off than I am. I keep a healthy and balanced perspective." Someone once told her that in tough situations, she could become bitter or better. "I would like to think that I'm becoming the latter."

The predisposition of people with concealed illness determines how well they handle sudden, new restrictions and changes. Were they spiritual before becoming ill? Did they have a deep faith despite the prior twists and turns in their lives? Were they always cynical by nature—seeing the glass half empty rather than half full? Were they people who were abstract and creative in their ability to solve problems, or were they concrete thinkers in need of concrete responses?

"Abstract thinkers accept chronic illness or pain more easily," reports Yaffe.[2] "This expansive thinking can incorporate paradox and inconsistency, such as the ups and downs of health problems and flare-ups. They are more apt to accept the struggle as ongoing but dynamic. For the more concrete thinkers, pain and illness thrust them into a world of chaos that they cannot control. Linear thinkers will often assume, If I do A, then B will happen. In the world of silent illness, life becomes nonlinear. Actions no longer guarantee anticipated results. There is a non-linearity to this journey, and people inclined towards the abstract will look to new formulas for quality of life.

Life can newly blossom with the solace that comes from connecting with others, from prayer, and from being able to let go rather than clutch desperately."

Laura H. is a vivacious and colorful senior citizen. She was a joy to interview while conducting research for this book. In her youth Laura had been a singer and involved in theater. An early bout of polio had left her with significant swallowing problems. This handicap was never evident to others but was one that Laura had to remain aware of each time she ate or drank. "I have difficulty swallowing. I also lost my ability to sing more than three or four notes. I could no longer make the sound of laughing or crying, and I coughed and sneezed in a funny way. I could not drink at a fountain because the water would come out of my nose since I lost the ability to close off my throat. I had to be very careful to chew my food thoroughly. If I were not careful, I would choke. I also had difficulty catching my breath."

When I first met Laura, she was living in the same tiny 1920's bungalow where she had raised her children. Laura's daughter is now an actress and has inherited her mother's theatrical flair. She flies in and out of town in-between shows. Laura has turned her daughter's old bedroom into a wardrobe closet full of her old costumes from her glory days on the stage. Laura seemed lonely but strangely content. "I'm actually quite proud of myself," she said with great confidence and conviction. Post-polio syndrome has not gotten the better of her but rather made her stronger, more humorous, and more grateful for what she did have. "I've accomplished a lot and feel I have led a full and satisfying life. I have had more than my share of adventures in the states and abroad. I have seen what I wanted to see and accomplished what I set out to do. My kids are fine, I have many good friends, and I went to my fiftieth high school reunion. I don't let things get me down. I don't worry about things I have no control over. I can laugh at myself, and my saving grace is a sense of humor despite living with post-polio syndrome."

When Kristen B. and I first met for our photo session, she was living in a small apartment in student housing. Kristen was a soft spoken and petite young woman, which made her story that much more poignant. She has lived with a concealed chronic illness since early childhood. Kristen was all too familiar with going on and off steroid treatments and being in and out of hospitals throughout her young life. Now, life was good for her despite the pitfalls of her illness' periodic flare-ups and setbacks. Her demeanor was positive, and she looked forward to a brighter future. Her faith seemed to bring her great comfort and peace. "I always try to keep a positive attitude and think of the good times."

Rita N. is newly married and coping with a recent diagnosis of Crohn's disease. "I sometimes like to think that I was chosen to deal with this disease because God knew that I was strong and I could handle it."

"I have worked with clients from every major religion," said Bejai Higgins.[3] "Some folks have a strong faith in God, and some have no faith. Have you noticed that people with no faith have a harder time? There are no rituals. There are no special holidays set aside for these people. It is much harder work. Their process is fundamentally different. Their focus is on living the life they have before they leave this world. They want to do a lot of work around their relationships and goals they have set for themselves and around things they want to see and do. So, we begin problem solving. One client without strong religious ties wanted to see Africa, so we found a tour company that assisted medically-fragile travelers. We did all sorts of problem solving such as renting recreational vehicles instead of cars so he could be driven around and lie down when needed. That is what he wanted. There wasn't any afterlife for him, so the focus and urgency centered on the time he had left."

Harry K. has suffered many years with frequent surgeries and high doses of steroids for his Crohn's disease. In the process, he has moved closer to his Catholic faith. "In the beginning of my illness, I felt angry. I kept asking, 'Why me, God?' Of course, the answer came back loud and clear. . . 'Why not?' My priest and the good friends I spoke with helped me through the tough times."

One woman finds that her emotions swing, sometimes violently, as her pain and other symptoms wax and wane. "I still have days when I feel very upset. However, I have developed an inner peace that keeps my spirits up as much as possible no matter what life hands me. I have become even more spiritual over the years as I constantly look for meaning in my life and wonder why I have had to deal with this pain and illness. I remember to be thankful for everything I still have. I remember that in battling this illness, I still have a lot of fight left in me."

Dr. Michael Wrobel feels that many people initially lose their faith and religious feelings when dealt the initial blow of a chronic health condition. However, after going through the normal stages of grief, people tend to regain their faith and even stop and smell the roses in a new and more profound way. "Some people may be helped by considering that God is also a bit frustrated and angry at the notion of a chronic illness, too."[4]

In the end, nothing can compromise your spirit. You are not your pain. You are not your illness. Look at your physical state of health as the movement of the ocean. "There will be rough waves," warns Jan Yaffe, "but the tide will also recede, and there will be calm periods where you will find relief. The good news is that we have the capacity to make some issues foreground and some issues background in our lives. This is a dynamic choice that we make all day long throughout our lives."[5]

What part of your illness can you put in the background, if only for a short while? Have a visit with someone you love. For that moment, you can welcome your joy to the foreground, even if only slightly. Keep inviting those inspiring, meaningful experiences into your life. Most of the time, life is all about these small and precious moments.

Conclusion

Do we truly get better, or do we simply get better at dealing with illness? Why does one person become chronically ill while another recovers completely and effortlessly? We will never know the reasons for many of life's mysteries or the answers to probing questions about the nature of illness and pain. Who gets sick and who gets well does not, and may not, ever seem fair or reasonable to a logical mind. Nevertheless, we all need to make peace with our state of health, the limitations of our own bodies, and the ebb and flow of symptoms. We all have a wondrous, yet often fallible, machine—the human body—to take us through an entire lifetime.

In the case of chronic health disorders and medical challenges, the destination or goal is not necessarily to become well, but to learn to accept what life has handed us. It may not always be a welcome gift—this one of chronic symptoms and unpredictable days—but it can be an opportunity to learn more about our inner strength and the importance of the people in our lives. It is also a chance to use the gifts within that would have otherwise sat dormant. Sometimes, learning to be compassionate with ourselves is a far more difficult assignment than caring for others. Fortuitously, chronic physical pain or symptoms often force us to care for and about ourselves in new and profound ways.

Our individual differences as human beings pale when compared to our shared experiences and feelings. This bond can provide exceptional comfort to those who suffer in silence and feel isolated. Sharing extraordinary experiences and feelings and obliterating barriers that are part and parcel of illness and pain are addressed in the final section of this book.

Each person and every face featured here has a vital tale to tell about their journey. You have to look closely. Read each individual's testimony and study the true story that lies behind the mask. Most feel obliged to present to their family and friends (and sometimes themselves) an appearance of good health and normalcy. Seldom, however, do facial expressions correspond to an illness' devastating trials and challenges. Pleasant demeanors projected to the world are often in direct conflict with a turbulent internal experience.

"Being chronically ill is often a humbling series of lessons in dependence and learning how to ask for help," says Bejai Higgins.[6] The psychosocial ramifications of these experiences are immense. People with chronic disorders must learn to interrupt the downward spiral of isolation and depression. They need to find ways to discuss changing roles within the family and in relationships with friends and coworkers. It is important for them to learn to become advocates for themselves when dealing with healthcare professionals. And they must fight for their quality of life in the daily battleground of career, relationships, and self-fulfillment. The exact nature of challenging chronic conditions notwithstanding, these issues must be approached at some stage on the wavering journey to acceptance.

Larger communities and organizations of people who live with chronic disorders are renown for a multitude of worthy goals including lobbying and educating the public about the special challenges of such disorders. Isolation can easily be reduced by joining forces and reaching out to others in similar situations who are confronting comparable issues.

Illness can be a significant catalyst for change, for enlightenment, for new beginnings. If nothing else, pain and illness can interrupt the flow of everyday life with a startling but worthy wake-up call. It can alert us to the frailty and importance of life. It can rattle and remind us of our limitations, of the preciousness of time, and the wondrous opportunities we have to relate to one another. Illness and mortality are straight shooters; they can put us on notice that life is short—sometimes sweet, sometimes bitter. Health challenges can force us to reexamine priorities and the way we spend our time. Challenges can prompt us to take stock of friends and family and their value in our lives.

No one chooses to have a chronic illness or experience unyielding pain. When struck with a disability, people usually feel compelled to return to their former selves and rejoin previous routines. Almost primordial in nature, we intuitively ache for a bygone era when life was predictable and comfortable. To accept a new and limited way of functioning is not very appealing. Why should a person want to live happily in a body that is out of order? There are many who fight illness, pain, and a cockeyed condition that seems resistant to interventions. Some become gifted at taking flight. They ignore and run from a chaotic set of symptoms that has shattered their habitual schedule. Despite the frustrations and various stages of grief, most people eventually move on and coexist in relative peace with their disorders. They ultimately learn to make space for a new reality—from the inside out. They learn to dance with the pain using new steps and discover what they can now do rather than what they used to do. Having lost the ability to kick up their heels, they learn to tap their toes to a new tune, perhaps a bit closer to the ground.

Disease and pain are turning points that steer us inward, not outward. We tend to view disease as evil, but in fact it can turn us back to ourselves, to where we truly live and where we eventually learn, grow, and flourish. There is an old Chinese saying: "In crisis, there is both danger and opportunity." Pain can prove a sterling teacher; it can challenge and guide us through periods of unprecedented change, growth, and reevaluation. Perhaps the greatest lesson we can learn is to focus on improving ourselves and our own situation despite our limitations. Many regard pain as the point where the rubber meets the road, where we decide to concentrate on ourselves rather than compare ourselves with others. Difficult to do though easy to say, the commitment to engage with rather than repudiate our disease is indeed a defining moment.

One of the most profound opportunities we have when faced with a concealed chronic health challenge is to begin to examine our flaws and cultivate unconditional love for ourselves despite physical disabilities or psychological scars. To accept and care for our bodies or psyches as they are now is perhaps the biggest challenge and greatest achievement. Illness cannot be vanquished by power of sheer will and determination. In fact, some do more harm than good when they push themselves unreasonably. Learning to honor limitations is a massive accomplishment, and each person has daily opportunities to attain this worthy goal.

Change is difficult, but there is comfort in knowing that as we stumble through the process of change, so do millions of others. We must learn to listen to the internal as well as external voices of change. We must learn to pay attention to one another, to look beyond the guise and into the story that lies behind the facade.

Learning to trust and feel centered in your body and in yourself, even if others make judgments about your physical failings and pain, is what life is all about. Maintaining hope and learning to trust in your strength, the kind that exists beyond physical endurance, will help you handle whatever life hands you. Illness often leaves a person looking back longingly at the way they used to be, when health issues and challenges were less complicated or nonexistent. Despite what pain and struggle lies ahead, it is critically important to remain focused on the possibilities of both a vibrant present and a hopeful future and to summon new-found courage and resilience.

The only constant in life is its unpredictable and changing nature. A concealed chronic illness or condition does not have to be life's sole focal point. At times, it will roar like a tornado that refuses to be ignored; alternatively, it can fade to white noise that hums like a slow distant wind. Acceptance means riding out the cycle of change rather than allowing defeat to become one constant chord playing throughout the day. Life truly is a symphony filled with soaring highs and dispiriting lows. Learning to endure what you can and reaching out for assistance to help you contend with what you cannot is the most constructive and courageous way to live with concealed chronic illness or pain.

Today, there are more beneficial treatments and resources for chronic disorders than ever before. Support groups for specific diseases meet regularly, both in person and online. Camaraderie and information are only a mouse click or telephone call away. Numerous organizations for particular illnesses and conditions, such as the Arthritis Foundation, Crohn's and Colitis Foundation of America, Headache Foundation, and countless others, provide educational information to those with health challenges and to their family members. There is also a vast amount of research underway. Medical scientists and alternative healthcare professionals are learning to recognize, control, and in some cases prevent, a host of chronic disorders.

But, what can you do today? You can learn as much as possible about your illness or condition and how to control some of the symptoms. Locate a considerate and knowledgeable healthcare team; realize that you are more than your health challenges; use what you have learned about your illness or condition to assist others; pay attention to your limitations and honor them. In other words, worry less about maintaining an immaculate kitchen or simultaneously spinning ten plates in the air. These challenges are tall orders, but they are also goals that are well within reach. Learning to feel hopeful is perhaps the most effective treatment for all chronic conditions.

Acceptance and hope are two of the most critical skills that are learned over time—often through trial by fire. The faces featured on the following pages have achieved, or are in the process of building, a new level of acceptance and hope into their everyday lives. Each of these individuals is at a different phase of adjustment. Some are newly diagnosed. Some have lived with their disorder since childhood. Each person's viewpoints and experiences are worthy of examination because each phase is an important piece of the puzzle. All individuals must learn to adjust and cope with an ever-changing landscape of symptoms and emotions.

Everyone knows someone—a family member, coworker, friend, or acquaintance—who is living with easily concealed but challenging symptoms. You do not have to look very far to locate those who live with a chronic illness or condition—but more than likely, you will not be able to detect the problem in their eyes, in their voice, or in the way they carry themselves.

It is my paramount wish that this final section will resonate with those who have chronic or painful conditions as well as with those who care for or treat them. Examine both the portraits and their associated stories and you will find practical and spiritual insight, assistance, tools, and comfort that serve as prelude to the courage and resolve that are essential to an enhanced quality of life.

Ten

Looks Can Be Deceiving

Ordinary people are faced with extraordinary challenges
every day. All of the individuals featured in this book have, at some point in
their lives, found themselves immobilized at an unfamiliar stop along life's
highway. A bit dazed and confused, these courageous people are now in the
process of dusting themselves off and getting back on track—perhaps taking
off in an alternate direction or on a different path altogether.

Challenges, reflections, coping mechanisms, emotions, and experiences
are all candidly discussed in the following pages. Each person's experience is
a valid and valuable one. Interestingly enough, whatever form of illness or
pain has manifested in the bodies of these individuals, the same issues, con-
flicts, and feelings arise in their discussions. It is critical to show these common threads, even at the risk of repetition. It is also important to feature those
who are at the start of their journey, or stumbling on a bump in the road, and
may not necessarily have effective coping skills or wisdom to share just yet.

The readers of this book who find themselves contending with their own
chronic symptoms may likely see a part of their own story reflected in these
pages. Perhaps they once had similar questions and concerns. Every view-
point and perspective is significant and valuable in its own way. Every story
deserves to be told, and each stage of coming to terms with an illness or
condition is worthy of examination.

The photographs on the following pages remind the reader that a picture
does not always disclose the entire story. A facial expression can offer an
impression that runs contrary to the reality of an inner world of experiences
and emotions. These pictures are not worth a thousand words. In fact, they
require words to tell the full story. I hope that you will view these photographs and consider the tale that lies beyond outer appearance or demeanor.
Looks can be deceiving, even to the most penetrating and perceptive eyes.

Laurie E., Artist

Mastoiditis, Migraines, Chronic Lung Disorder

My physical challenges include balance and hearing problems as well as frequent migraine headaches. The most common statement I hear from others when I tell them about my health challenges is "Well, you look good." They seem to be saying that physically looking good should somehow make up for the pain I live with. Some people make me feel as though I am lying to them, or I am faking it because they cannot see evidence of my symptoms. Society is conditioned to believe that an illness is something that must be seen. Many people seem to require some sort of proof that something is wrong with you.

My friends and family are supportive because they know what I have to deal with on a day-to-day basis. People I do not know well are the ones who treat me differently. When I explain my illness, my surgeries, and my pain, I can almost see the wheels spinning as they are giving me the once-over. It is as if they are trying to see my pain, as if the pain must be seen to be real.

I have been fortunate to have good doctors who understand my health challenges. At the same time, I know their knowledge and skill are stretched to the limit. They try to help me cope with my pain and other symptoms, but they have few answers to my questions. I have been dealing with this illness since 1994. I have good days and bad days and everything in-between. Over time, I have gradually had to give up activities and many things that I enjoy because of the illness. I cannot always plan things in advance, since I don't know how I'll feel on any given day. When I do plan something, I realize that I may have to cancel if I am not feeling well enough. I have been unable to work full-time for the past few years. This year, I have been living on disability insurance. I hope that I will be able to work again soon.

I have reduced my physical activities to practically nothing. I have been unable to participate in sports and other physical activities for an entire year. During the course of this illness, I have seldom dated and have only maintained very short-term relationships. I currently have a boyfriend, but it is very difficult to have a relationship because I spend most of my energy trying to find ways to get better from my illness. I spend less time with my friends in person and more time with them on the telephone. I have reduced most of my social activities. Last summer, I joked with my roommate that I was beginning to feel like an eccentric recluse.

One of the most important things I have done to improve my health is to use nutritional supplements. I do a great deal of research to find the ones that are right for me, and I consult alternative doctors for guidance. My health

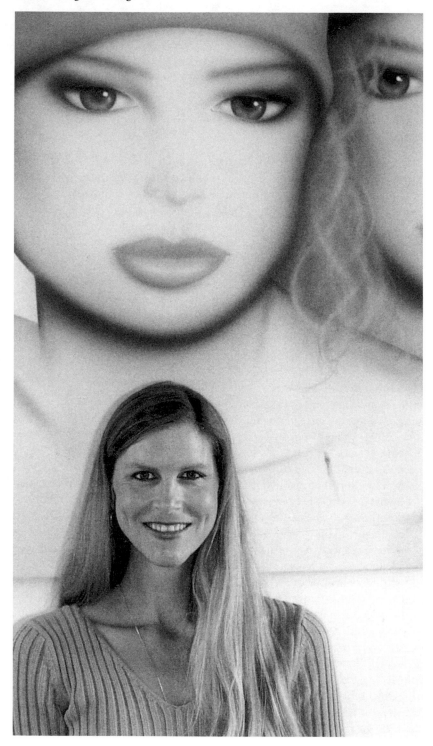

problems include mastoiditis, ear infections, and upper respiratory infections. As a result, my immune system is constantly challenged. I have relied heavily on nutritional and herbal supplements to keep my body as healthy as possible. I believe that the body can heal itself when given the proper support. I had a chronic infection in my lungs that traditional medicine was not able to help. I read an article in an alternative newsletter that talked about a natural product for people with chronic infections. This product was able to finally clear my lungs. Through the combined help of medical doctors and natural medicine, I've been able to deal with my illness and pain much better.

My friends always ask me how I am doing. It is always part of our conversation. When I talk to my family, it is always part of our discussion as well. Talking about my condition is a part of my daily interaction with others. People want to know how I feel that day and what the doctors have to say about my conditions. People who do not know me well will ask mutual friends how I am feeling. Sometimes I feel as though I'm living in my own soap opera.

When I meet someone new, the discussion of my illness may or may not come up. I do not automatically talk about it. I like to have conversations with people who have no idea that I am dealing with an illness. If it does come up, I answer all of their questions. I often find that people are curious and have a lot of questions. Other times, they do not want to get too involved.

I wish the legitimacy of an illness were not judged on the basis of its visibility. . .

As each year passes and I am still dealing with my illness and chronic pain, I have begun to envy healthy people. I feel that many people are not completely thankful for their good health. They take it for granted. I have become very sensitive to others who abuse their bodies, as if it is no big deal. I do not understand how someone can abuse himself or herself physically with smoking, alcohol, or drug abuse. I want people to understand how important their health is and to treat their bodies with the utmost grace. I get irritated if I hear someone complain about his health when he has been abusing his body with drinking or smoking. When someone is complaining about a hangover, for instance, I think of how hard I struggle to just feel well. I don't want to watch someone else destroy his or her own body. My illness did not come from being careless with my health. Each day I do everything possible to live the healthiest life I can, so that I can feel the best I can. I envy those people who never have to give their good health a second thought. I have difficulty being supportive of someone who has a headache for one day, when I live with headaches on a daily basis.

Hearing how great everyone else's life is can be difficult for me at times. I wonder why I have to deal with my illness while they are having fun and working and doing all of the things they enjoy, which are the things I once enjoyed. I also understand that my friendships should not revolve around my illness. Everyone else's life shouldn't stop just because I have this to contend with. Therefore, I work hard to stay involved with other people and ask about what they are doing. I encourage and support them just as I would if I were completely healthy.

I can secure periods of peace when I happen to have a day where I feel good and somewhat normal. It reminds me of the possibility that I can live without illness and pain. It makes me believe that there is a key to unlock the door of my pain and my unanswered questions. I have learned how to simplify my life and to keep focus on what is most important. I work hard to understand what I am learning from this experience and how I can still be the same person I have always been. I try not to let my illness get the best of me by turning me into an angry and bitter person. I spent a great deal of time this summer planting flowers and working in my garden while I was recovering from surgery. It made me feel better to take care of other things. It gave me a focus on something other than my illness.

I spend a lot of time learning about the world around me and discovering new things. This also serves to keep my mind focused on things other than my illness. I have always had a strong spiritual philosophy, which is my strength. I have developed an inner strength, which helps me get through the many challenges in my life.

My emotions go up and down, and I still have days when I feel very upset. However, I have developed an inner peace that keeps my spirits up as much as possible no matter what life hands me. I do not want my illness to have total power over me. I have become even more spiritual over the years as I constantly look for meaning in my life and wonder why I have had to deal with this pain and illness. I spend more time talking to God. I pray more. I remember to be thankful for everything I still have. I remember that in battling this illness, I still have a lot of fight left in me.

I want people to understand that this inner pain is not visible. I think that illness is illness, and a disability is a disability, whether visible or invisible. I wish the legitimacy of an illness were not judged on the basis of its visibility.

The will and strength I have developed as a result of this illness have made me very resilient. If I have a bad day, I always tell myself that tomorrow will be a better one. I have the support of my friends and family and that helps me a great deal. I talk to friends. I work on art projects. I focus on the things I can do instead of focusing on my limitations. I always tell myself that I can get through this no matter what. I try to remember the saying that God doesn't give us anything that we cannot handle.

I have a drama and an acting background, so some of the skills of presentation are easy for me to do. It takes the focus off of my pain, making it easier to ignore. Since I have been dealing with this for about eight years now, I have learned how to present well. I take on the role of someone who feels great. I focus on other people and take my mind off of myself. If I expend a lot of energy on others, however, this can take a toll on me and I require some time to recuperate.

An advantage of having a concealed illness is that I can move about the world as though nothing is wrong. No one knows that something is wrong with me unless I tell them. I can walk into a room and no one feels sorry for me because of whom they see in front of them. However, if I am having a bad day with my illness, I cannot tell anyone, and that is a huge disadvantage. They may sense that something is wrong, but they cannot see what is wrong. Some may feel that I am exaggerating my symptoms in order to have them feel sorry for me or to get special treatment from them. Since they have no proof of my illness, they only know what I tell them. This can make them unsure about the validity of my illness.

Having a concealed illness is challenging. Since my illness interferes with many of my activities, I get tired of having to explain to others why I cannot do this or that. Sometimes, I think that if one more person tells me that I look great when I am feeling awful, I will scream! It gets tiring when I feel that I have to explain myself all of the time.

Sometimes I wonder if my friends think I am using my illness as an excuse so that I can get out of doing things with them. This is not the case, but I sometimes see the doubt and scrutiny in their eyes. I often think that others look at me and must wonder why I haven't done more with my life. They don't understand what I go through each and every day. Dealing with a concealed illness certainly helps you learn who your real friends are.

I cope by always holding onto the hope that I will get better in time. I use music to change my mood; I spend time in nature to help me feel better; I work on developing my mind; I stay strong so that the illness does not win. I examine the lessons I have learned and what I have gained by going through this experience. No matter what comes my way, I will get through each day.

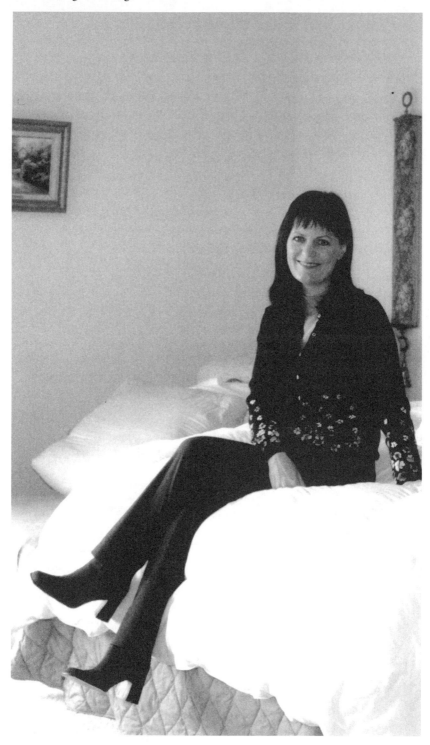

Diane M., Social Worker, Health Educator

Chronic Fatigue Immune Dysfunction Syndrome,

Migraines, Mitral Valve Prolapse

When I first became ill, I was desperate to find out what was wrong with me and what I could do to get better, because I was suffering terribly. I lost confidence in my physical ability because I had become so weak, dizzy, and sick. I had to learn how to survive each day and take comfort in the fact that my existence was worthwhile aside from what I could accomplish. Taking pride in whatever I could successfully accomplish has helped my own sense of satisfaction, even if the task seemed small and trivial.

I've learned that sometimes I have to slow down and take each day as it comes.

I have had to learn to pace myself because of my illness. This has been very hard for me to do, because I have always had tons of energy. My life, as I knew it before, came to a screeching halt when I suddenly became ill. I had to leave my wonderful new job, leave school, and stop doing my aerobics classes. My social life disintegrated. Friends drifted off when I could not make plans. I could not take care of my family and do the normal chores and errands. It was very difficult to have anyone working in our house because I needed peace and quiet.

Living with a hidden disability adds to the distress of the illness itself, because it adds a layer of disbelief from others. Having to prove my illness when I am already knocked to the ground drains my energy. I feel that others think I am lying or that they are disparaging my character by thinking I am a hypochondriac or a malingerer.

I never know exactly who is questioning the real nature of my illness. I wonder if even those close to me sometimes have doubts. It is not a good feeling. I have to hold onto a firm sense of self and to hell with those who don't support me!

I have never wished to look more physically disabled. I feel better emotionally knowing that, with a little blush on, I can look pretty good. I try to stand up straight and walk with purpose (if I have energy that day). This gives me confidence and a sense of power—real or imagined. I also feel better emotionally if I look better, so I put on makeup before I go out. I feel better if my hair is clean and looks nice. I continue to read magazines and try to keep up with the latest fashions.

155

People would be more sympathetic if I looked disabled, but I wouldn't want their pity. I wish doctors, lawyers, and judges believed that it is possible to appear healthy and still be very sick and disabled. The burden of proof lies much more on the ill person, which is just another frustration that brings on more stress. I have had people of all ages yell at me for parking in disabled parking spots, even with my handicap placard visible. I only use my placard when I really need it. I have learned to say, "I don't care to discuss my disability with a stranger." It hurts my feelings and embarrasses me in public when this happens, but there are a lot of people with personality disabilities and rash judgments out there.

Sometimes I envy the vitality and good health of others. I do not always want to hear about my relatives' wonderful trips, and my friends' fabulous new jobs, and fun activities that I wish I could be doing. My husband once went to a close friend's wedding in Hawaii without me because I could not travel that far. I loved seeing the pictures, but I was sad that I wasn't in them. It hurt.

My husband enjoys wonderful health. It is not fair that he married someone who has become so ill for so long. On the other hand, I didn't sign up for this either. If he had to live in my body for one day, he would know what a good sport I am most of the time.

My faith has helped—especially believing in the afterlife. Even though I am suffering desperately now, I will be in no distress and will be happy forever at a later time. I have a great faith, even though I can get very angry and frustrated with not understanding why this is happening to me.

I picture my spirit as a garden. When I'm feeling my worst, the garden may be down to one rose, wilted at that, but it is always alive. When I start to feel better, that one rose lifts its head and becomes strong. On the best days, I have a whole garden of flowers, vibrant in the sun. Having this image cheers me and keeps me grounded and hopeful. When I feel my worst, however, I desperately beg God for good health. Unfortunately, my spirituality seems to go to the back burner when I feel better and am having a good day. I want to remember to remain spiritual all the time, regardless of my health status.

My husband has been very supportive and sweet. He is very easygoing. I don't know if I would be as understanding if the circumstances were reversed.

One advantage of an illness that is not easily detected by others and is virtually concealed from sight, is that a person is treated normally without deference or pity. This is a good thing. I am not treated a certain way because someone feels sorry for me. Also, I do not have to continually explain my illness to everyone. I get sick of talking about it. On the other hand, a disadvantage of having a concealed illness is feeling others do not believe me because I appear perfectly fit and able. When one has a concealed illness, one may have to be his or her own medical expert because the illness is not well known or accepted (and half the time one is educating his or her own doctors). Since this illness is largely diagnosed on symptoms, if I look healthy, even my doctor may think I am lying.

Another disadvantage is the denial of deserved disability insurance payments. Not only does this deny my livelihood, but also threatens my quality of life. I cannot work, but I'm not allowed the disability benefits I paid for, so how am I supposed to live? It is very tough. Thank goodness I am married. If not, I might be homeless. Unfortunately, without my income, our family's financial status decreased considerably, and we now have to sell our house.

My elderly mother has been very generous financially, but she shouldn't have to be. It is frightening. Many people with chronic illness become divorced because of the stress of the illness on the marriage. Add to that no disability insurance payments and a physical inability to work—it is a horror story. No one should have to deal with these stresses while dealing with a debilitating illness.

What is it like for me to live with this illness? I can answer that question in ten simple words: I want my life back—I hate having this illness. I vacillate between anger, frustration, sadness, and acceptance. I do what I can and enjoy what I can. I remember to do favors for myself.

It is hard to come up with a benefit of being ill. I'd like to think I have learned to be a nicer or more considerate person. I can empathize if someone is ill. I have adapted my schedule to what works for me. I have insomnia a lot, so I use my time at night for creativity, and then sleep late in the mornings. My friends and family know this. For others, I just say, "I work at night and need to sleep in the morning." No other explanation is necessary.

Not all alternative treatments were helpful for me, but reflexology and the use of various Chinese herbs gave me a sustained boost of energy and feeling of well-being. I couldn't use a personal trainer as I was too weak to exercise. Tai chi was relaxing, but difficult to do for long periods of time because of my extreme fatigue. I found that getting regular massages was not only relaxing, but alleviated a great deal of my muscle pain.

The counseling I sought was with a therapist who had the same illness I was dealing with. She always knew what I was talking about because she had been there and could share resources for coping. Keeping a journal of my feelings, frustrations, and hopes helps me to cope with this illness. Also, having hope and listening to what my body and spirit want at anytime and responding accordingly, gives me a sense of control.

I really appreciate the good days and have a sense that I am healing, although very gradually. I have learned that sometimes I have to slow down and take each day as it comes. There is always tomorrow. I appreciate all the small things. There's tremendous joy and beauty and peace in nature, and nature is indifferent. It doesn't care what you've done, or who you are, or how you are feeling. It is just there for you.

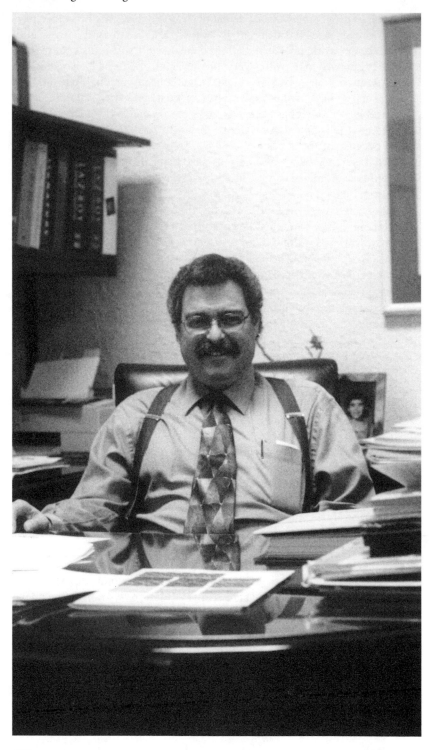

Stuart G., Sales Manager

Crohn's Disease

I'm a firm believer that you should be in control of your life as much as possible. There are times when my disease can take over, but I take a proactive approach to get back in control as soon as possible. I hate the idea of walking around feeling like a victim, so I don't. Having had this disease for over thirty years has given me the opportunity to develop an attitude and a perspective that enables me to be positive. When I think how Lou Gehrig stood in front of the whole world, knowing he was suffering from a fatal disease, and said he was the luckiest man in the world, it makes me pause and count my blessings. So what if I have to go in for infusions every eight weeks? So what if I have to take handfuls of pills every day? So what if I have to special order at almost every restaurant? So what if I don't make it to the toilet every once in a while? I still have a wonderful wife, a wonderful daughter, a job, and a nice place to live. I volunteer, and I make a contribution to society. For crying out loud, I'm pretty lucky too.

I have a better understanding of what I can handle. Even if this flares up, I will survive and get better.

My spirit has been strengthened in many ways through having this disease. I have a much better understanding of what I can handle emotionally and physically. I know that even if my disease flares up, I will survive and get better.

I am a salesperson and need to be at my best when a customer calls or comes into my store. Often, I just have to hide my symptoms. Just the other day, I had to visit a client and had to measure their space for new furniture. About halfway through our meeting, I started to realize I had to make a quick trip to the bathroom or else. It's very awkward to excuse yourself when you are trying to sell your product. So I just kept a smile on, and fortunately I didn't have an embarrassing emergency that time.

I believe my disease has affected my career path. I have taken a conservative approach and not taken any risks that would affect my health insurance. I have stayed at my present job for over fifteen years.

I become more quiet and withdrawn if I feel ill when I am at home. Usually my family is very conscious of my emotional state. I'll usually just go off to my chair in front of the television and try to relax. Sometimes, I tell my wife that something just doesn't feel right.

I have no desire to appear disabled, because I don't feel disabled. However there are times when my disease flares up and I am unable to fully express what is happening to my family and to the medical staff. At those times, I just wish I had a big sign on my forehead that would show everyone what was going on so I wouldn't have to explain it over and over again.

There are times when I wish that I could eat like most other people. A nice big Caesar salad would taste real good right now. I wish I could vary my meals more. But when I look around and see all the strange diets normal people are on, mine doesn't look so bad.

I always hear from people who heard about someone who did this or that and were able to go into total remission. These are always anecdotal stories. I told one person who kept trying to give me advice, that it was a well-known fact if you give a bunch of sick people sugar pills, approximately 10% are going to feel better. I finally said to this person, "Get me some evidence that it really works. Until then. . . "

My family has given me the most security in my life. My wife always has her eye on me and that gives me a tremendous sense of assurance that if something happens, she will always be there for me.

Knowing that the people around me understand my condition enables me to spend time in a home that is insulated from the worries that follow me in public.

Lynn E., Licensed Clinical Social Worker

Chronic Fatigue Immune Dysfunction Syndrome (Myalgic

Encephalomyelitis), Fibromyalgia, Myofascial Pain Syndrome

Because I have a hidden illness, people assume I am able to live a life similar to theirs—unless they can be convinced otherwise. People often doubt or scrutinize my symptoms or view me as a malingerer. It is much more difficult to obtain not only emotional support and understanding, but also physical assistance. If physicians don't yet truly understand fibromyalgia and chronic fatigue immune dysfunction syndrome, how can laymen be expected to appreciate the enormous complexity of these illnesses? Would anyone ever tell a cancer patient that they couldn't possibly be that ill because their cancer is not visible?

I sometimes envy people who are well enough to work full-time, have a regular and active recreational life, and earn decent money. However, what I find even more difficult is having people complain they aren't earning enough, or that they are taxed too much. Even turning on the television often drives this point home. The news has featured countless stories about wealth. Advertisements never address the difficulties of the disabled, but speak only to the marketing power of the affluent.

Those who have a pet may relate to the immense therapeutic benefits of an animal. My closest and dearest friend Chelsea, my Golden Retriever, has been there for me in a way that no human being ever could. She showers me with love whenever she senses I need it. If I need to crawl in bed and have a good cry, Chelsea is eager to share my pain. Yet, in an instant, she can make me laugh with her superb canine wit and beguiling ways. Just looking at her reminds me that there is still something important to live for. The bond with animals can be immensely powerful. For people who are chronically ill and primarily housebound, this bond can be so profound that it takes the place of unavailable human companionship and provides a purpose for living when careers and human relationships have been stripped away. How truly tragic it is that our society does not provide financial assistance for disabled and elderly people to support their animal companions.

Not long ago, my dog became certified as an Assistance Dog. Of all the encounters I have had since becoming disabled, the experience of being in public with a service dog has been the most revealing. Chelsea wears her blue assistance cape with pride when she accompanies me to restaurants, shops, and doctor appointments. Since I have never sought public attention, preferring not to be conspicuous, this has been a challenge for me. One time, while we were waiting in an airport, countless people approached us with probing

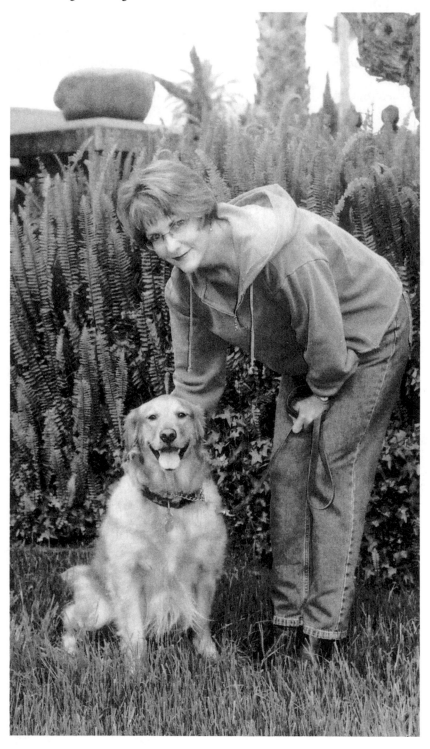

questions, such as, "Is she a dog for the blind?" However, the resounding question was, "Is she in training?" This question implied that she was in training to be someone else's service dog. If I answered that question honestly, explaining that she was not in training, but was my service dog, my response was met with tremendous confusion. I was then placed in a position of explaining that she was, in fact, my own service dog. This was like opening up Pandora's Box. People asked, "How does she assist you?" By nature, I am most comfortable being candid and honest. However, my disabilities are my own private business. Moreover, the mere energy this discussion requires is extremely exhausting. People assume that if one is not in a wheelchair, or blind or deaf, one is not truly disabled. The positive side to this situation is that having a service dog has given me a unique opportunity to educate others. Therefore, when I have the energy and patience to engage in full conversation, I assume the role of advocate, creating awareness for many people that disabilities may, indeed, be invisible.

I don't want to be seen as lazy. By nature, I am a very ambitious person. Therefore, I often attempt to do things that I shouldn't. Sometimes I do not want to fully acknowledge that I am disabled. I want to be normal. If I look okay, I can sometimes even deceive myself. It makes it much more difficult to accept my illness and disability on an emotional and psychological level. Furthermore, a person telling me that I look great

People have a hard time believing that someone who seems so competent can be truly disabled.

also contributes to my inner conflict about how disabled I truly am. It took four years for me to apply for a handicapped-parking placard due to my own fears and sense of guilt about how others would see me when I got out of the car.

Since my illness, I have had to create an entirely new life. In being unable to maintain regular employment, my biggest adjustment has been trying to survive financially. Most people are worried about earning and saving enough money for their retirement. Such worries now pale in comparison to the difficulty of not knowing month-to-month if I can survive as a single, disabled person, especially after exhausting all savings. The forced change of income has meant not being able to afford to leave town, go out to dinner, buy new clothing, pay for recreation, etc. Excessive medical bills, high premiums, and a lack of prescription medicine insurance coverage have forced me to sink into increasing debt as time goes by.

Before I became disabled with this illness, I could hop in the car after a full day's work and run two or three errands. Now, a good day is having the energy to run any errands at all. When I was well, simple things like trips to the laundry room were taken for granted. Now, I must often return to bed for brief periods of rest during and after the laundry chores. I used to work forty-five-plus hours a week, lead a relatively active social life, walk my dog in the morning and evening, exercise regularly, and make plans to see friends. Now, in spite of not working, it is challenging to exercise the dog, let alone me. Because of debilitating fatigue and malaise, some days do not permit any activity whatsoever. I frequently tell people that the hardest part of all of this new life is not getting anything accomplished. On bad days, it's a challenge just to stand and make a quick meal, like a sandwich.

Time has become synonymous with energy. I have had a very difficult time learning to live with a cluttered, dirty house, piles of important papers everywhere, waiting to be filed. Since I am neat by nature, I had to learn to accept that I cannot be that tidy person anymore. Previously active, my life's motion has been reduced by two-thirds. Simple events such as grocery shopping must now be planned. It's as if I am given a quarter tank of gas instead of a full tank for the day. Each morning I ask myself, "What will that quarter tank allow me to do today?"

Because of my reduced energy, I have had to get used to spending most all of my time alone. Socializing is too draining now, and activities are unaffordable. Dating has become less frequent in recent years. If I were to become engaged in a long-term relationship at this time in my life, it would have to be with an individual of enormous depth and compassion.

I feel constantly challenged by the physical adjustments to pain. Bending over to brush my dog was not previously an activity I had to agonize over. Some days, even walking has to be avoided due to the accompanying pain. The fact that I am highly verbal and present intelligently can also be deceiving to others. People have a hard time believing someone who seems so competent can be truly disabled. Those who see me slowly walking my dog in the neighborhood don't have a clue as to what I am going through on an hour-by-hour basis. They can't actually see my pain, dizziness, or nausea when I bend or squat to play ball with my dog. Nor do they know that I have to spend time in bed both before and after most walks outside.

When it all becomes too much, the first thing I do is go through my date book to cancel and cross off all possible plans I have made, from errands to doctor appointments to doing the laundry. This relieves the pressure. My life's motto has become "Less is more; more is less."

The adaptations are endless, but I believe the emotional and psychological adjustments have actually been the hardest. I never want to believe I am disabled; I never want to accept that I won't be healthy again.

Sallee S., Financial Analysis Manager

Interstitial Cystitis, Irritable Bowel Syndrome

Since I am young and people cannot see anything wrong with me, they assume that everything is fine and expect me to act that way. The fact that little is known about my chronic condition, called interstitial cystitis, only makes it worse. When I tell people what I have, they usually do not know what I'm talking about. They assume that since they have never heard of it, it cannot possibly be that bad to live with. People say things like, "Just buck-up, be strong, and take it." They have no idea how challenging it is and what I am truly dealing with.

Everything in my life has changed. My whole life now revolves around my illness. When I leave the house, my time has to be planned around my health needs, as does my schedule at work. I hesitate to plan occasions that require being away from home for long periods. I carry a briefcase full of medications everywhere I go. I limit my activities after work and on weekends so that I have some downtime.

I feel limited as to what activities I can handle these days, so I hold back a lot of the time. I often do not feel up to going out with friends, dating, vacationing, going after a promotion or better job—all of the normal things people do without a second thought. I've always wanted to go back to school for my master of arts degree, but I know I cannot handle the long days. Most of all, I envy other people's happiness and contentment. On the other hand, being ill has made me realize what truly matters in this life.

I don't want sympathy; I just want understanding. For a while, I was very depressed in trying to deal with this illness. No one can possibly understand what living like this every day is really like. But, of course, I am not allowed to actually say those things out loud, and that is what is so hard. The medical professionals tell me to talk about my condition because this will help me deal with it, but most of the world does not want to hear it.

My advice to others with a concealed chronic illness is, only do what you can do, and try not to worry about everyone else or what they might think. You have to be self-disciplined; you have to learn to say "no." You cannot always do everything with everyone all the time. Take some of the pressure off yourself. That is a huge relief.

I used to try to appear normal, hide the illness, and not talk about it. Now, I don't really care. Eventually I got to this point because my body and mind could only take so much. Hiding it becomes more of an effort than being open and honest about it, and the last thing I need are more obstacles. The people

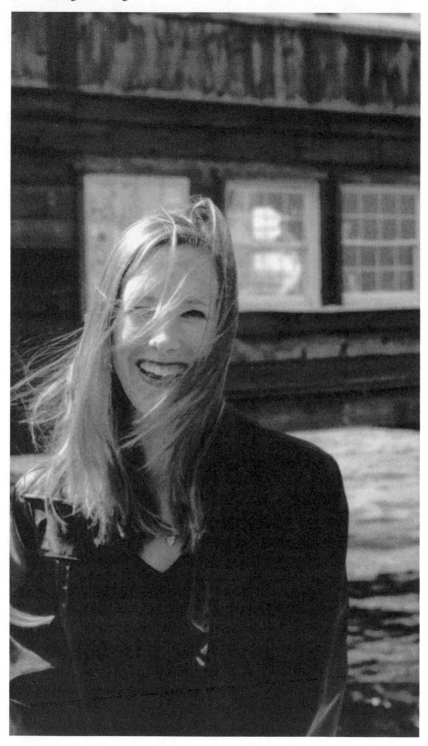

closest to me can take one look at me, or know from the sound of my voice, when I have had a bad day.

The positive side of having a concealed illness is that people do not treat you differently, because they cannot see anything different. Perhaps there is not the same judgment that goes on with a concealed condition as there is with a visible disability.

When one has a concealed chronic illness, relationships are difficult. Balancing everything in my life is hard enough, so I tend to stay away from the roller-coaster ride of relationships, not to mention the difficulty of asking someone else to put up with all of my health problems.

I worry a lot about the future, because if I am like this at age thirty, what will I be like at fifty and sixty? I try to tell myself that there is always the hope for new medical developments in the years ahead.

This illness has changed me and my attitude towards what others may be carrying around. The more I talk to people, the more I find that everyone has their own challenges to overcome. People go about their lives every day, but they probably have some sort of struggle going on inside of them, too. This is a valuable lesson, that we are all in the same boat and we need to have respect for one another.

People say things like, "Just buck-up, be strong, and take it." They have no idea how challenging it is.

I pray almost every day—not that my illness will go away, because it will not—but for the strength and trust to deal with it. This has given me some peace. Talking directly with God about my feelings and my illness has helped me cope. In prayer, I can talk about exactly how I feel, without leaving out any of the grim details. Talking to friends and family also helps. Sometimes I feel better after I allow myself to get really mad. Sometimes I just need some sort of release to purge all the feelings that are building up inside.

I realize that there will probably be a lot of bad times, and they may last a while. I remind myself that we are not here to suffer and be miserable. We are here to experience life and make the best of what we have been given. I remind myself of this to keep things in perspective each and every day.

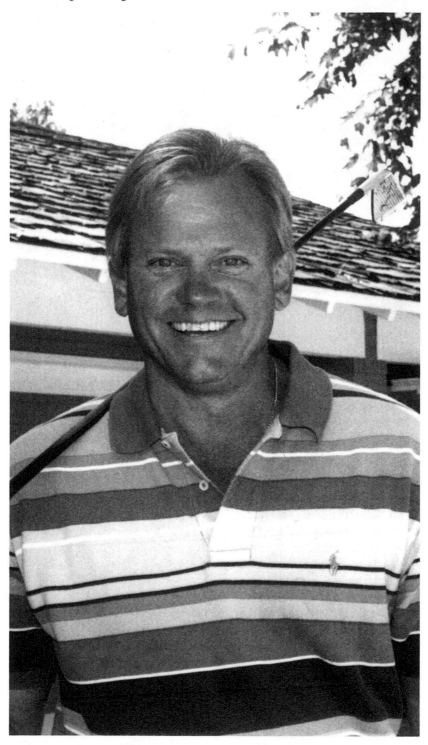

David K., Vice-President of Operations

Rheumatoid Arthritis, Scoliosis

The power of positive thinking, which was instilled in me at an early age by my mother, is the most powerful thought process for overcoming any negative situation. But, to break that down a bit, it is easier to remain positive if you look at every negative situation as temporary, because everything is temporary. Pestering diseases are temporary because we're temporary. Even a day-long aching joint session of rheumatoid arthritis is temporary, because eventually one has to go to sleep.

It is also vital to maintain a sense of humor about yourself and about life. Maneuvering through airport security is always interesting. An iron rod, which has run along the length of my spine since a spinal fusion surgery for scoliosis, does not set-off the big metal detectors. However, it will light up a hand wand metal detector. During a routine search the wand lit up, and with dozens of other passengers within earshot, I politely asked the

I never feel envious of other folks because most people have their own cross to bear.

security woman if she wanted to "feel my rod." She grinned, and the people around us laughed. I proceeded to tell her it was my favorite pick-up line in college.

My scoliosis and rheumatoid arthritis have not affected my married life. However, there was a period immediately following my spinal fusion surgery when my dating life was significantly altered. I've always been a believer in taking a negative situation and turning it into a positive one. After my surgery, I had to wear a body brace for nine months. In this cage, I expected to be dateless. After all, I could not take it off and could only sponge bathe. I had a surprisingly good time then because women seemed to flock to me like bees to honey. I suppose my ugly body brace attracted their motherly/sympathetic side. Of course, all of this good dating unfortunately ended when the brace came off. I outgrew it and couldn't get it back on again.

I never feel envious of other folks because I am fully aware that most people have their own cross to bear. My health issues stemming from scoliosis and rheumatoid arthritis are relatively minor in comparison to the laundry list of things that can cause people to be unhappy in this world.

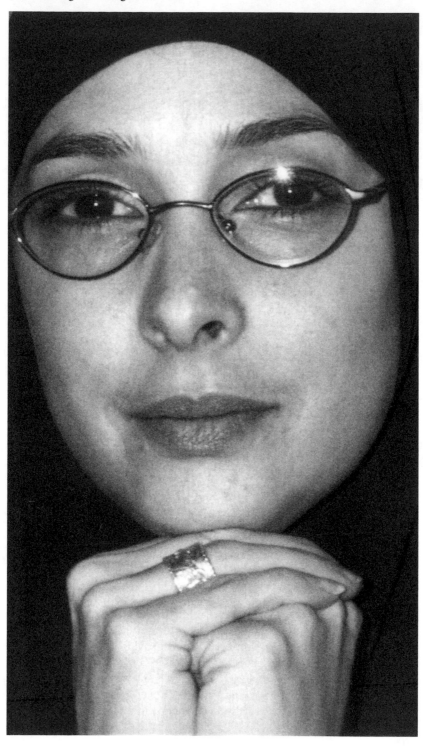

Sahar A., Domestic Violence Counselor

Crohn's Disease

When people think of illness, they expect to see the results of that illness manifest in some visual way so they can compartmentalize it, justify it, and eventually accept it. We humans have always depended on seeing with our eyes before believing, except when dealing with faith-based concepts.

A concealed chronic disease such as Crohn's disease, which for the most part is visually hidden, leaves the patient actually questioning the existence of their own disease. Despite my test results, which were conclusive, I still continually question what is making me feel so ill. My mind cannot consider that Crohn's disease is the culprit. If I am having this much difficulty accepting these parameters, I can only imagine the frustration my loved ones are having when trying to console me through a relapse that they themselves cannot visually see or comprehend.

> *We humans have always depended on seeing with our eyes before believing, except with faith-based concepts.*

I started to become seriously ill when I turned seventeen-years-old. Before that time, I had no symptoms and prided myself on never being sick or missing school. At this young age, I attributed my bouts and body pains to the stress caused by living on my own. Coming to that conclusion made sense at the time. I was a seventeen-year-old, so I didn't have a lot of pocket change. Since I was barely able to make ends meet, going to doctors for tests or checkups was impossible. I hid my pain and my disease and never mentioned my symptoms to anyone. People around me actually thought that I never ate because I was so slim, but they never considered a disease to be the cause of my weight loss. Why? Because I myself didn't think my weight loss was caused by a disease.

Prior to becoming so ill, I was healthy, strong, and athletic. When I became ill, I found myself becoming fatigued easily and self-conscious about going out to eat or going anywhere that might not have an available bathroom. Working every day was also difficult. I never ate anything until I got home from work, as I feared having an embarrassing attack (that's what I called them) at work. I began equating food with pain. Eating, which was something I used to take pleasure in, became my enemy. At this particular time, and for a very long time, I ate only to survive.

When I was nineteen-years-old, I lost my gallbladder. I was a vegetarian at the time, weighed 110 pounds, didn't smoke, drink alcohol, nor do drugs. Yet there I was, on an operating table with my gallbladder ready to pop. When they took it out, I thought, "Okay, that was the problem. Now I am cured." After a few weeks, however, when I obviously should have been feeling better, I wasn't. When I refused to go out to eat or go any place at all, those around me thought I was just being moody or had premenstrual syndrome (PMS) or something. I let them think and believe whatever they wanted so they wouldn't think I was a hypochondriac. I was so absolutely embarrassed by my disease, which was still not diagnosed. I allowed people to lecture me about eating better, ingesting natural herbs, exercising, and anything else they could come up with. I was very willing to try almost anything that had a sound medicinal basis. Everyone around me had a cure to suggest. When their suggested regimen did not work, I am sure they thought that I just didn't want to get better.

I would sweat so much at night that my clothing would stick to me like a wet rag. I had fevers and chills and became so ill that my husband once thought he was going to lose me. He took me to the hospital where I was told that I was under stress and needed to relax myself. In a nutshell, I was told that I was making myself ill. I will always remember feeling small and stupid because of this. That doctor's seemingly innocuous diagnosis haunted me for years.

While my husband was always kind and tried desperately to understand when I was having a bad time, inside I felt like a fool. I felt as though I was letting my family down by not being able to contribute to the household. After all, I was the one causing myself to be ill, or so I believed. What kind of woman was I to make myself so sick? What a weak individual I was becoming! Absolutely pathetic! Was I looking for attention, as one family member once commented? I couldn't, for the life of me, figure out a way to make my symptoms stop.

I will never forget the moment my doctor called to confirm the diagnosis. I never thought I would ever know what the cause of all this pain was, especially after the many invasive tests I had undergone for so many years. I can remember feeling a moment of relief that I wasn't a nut and that there really was something causing this to happen to me. I wasn't making myself ill because of stress after all. Imagine that! All I knew at that moment was, I wasn't crazy and I didn't cause my symptoms. I do remember asking a doctor how I got this illness and what I had done to make it become so bad. When he said "Why, nothing!" I went into shock. I was thirty-seven-years-old and had carried around the guilt of self-induced illness for over twenty years.

I don't try to hide my disease any longer, although I don't announce it when I enter a room either. My family works around my needs, never trying to make me feel bad because I have to run unexpectedly to the bathroom in the middle of an activity, or when I relapse and I need to be in bed or on medication.

My husband is incredibly fit. He works out on a daily basis despite a long and arduous workday. Most of my children are very athletic. My family mountain bikes, plays football, basketball, hikes, you name it. I try to encourage them, but inside I feel left out because I cannot participate with them on a regular basis. When I can join them, I make the best of it and I enjoy every moment I have with them.

Sometimes I envy other people because of their good health. I actually find it harder to hear about the accomplishments of others outside my family circle, because I can somehow allow myself to feel the jealousy I wouldn't indulge in otherwise. I wouldn't wish this on anyone, but to hear of the activities and successes of others becomes difficult to listen to, especially when I am having a relapse and experiencing pain. I become quiet and build a wall around myself and am unwilling to share what I'm thinking.

I am an avid reader. I can travel in my mind to places that I cannot physically go. If I cannot exercise my body, I exercise my mind. I also homeschool five of my children. That is a job that does not allow you to feel sorry for yourself for very long. I also am earning credits towards completing my master's degree in health and wellness promotion (there's an irony in there somewhere) and in health administration. I have a bachelor's degree in psychology and education, a certificate to be a domestic violence and sexual assault counselor, and a certificate in community health. I also enjoy writing for a local newspaper. Lately, I have been too worn out to go back to work. I used to work a twelve-hour shift. Now that is impossible.

I am a Muslim woman with a strong faith, which has helped force me to get past self-indulgence and accept this situation for what it is. I know that this struggle is something I must face, and I know there is no room for compromise. This is my path, and like it or not, I am on it.

What has helped me to deal with this illness are prayer, motherhood, and being a wife and companion to my husband. These are what get me through it all. When I reach a point where I feel depressed, I pray. I cry to my Creator and make dua (request to Allah) for strength and guidance. I am a stubborn woman, so this too has been a hidden asset. I absolutely refused to give in to this disease. It may win once in awhile, but I am still going to have a life.

My sense of humor also helps me to cope. I joke about most of these illness-related woes. When I do break down and cry, it scares my family because they are not used to seeing me like that. Frankly, I haven't been all that great at hiding my pain recently, and they have been extremely loving and supportive. This is a double-edged sword for me because I hate to feel like a burden to them. I pray that I will go into remission soon and bounce back. I hate calling my doctor when a relapse of the illness occurs. I feel like a pest, although he has never makes me feel like that.

I try to stay busy. If I am in pain, I try to hide it and do what needs to be done anyway. I will go to the bathroom nine times and still clean house, teach the children, and go food shopping. I play it off, but my husband can always tell. He knows how to read me by the look in my eyes. I can't fool him very often, or for very long.

When you do not look the part of someone who is ill, people think you're being dishonest about why you don't wish to participate in something or be somewhere. You feel almost forced to reveal your health issues to strangers just so that you don't appear to be lazy or a liar. Rather than reveal it, I push the envelope and usually pay for it in the end. If those around me could see that I was ill, I'm sure they wouldn't expect so much from me all the time.

I just went on a camping trip last summer. I arranged everything because I knew I had to be near a bathroom. Had I let the others pick the cabin, who knows how far from the much-needed restroom I would have been located? (I even bought a port-a-potty but couldn't find a private place to set it up.) Instead of revealing my illness, I volunteered to set up and arrange the entire trip. During one of the days there, I became so ill that I had to run to the bathroom over fifteen times. I was exhausted. I knew I shouldn't have gone on this trip, but I desperately wanted this to be a part of my daughter's life and for her to have this memory. A few times, I even bought items at the company store located next to the bathrooms so that the group would not know I was running to the bathroom once again. When one person saw me taking an antispasmodic medication in the cabin, I felt compelled to tell her what was up. The look on her face when I told her I had Crohn's disease was one of shock. They even told me they would have never have guessed, because I always looked so pretty and together. Explaining this illness to others is a burden. I feel ridiculous, especially when they look at me with a look of surprise or flat-out disbelief.

I am also concerned with my professional life. For instance, do I still have one anymore? I can do so much to help my community, but the pain and discomfort have left me wondering about where I am going with all of these cumulative degrees I have hanging on the wall.

Alain L. Piano Teacher

Neuropathic Pain, Peripheral Blindness, Sensory Impairment

Over the past fourteen years, and on a day-to-day basis, I have learned how to cope with my physical challenges following a cerebral hemorrhage and coma. It has been quite a learning experience.

I still do not have peripheral vision, so I often don't see people or objects approaching me from the left. This has made for some creative accidents, especially in the kitchen.

When I came out of the coma, I made an important decision: I decided to make my recovery the greatest experience in my life. Everything following that moment supported my goal.

Today, that goal still helps me lead my life. Part of my goal was that I didn't want to be limited by what had happened to me. At the time, I was in a wheelchair, unable to walk, and generally very confused in my thinking except for the focus I kept on my goal. This was part of healing and finally getting better.

Setting goals and being committed to these goals still helps me cope with my condition. This daily experience of commitment helps me to get better and to achieve many other successes.

Having goals was vitally important, because it helped me realize I was not my condition. I was so much more than just a person with a physical condition. I was a human being like any other human being who works and has relationships. I examined my own state of emotional distress before the hemorrhage to determine what it was that brought on this series of events—hemorrhage, coma, and healing. I had to learn to redirect my actions toward goals that go beyond myself and my own needs.

The support of my partner was extremely important and a significant element in my progress. Once goals are established and there is a strong commitment to these goals. Having support and learning to be supportive is key to making progress.

Support may come from friends, family members, or support group members, but it's vital to be able to share and support one another through recovery.

My conditions greatly affect my ability to travel or go out, because I cannot drive any longer. Living in Southern California without a car is a great handicap. Furthermore, because my pain medication is effective only during the day, I have to take additional medication at night if I choose to go out.

I tried just about everything to feel better. I investigated many choices

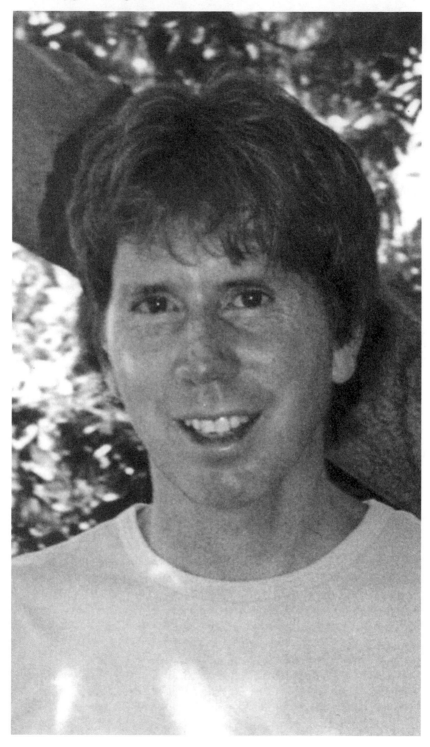

and tried a lot of useful treatments including alternative medicine, tai chi, and qigong. A few months later, I was encouraged to start running—just around the block at first.

This was hard for me to achieve at that time. But, since intellectual activities were really hard to do because of the condition of my brain, I tried running. After a few days of running, I began to really enjoy it.

Running became my favorite activity; I had never run before. I began to enjoy this type of exercise because, when I was running, I felt my body come alive again—a body that had almost expired just a few months earlier. Within seven months, I ran my first ten kilometer race. I have run five marathons since getting out of my wheelchair in 1989.

Involving myself in any kind of exercise remains the best way for me to manage my pain. Exercising releases endorphins which are natural painkillers—painkillers with no side-effects.

Meditation helps me feel better and cope better with the physical state of my health. It also helps me to focus on my goals and to obtain spiritual help when I need to make decisions.

Setting goals and being committed helps me cope with my condition.

Meditation helps me attain a more neutral emotional state which is important because emotional distress weakens the immune system.

In my case, since the neurological pain is due to irritation of the injured nerves in the brain, meditation helps me to reduce the level of pain.

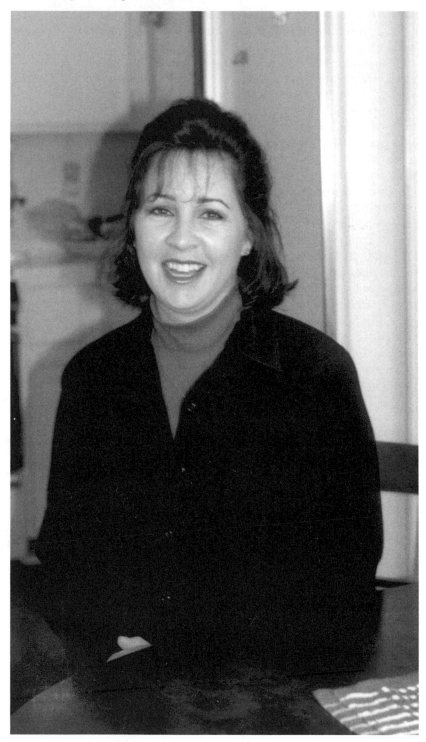

Kathleen H., Court Reporter

Repetitive Stress Injury, Myofascial Neck Pain,

Thoracic Nerve Paralysis

I am just beginning this journey. I have been in limbo—not able to work and barely able to function—for eighteen months. I was not really focusing on anything but getting well enough to go back to what I was educated for and love, which was my beloved career as a court reporter. Now that career is no longer a possibility for my future. Trusting myself, knowing myself, and believing in myself is going to pull me through this. That is the core to my survival. That is what I have to get back to. I lost that somewhere along the way, or maybe I just misplaced it, temporarily.

> *I don't want to appear disabled. I just want to be taken at my word.*

Others have told me that I appear to be independent and strong. Consequently, when I go to the doctors, I am sure they read me that way too. When they ask about my condition, I tell them succinctly and directly. Sometimes I feel that, because I'm not sobbing from the pain or going on endlessly about the symptoms, they doubt my credibility. I do not want to have to do that. That is not the person I am and not the person I want to be.

The most difficult aspect of the situation is that I am not the type of person who wants anyone to feel sorry for me, so I downplay my injury. I tell only close friends and family and only those I have to. I have great difficulty asking for help. I don't know why. I'm finally learning that I have to limit what I do and that I have to explain to others what my limitations are. It is very uncomfortable, and it is an ongoing process. I have to constantly work on that. I have learned that if I do not let myself ask for help, I am only hurting myself more. It has been, and continues to be, a big adjustment to make, but has also taught me a lot about myself.

I don't envy others and their good health. I am normally a very content person. I am happy for others when they are doing well. At this stage of my injury though, I'm disappointed that my own body is failing me.

Having a concealed illness or condition is definitely different from contending with one that is visible to others. Although you may explain to others that you have an injury, over time they tend to forget because there are no visible signs of an injury or illness. With a broken arm or leg, you wear a cast and use crutches; when you cut yourself, stitches are visible.

The biggest adjustment I have had to make is to accept my new self. I have had to accept that my body is no longer the same and likely will not be again. I have had to exercise extreme patience with everyone. I have had to listen to everyone's solution on what they are sure will cure me. I probably will never return to my previous profession, which I loved. That will be, by far, my biggest and most difficult emotional adjustment.

I have also had to make personal adjustments. In every area of my life, I have always been a pillar of strength. Because of that, when this injury occurred, I found that others were not quick to respond to my needs. I think that it scared all the people I was close to because they had not seen me in a position of weakness before. They did not know how to react. I was extremely hurt by this at the time, but I have thought over the whole process and have come to realize that I rarely asked for help in the past. Consequently, I have had to learn to ask for help, to be very clear to those close to me that this is a real situation that will be with me for a long time, and I have to take care of myself first. This has been a difficult process, but one that has to be done. I had to learn to change a cycle that had been in place for as long as I can remember.

The only person aware of what it is truly like is the person living with the concealed condition. The medical community had a difficult time believing my particular symptoms were real because various test results, such as Magnetic Resonance Imagery scans, nerve conduction studies, and others came back with negative findings.

I made enormous adjustments once I was finally able to accept that I had a chronic concealed condition. With my particular injury, I have tried to become left-hand dominant since the right arm is injured. I have someone clean my house. I never wash my own car. I have had to rely more on my teenage daughter for housework. I have groceries delivered. I sleep in a different position—that is, when I can sleep. Any tote bag, suitcase, or backpack I use has to have wheels on the bottom. I never carry anything over my right shoulder. I have changed mattresses, bought a pillow with magnets, and have had every kind of therapy there is. I have used an electronic nerve stimulator for chronic pain. I have been on numerous kinds of medication and have had to deal with all sorts of side effects. Nothing has been helpful.

I don't want to appear disabled. I just want to be taken at my word. People ask about the injury; and after explanation, they do not have any doubts. They also know the kind of person I am. The courtroom judge with whom I worked with for eleven years, after I complained to him on some issue, said to another employee that I had never complained to him the whole time we had worked together, so when I did, he took it very seriously.

The most significant factor in finding some peace about my situation is talking to others who are in a similar position. They are out there, and I seek them out. Being able to communicate with others about my feelings and to have them listen, understand, and relate, is soothing to my soul and keeps me from feeling isolated. I also locate other people who are in a similar situation to mine and talk to them and try to prepare them for what may lie ahead based on my own experiences. I went into my situation unaware and uninformed. The more facts one has, the better decisions one is able to make. I try to help people in that way. My involvement in this book on concealed conditions has been extremely therapeutic to my own process of healing.

The disadvantages of having a concealed condition are numerous. First of all, of course, is my credibility: I tell the same story over and over again because the condition is unseen. Naturally, people are skeptical of things they cannot see. I have to say that I am a bit guilty of these types of assumptions myself. I have certainly learned not to be so quick to judge anyone.

Having a condition not easily detected by others also threatens my mental and emotional stability. I even start to question myself. I am aware of what is going on with my body, but that is so hard to convey it to others. I may need to ask for help under certain circumstances. That may bother people. They may resent me. They may question me.

Getting help from the medical community can be difficult. My credibility is in question. Test results may reveal little or nothing at all about my condition. My diagnosis can change from doctor to doctor; therefore, different forms of medications and therapies may be given that affect mind and body.

Having this disability has really rocked my entire world. I have experienced an emotional breakdown over the inability to function and to work. It has also changed many of my personal relationships. It has made me question and doubt the medical community. It has tested my strength. I have also learned a lot about myself. After having a breakdown of sorts, I resolved to become much more proactive with my medical care. This is definitely an ongoing learning and growing process.

I have had to make physical adjustments and give up certain activities I have enjoyed in the past. I've had to become more patient with myself. I have learned that self-love or self-care is not the same as selfishness. I'm coping the best I can. I must stay involved in life and realize that major changes are happening, whether I am ready for them or not. I try to stay educated on my particular condition and seek out new treatments that might help. I have sought out counseling to help me through this entire process. I'm trying to move forward.

I have worked very hard not to consider myself a victim. I am very proactive about what happens to me. These have been challenging times, to say the least. I have to find a positive in this negative situation.

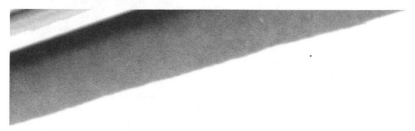

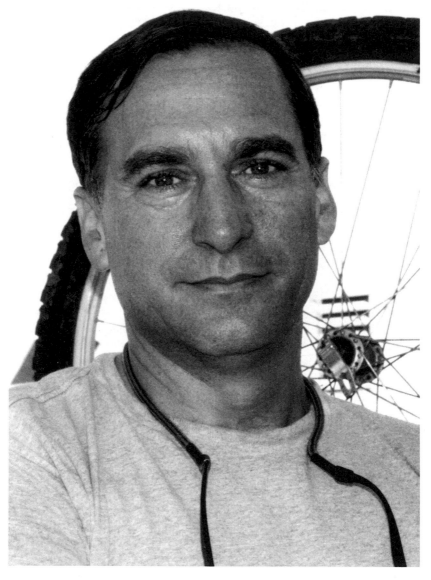

Rick D., Engineer

Chronic Ottitis Externa, Lichen Planus

When I returned from the Gulf War, I came down with a hearing problem that was initially diagnosed as Gulf War Syndrome. Eventually, The doctors determined that my problem didn't fit the usual pattern for this syndrome. I have ottitis externa, which is a chronic ear infection that causes hearing loss. Exposure to mold causes my condition to become much more severe.

I was in the Gulf just prior to the start of the first Gulf War and then went back again a few years later. I noticed the first symptoms within a week of returning from my last trip there. During both tours, I was flying surveillance missions from an aircraft carrier as well as working daily on the flight deck. There were many times when sand storms would cover everything on the flight deck with sand and dust, and I flew through a couple of sand storms. The only thing that doctors could determine was that there could have been something in the sand that affected me at a time when my immune system was vulnerable and stressed. I also used to fly in Navy land-based patrol planes all over the Pacific, to places like Alaska and Tahiti, so I may have been exposed to something that took a long time to manifest itself, or was just waiting for a moment of weakness in my immune system.

The intermittent nature of this condition has led to an endless cycle of hope and despair.

When you have a condition that is not immediately noticeable, people expect you to be 100% responsive and have no limitations in your social or work setting. A more visible and obvious condition causes other people to adjust their expectations.

Fortunately (if it is at all fortunate), my hearing difficulties seem to affect only one ear at a time. When jogging along with friends, I try to place them on my good side, so I do not have to ask them to repeat themselves too much. I do the same thing at meetings whenever possible. I also find myself trying to read lips, especially in a high noise environment. I also do not swim anymore since the chlorine and pool water can cause a severe flare-up. Swimming used to be one of my main exercise activities. I do not go hiking or climbing as often as I used to, because the mold that causes flare-ups seems to be prevalent in those areas. Another adjustment has been my loss of fingernails.

You do not pay attention to how many day-to-day functions require fingernails until you do not have any. I cannot open soda cans, peel an orange, pick
up coins from a flat surface, or open a pocketknife. There are many other
things, but you get the idea. I envy people who can listen to television, speak-
ers, or anything at normal levels. I also envy those who do not have to try and
hide their fingers because of an unsightly condition.

I sometimes wish I appeared disabled. People might be more sympathetic. I wish people knew that I cannot understand speech unless I am looking directly at them. People often talk while looking away, speak from across
the room, or even from another room, and expect to be heard and understood.
All I can hear under these conditions is mumbling, if I can hear anything at
all. I suspect that I often appear rude to others in a social gathering when
there is a great deal of talking and background noise, because I am non-re-
sponsive. I wish they could intuitively know, in some magical way, that I'm
not slighting them, I just can't hear them.

One of the behaviors I engage in that helps me to cope, is exercise. I run,
mountain bike, lift weights, and sometimes rock climb. With the exception of
climbing, I can do most sports by myself. I prefer to do these activities solo
when I'm experiencing significant hearing loss. I have less stress and they're
more enjoyable when I don't have to worry about what I'm not hearing. Sometimes I have several days to weeks without a flare-up, and that always gives
me hope that maybe this is going away. Then a flare-up happens and I get
pretty depressed. I always feel so elated when I can suddenly hear normally in
both ears. The feeling is hard to describe, but all of a sudden my mood is
much brighter.

Communication can be a big guessing game for those who are deaf or
partially deaf. I never expected to have to deal with this challenge, especially
at this young age. I often have to pretend I have heard something when I
really have not. This often happens in meetings. Many times, someone will
lean over and whisper something during a meeting. Since I cannot hear them,
my technique is to smile, nod my head, and hope that I can deduce, from body
language or the context of the meeting, what is being said.

One huge disadvantage to having a concealed chronic condition is that
everyone expects a fully functioning human being. Why? Because you appear normal. For example, I was asked to sit in on a conference call a couple
of weeks ago. The telephone connection was poor, and I could not hear the
people on the other end. I could not be sure if it was the telephone equipment
or me. Another disadvantage is that some people naturally speak very softly.
I have seen these people talk louder or more forcefully when in the presence
of someone wearing a hearing aid; however, it is never obvious to others that
I cannot hear them. Depending on a situation, I will sometimes offer a brief
explanation that I have difficulty hearing and ask them to please speak louder.
However, I rarely do this.

Having this hearing condition is very unnerving for me. I never know
when I go to bed if I will be able to hear when I awaken in the morning. I have

lost a lot of sleep worrying about this. I worry during the night when I have an important meeting the following day or have to travel for business. I find myself waking up several times during the night to test my hearing. If my ear is plugged, I tend to have a minor panic attack. I sometimes lie awake for hours until the alarm sounds.

I think the lack of a peaceful sleep is one of the most upsetting aspects of this condition, as I become moody and depressed during a major flare-up. I know this is hard on my family. I have been working to accept my condition and just get on with life. The intermittent nature of this condition has led to an endless cycle of hope and despair.

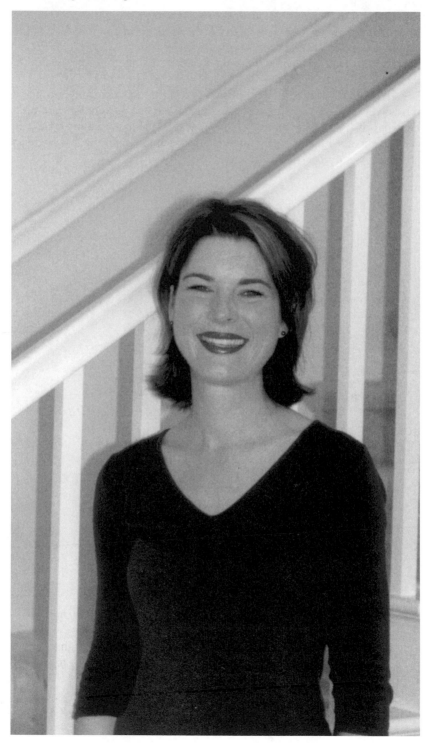

Cari D., Pharmaceutical Representative

Crohn's Disease

People do not question my illness; they simply forget I'm sick because I normally appear healthy, even while dealing with pain and other symptoms of my disease. And that is perfectly fine with me until severe symptoms rear their ugly head. I have to admit that I occasionally feel jealous of others who have good health. I don't have a problem hearing about their accomplishments, but I do envy their healthy lives, which are unfettered by medical issues. Most of my friends are in their late twenties and simply do not have to deal with what I do, such as frequent fevers, having blood tests every couple of weeks, rectifying insurance problems, colonoscopies, x-rays, medications that may cause cancer in the future—the list is endless and quite scary at times. I envy those individuals who do not have to face these problems until they are well into their eighties.

. . . the reality is that bad things happen and we have no control over it. The only thing we can control is our reaction to it.

Living with a hidden illness is definitely different from contending with one that is noticeable. I will never forget returning to work after being newly diagnosed with Crohn's disease. I had spent six days in the hospital in extreme pain and had been through CT scans, an MRI, a colonoscopy, numerous medications, and a great deal of emotional strain. I went back to work several weeks after the initial onset of my symptoms. Since I had not been able to eat for several weeks, I had lost about ten pounds, my skin was clear, and to be perfectly frank, I looked good! Here I had been through hell, but I looked like I had just spent two weeks relaxing at the beach, minus the tan. I'll never forget trying to explain to others what I had been through. It fell on deaf ears.

I feel that the benefits of having a concealed disease outweigh the disadvantages. The compassion and understanding are more difficult to come by when dealing with a hidden disease, but on the days that I'm feeling well, I don't have to think about having Crohn's disease. There is nothing about me that would make people think I am sick; therefore, I don't have people feeling sorry for me, thank goodness. I crave compassion when I need it, but I never want to be pitied. I quit my job as a manager with a Fortune 500 company and sought a job that would give me more flexibility for my doctor's appointments and less stress to aggravate my illness.

I do not believe that suffering is necessarily a bad thing. Oh sure, I have had my share of pity parties and have experienced times of great depression and feelings of being all alone with my illness, but the reality is that bad things happen —disease happens—and we have no control over it. The only thing we can control is our reaction to it. I try to appear normal and in good health. I do not like being perceived as a sick person. Perhaps it is a bit of denial or self-preservation on my part. I do not like thinking about my disease when I do not have to.

I know I am not supposed to stay up late and have a beer with friends, because it injures my immune system, but I feel so silly going to bed early on the weekends when everyone I know is going out. I actually have made myself sick by pushing myself beyond my physical limits in order to appear to be a normal and healthy single twenty-something woman. I think there is a balance. I should not be pushing myself to stay up too late all the time simply to have fun or appear healthy, but just as importantly, I do not stay home all the time and limit myself. There is a balance to be found, like most things in life. Perhaps I am still trying to find the right balance.

A good portion of my life is consumed with fighting this illness. I receive sympathy from friends and family, but no one really understands what this portion of my life is like and just how all consuming it is. Not only do I take medication daily, go in for blood tests every three weeks, visit the doctor every four to six weeks, but I have to realize that I am not getting any better. There are stronger medications and possibly surgery in my future. These are scary things to deal with, and sometimes I feel quite alone. I never know when a flare-up of the disease is going to occur. When it does, I feel very weak and run a high temperature. During these fevers, I have had to go to the hospital for CT scans to see if there are any abscesses in my intestine. I am in my twenties and I actually feel comfortable in hospitals. Goodness, I have preferred veins for IVs. That is not normal!

Only my friends and family know that I am ill. If I have to miss work, my coworkers assume that I have the flu. I missed about ten days of work last year due to this disease. I hide it because I do not want to be viewed as a liability. Besides, I look healthy, so I cringe at trying to explain the severity of the disease. I cope with this illness by taking life one day at a time. A better treatment could be just around the corner for me. I am very hopeful and very thankful that I live in a time of great strides in modern medicine. I cope with my illness by remembering that there is always someone better off than me, but there is also always someone worse off than me. I keep a healthy and balanced perspective. Someone once told me that in tough situations, I could become bitter or better. I would like to think that I'm becoming the latter.

Peter S., Recording Engineer, Jazz Guitarist

Psoriatic Arthritis

Psoriatic arthritis is in the same family as rheumatoid arthritis in that it is a systemic autoimmune process where the immune system is attacking itself. Even joints that aren't overused have problems, because the whole immune system is involved. Every joint in the body can hurt: hands, feet, ankles, hips, shoulders.

Walking far is not good for me. I used to be a runner and noticed my first symptoms of psoriatic arthritis at that time. Getting a diagnosis took a long time because several other illnesses, such as Reiter's syndrome, have similar symptoms. At first, I had minor symptoms, but the turning point was developing tendonitis in one of my fingers. It looked like a direct link to overuse, and I thought it was simply from playing guitar so much. I took six months off, didn't play, and then all of these other symptoms started developing in other fingers, in my jaw, feet, etc. That's when I started having tests and seeing doctors. There was an enormous lengthy ride of trying to make my life work with this new set of symptoms that were causing parts of my body to not work very well.

I come from a background of holistic medicine so I explored a great many possibilities within that realm. The one thing that has had the biggest impact on my disease, other than the traditional medication I take for this condition, is yoga. I still practice yoga and meditation and they remain powerful and hopeful practices in my life. The basic daily struggles start in the morning when I'm stiff. Yoga is very good for every part of the body. I do an hour of yoga a day. It reduces stress because it is a gentle motion that you have to be present with; you can't drift because you must focus on what you are doing. It's sort of like exercise but done in a gentle, thoughtful way. I have been doing yoga since I was twenty-years-old, long before my arthritis started. It feels natural to me and seems to have a big impact. I feel measurably better after my yoga routine. Also, I feel as though my overall health is better than if I didn't do yoga.

I eat a vegetarian diet and watch what I eat. I don't drink alcohol and never really did, but this has turned me further away from drinking. I take medicine for this condition that shouldn't be combined with alcohol anyway. When I look at my disease, I want to take responsibility for it. I don't want to be one of those people who says, "Why me? I don't deserve this." But I've certainly had a lot of those feelings. One of the biggest things I didn't do correctly is that I didn't always get enough sleep. My balance seemed to be

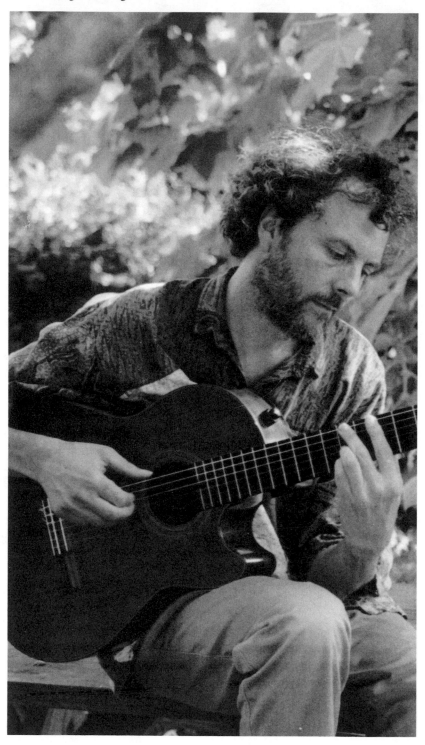

off because I did without sleep so often. I would play my musical gigs late at night and wake up and have a busy day, so I went without a lot of rest. I was tired a lot. I was working hard, physically and mentally. I was extremely disciplined in my musical career. My mind was so busy all the time that I stopped taking my physical body into consideration. Most people have a predisposition to illness or conditions in their genetic make up, and if things get too off kilter, these disorders can appear. For me, lack of sleep and proper diet played into it. I was out of balance.

I struggled for a long time believing that if I did the right things, I could become better again. I used various alternative treatments for six years. After that time, I was in a lot of pain and playing guitar a lot less. My hands were getting worse and worse. I repeatedly asked myself, "What am I going to do for a living that is related to music if I can't play music?" That's how I got into the recording aspect, which I now love. I'm still involved with music, and still making all these musical decisions and using all of my musical knowledge, without having to play instruments all the time. I now produce other artists; I write music for documentaries and put out my own music. I shifted the emphasis of my career from playing to recording.

You either view your illness and life in a way that it is a good thing or a negative thing. That's your choice every day.

Six or seven years ago, I decided to take the traditional medicine that I had known about and been urged to take. I was reluctant to do this for a long time because it's against my core belief. I got to the point where the suffering was so great and was forcing me to play less and less. Music had always been such a large part of me, not only in making a living, but for my own creative expression. The idea of letting go of music pulled me back to traditional medicine. My initial pivot point was: I'm suffering. I can suffer for the rest of my life, or I can take this medication, even with its side effects, and have a better quality of life. It's worth it to me to live a better life, than to live with every movement being painful and an effort.

When I finally decided to take the medicine, it made an enormous difference for me. Now I juggle the musical production, which pays far more than gigs, with playing live music. I am able to play a lot longer now on the medication. I am careful not to overdo it.

It's a spiritual experience when the music is right. It's a great moment when you are euphoric and free of the bad stuff of the world. Naturally, you want more of this good thing, so you cultivate all of these things to make playing more music possible. I had to let all that go for awhile, and it was so hard. I suffered. I went to therapy for many years and struggled with the idea of letting go of playing guitar. I am very careful with playing music now. I know that if I jeopardize it, I will again lose what I have. I don't take it for granted. I have a strong sense now that when I take guitar work, it has the potential to wear my body down. I have to make strong choices about this all the time now.

I get down because I am hurting. The sum total of all the therapy that I have had and what I've concluded in my little clip of wisdom: This is what is. You either view your illness and life in a way that is a good thing or a negative thing. That's your choice every day. Although it took a long time to get to this place, when I had that moment of wisdom and made that shift to realize I still have a lot and I'm going to do the best I can with what I have, it made a huge impact on my life. This view is rooted in me now. It wasn't before.

My hands do not look arthritic. I don't look like I have anything. Most of my colleagues completely forget that I have this illness. I'm not a big complainer. There is an amazing cloud that I go into when I play music, and the pain goes away. I pay for it the next day, but I don't feel it when I play. I can use music to take my mind off the pain and make it go away, at least for a time. Meditation is a good thing that helps in the same way. I feel that meditation and yoga have had an impact. I might have had the symptoms sooner had I not practiced meditation and yoga. My intent is to continue these self-help approaches to maintain the good level I am currently at with the progression of the illness. I never go to that place of if-only-I-hadn't-done-so-much, because part of where I am now with my career success is because of what I did and how I lived early on. It's my way to push hard. That's who I am and that's how I accomplished what I did.

The spiritual aspect of my life is always shifting and very unclear to me, but I'm cool with that. In yoga, there is the physical aspect, the meditation aspect, and spiritual aspect, and I was into all of them. I came to question a lot of the spiritual aspect along the way. I'm in a place where I don't know if I believe the same things as I used to, and I like that. I don't sit and say "I trust in God to help me out of this" or "God is looking after me." I am more of the belief of being a real doer. If I'm going to help myself out, I'm going to do yoga and help my situation rather than waiting around for things to happen or people to do things for me. A chronic disease takes away your choice, but do you want to give up this gift of life and be a complainer? I don't think it's the way to go. Smiling at someone or being kind to them on the phone can come from a suffering place as well as a healthy place. It's not easy, but it's possible, and I prefer it to being a complainer.

I feel as though my life is a wonderful gift. I might not have seen that without this disease. It hit in the midst of a good life. Things could be better, but you know what? Things could be a lot worse. The disease has shifted my career, but in a good way. I am not working as hard and I am making more money than I would playing live music. Now I do gigs that are artistic expressions. I cut out all the others that are not necessary. I have learned to appreciate my family and friendships much more, and the humanity and the value of being alive. Talking to my wife helps me deal with some of the tough times, and she offers comfort and a sense of hope that it won't always be this way. Sometimes I "gift myself" by resting. I just lie down, and that sure feels nice. Giving up can be a good thing. Give yourself the luxury of resting and not doing anything. Maybe life is about getting good at giving up.

The experience of life becomes much deeper when you know what suffering is. I go through days where I still have little pockets of time where I get down about my health, but overall I feel pretty accepting of it now. I'm not holding out for some magical thing to happen. I work hard at maintaining what I have. Doing an hour of yoga is not really fun, and it would be easier to sit on the couch and eat chocolates, but I do it. Yoga is beneficial and keeps me in the best shape I can be.

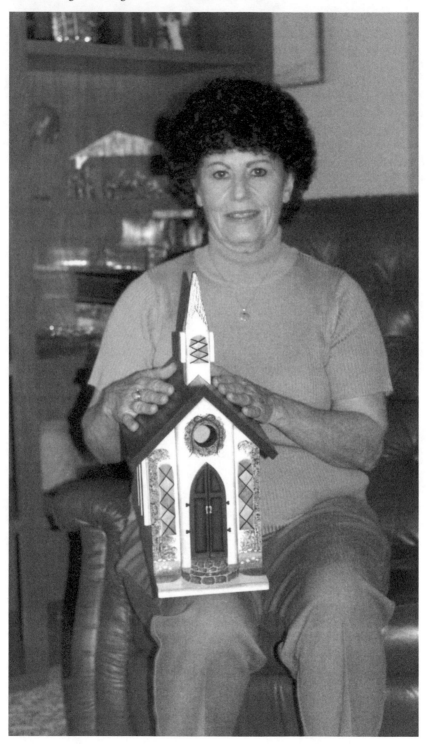

Marilyn M., Poet/Writer

Fibromyalgia, Chronic Fatigue Immune Dysfunction Syndrome

People do not always understand or accept my answer when I tell them that I am unable to function at the same level that I used to. When I have a cold, I have everyone's sympathy, because they are able to see and identify with it. But when I say that I hurt all over and am exhausted, their eyes glaze over.

My entire life is different now because of these two concealed illnesses. I can no longer pursue my career or many of my interests. I can no longer travel to visit my family or take care of my home the way I used to. I marvel at people's energy level. I have friends and relatives who are a decade or so older than me, and they are doing all of the things that I expected to be doing when I retired. This was not my dream for retirement. I was always a very active, athletic person, able to do several things at once. Now I have trouble doing only one thing at once.

Sometimes when people say to me, "You look just fine" I respond with, "I wish I felt as good as I look!"

Over a long period of time, I began to accept my condition to a certain degree. I now acknowledge that I am not the same person that I once was healthwise. I have lowered many of my expectations, which were perhaps too high to begin with. I refer to it as lowering the bar of my life. I have had to redefine myself within the framework of my present physical condition

At the beginning, no one had ever heard of chronic fatigue syndrome or fibromyalgia. I have received all kinds of suggestions that run counter to what I am able to do because of these illnesses. I would like to see more public education on the subject of fibromyalgia and chronic fatigue syndrome, so that there is more understanding and acknowledgement of the legitimacy of these difficult-to-manage conditions.

I used to try to hide my condition; I was always told, "People do not want to hear about your problems." Now I just try to be myself. Trying to be something other than what I am impacts my stamina and my symptoms. It is not necessary to dwell on my problems, or to be the one to bring them up, but if someone asks, I give them a very brief report and change the subject to something more stimulating. I ask them questions about themselves. Their perception of me will not be of someone who is sick, but someone they enjoy conversing with.

I became aware at an early age that most prescription drugs did not work well for me. I was highly sensitive, and if there were side effects, I usually experienced them quite severely. I have tried to keep an open mind about prescription drugs as well as about alternative treatments, although I have never ventured too far from the more common treatments.

Massage therapy is very helpful to me, but not affordable to those who are on disability and do not have insurance that covers these useful treatments. I have tried yoga and tai chi, and they were both beneficial. Gentle stretching is necessary for people with fibromyalgia, but both of these methods take a level of commitment to attend classes.

When you have something like fibromyalgia, planning ahead for classes, appointments, or anything else is difficult. There are days when I could not get ready to go to a spa or gym if my life depended on it. I highly recommend a lot of these alternative treatments, but most of us who are not able to work and bring in an income do not have the money necessary to receive these sorts of beneficial treatments on an ongoing basis. Therefore, I utilize cost-effective basic exercise methods, such as walking, stretching, swimming, and relaxation techniques.

Group therapy has been helpful to me. Talking to people who understand what I am going through has a positive effect. These groups offer tools to cope with illness or pain. There is a social component to belonging to a group that helps lower the level of isolation and depression often experienced with these illnesses.

Over and over, people ask what exactly is wrong with me. That is a very complicated question and there is no short answer. I can see people becoming uncomfortable and tuning me out as I go through the litany. Sometimes when people say to me, "You look just fine" I respond with, "I wish I felt as good as I look!"

I cope with my symptoms by sticking to a rather rigid routine, pacing myself, and getting as much rest as I can. I ask for help when necessary. I truly take one day at a time. The symptoms of this condition can get very scary; there are so many and they can change from hour to hour. Now I just tell myself, "It is just another fibromyalgia or CFS symptom" and I don't need to run to the doctor or have a panic attack. This has been a tremendous relief for me.

One of the worst symptoms is the ever-present exhaustion that prevents me from leading a normal life. I do feel down at times. That is when I call someone from my support group, and we discuss it. Although we have "whine not!" as our motto, we still feel free to vent our frustrations, and we all understand each other's bad days.

My father was a great wit; I always admired his sense of humor. I've tried to always keep my sense of humor and to pass it on to my children. I believe that I have succeeded. There are often amusing parts if you can see the irony in life and in your condition. It's a matter of attitude.

I have always had hope in my life. I refer often to the Emily Dickinson poem, *Hope is the Thing with Feathers*:

Hope is the thing with feathers
That perches in the soul,
And sings the tune without the words,
And never stops at all,

And sweetest in the gale is heard;
And sore must be the storm
That could abash the little bird
That kept so many warm.

I've heard it in the chilliest land,
And on the strangest sea;
Yet, never, in extremity,
It asked a crumb of me.

There are days, that this is the chilliest land and the strangest sea, but if I face each day with hope, I always have something to look forward to.

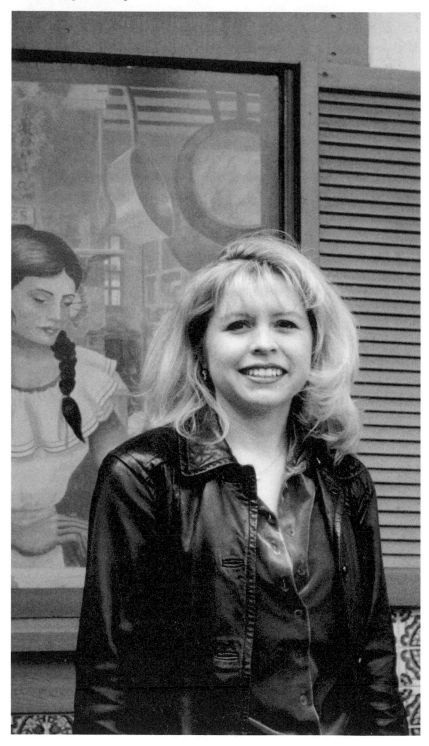

Rita N., Administrative Assistant

Crohn's Disease

I feel as though my illness doesn't count to the people around me, because it is not visible. When I was diagnosed, I had been in the hospital for a week and people did not know why. There were a few rumors about why I was absent, but when I returned, everyone assumed I was all better. I needed a year to find the right mix of medications to finally get my disease under control. When I experienced occasional inflammation in the colon, I was forced to stay home from work for a day. The inflammations caused me to lose fifteen to twenty pounds, but no one seemed to notice.

When I am with a group of people and suddenly get a sharp pain in my abdomen, I try to hide the pain. When I have pain at work and lose my concentration, I try not to make eye contact with anyone so that my coworkers do not see that I am in pain. One of the disadvantages of having a concealed illness is the feeling that people do not really believe that I am sick. If I have a lot of pain at work and I want

A disadvantage of having a concealed illness is that people do not really believe that I am sick.

to go home, I feel awkward saying something like, "I know that I looked healthy all day, but now, all of a sudden, I need to go home." Instead, I just end up staying at work the entire day, trying not to move too much, and hoping the pain will just go away.

There was a person I knew who had to deal with a visible illness. She constantly received cards and flowers to encourage her through the battle with her disease. In contrast, when I returned from the hospital, everyone assumed I was just fine. Even so, I feel that I have been very fortunate with my illness. My doctor has found the right balance of medications for my particular symptoms.

My parents had no idea what this disease meant, even though I landed in the hospital on numerous occasions. Sometimes walking a long time will cause pain in my abdominal area. I have to sit and wait for the pain to die down. I sometimes feel like I am in the way. I feel as though I am holding people back from what they want to do, because I have to sit and rest.

The most important change this illness brought into my life was not having children. My husband and I were ready to have children, but I was diagnosed the year before we wanted to start our family. There are moments when I am filled with guilt and sadness because I still have not had any children and I have been married for almost seven years.

My biggest concern during a flare-up is the location of the next restroom. On long drives, I worry about how long it will take to get to the next rest area. I have also changed my career focus because of this illness. I had always wanted to be a police officer, but with this illness, I had to consider and worry about whether I would need to suddenly pull over and run into a restroom while I was in pursuit of a criminal. As my condition continues to be controlled with medication, I have started to feel more confident. When I am doing better, I believe that I can still do the things I thought I would not be able to do again.

During the first year of my illness, before I was on medication, the most important improvements to my health came from my practice of yoga. The breathing really helped me relax into the pain when I was in the hospital. I have been doing yoga for three years, and I think that was the important added ingredient I needed to help the medication to work and help me heal. Yoga was not only wonderful exercise, but the meditation and breath control that go along with the practice are extremely beneficial. We were taught to find trouble spots in our bodies and to breathe them out. Those breathing techniques came in very handy during my two bouts with kidney stones. On nights that I was in a lot of pain, the breathing was about all I could do to control the pain. I am still amazed to see how much the mind can control some of the pain and symptoms.

Yoga has helped me on a physical level, but having an extremely caring and loving husband has helped me on an emotional level. I definitely could not have remained as strong throughout this process if it had not been for him. I sometimes feel guilty that he has to deal with all of this too.

I feel very fortunate to have this illness somewhat under control. I feel that my faith in God has really helped me to be a stronger person through this. Even though not everyone understands what I go through when I have a flare-up, the people who are closest to me have taken the time to read up on my disease and are very supportive. I think the disease has helped to bring my circle of family and friends closer together. I was also fortunate to have found a wonderful support group just after being diagnosed. I had no idea what Crohn's disease was or how to deal with it. The sharing in our support group helped me a great deal. I felt like I was no longer alone. If all of these people could deal with it, so could I.

I'm a very positive person and I try to find meaning in every part of my life. Having this disease has helped me to become more compassionate towards others who are diagnosed with an illness. It helps me offer other people words of encouragement. I feel that this disease has made me a stronger and better person.

Lisa V., Former Model

Lupus

Not a day has gone by since my diagnosis that I have not remembered that I have lupus. There are days when I am aware of it every waking minute. Taking my pills and putting on my medical identification bracelet are two things that I will do every day for the rest of my life. I will always be reminded of my lupus. That is too bad. I wish I could have just a day where I am happy and feel so inspired and healthy that I don't have to think about lupus at all. I worry about my security, about how I'm going to achieve all the things that I need to achieve, or at least feel that I need to achieve to be happy, content, and satisfied with my life. How can I do these things when I have this illness? Sometimes it is difficult to stay positive. But the question isn't how can I cope, but how can I not cope? Basically, no matter who you are, or whatever your problems and challenges in life are, your choices are two: either give up, or cope. So, I have to cope. That's all there is to it. Other people cannot imagine how I am dealing with the disruption of this illness, but if they were suddenly in my shoes, they would be coping just as well as I am. They simply would have no choice. They would have to.

Living with a concealed illness or condition is different than contending with one that is more visibly apparent to others. That is because people have been conditioned to prejudge people based solely on appearance. Usually, the first idea that a person has in his head about someone is based on visual signs. Therefore, if I have a smile on my face, or I have bothered to dress nicely, people have a hard time believing that I am sick. There are so many invisible symptoms one could be experiencing at any given time: headaches, nausea, arthritic pain, fatigue, and depression. An observer will be completely unaware of these problems, unless of course, they are told about the illness. Many people keep quiet about their pain because they simply do not want to sound like a crybaby.

I've had to make many adjustments because of my illness. For example, last summer I had to cancel what would have been a six-month trip to Europe because of my symptoms. Last September, I went to Seattle and Canada. After four days in Seattle, I was completely exhausted and spent the last day riding a boat so that I could rest. I had to change my ticket to come home early and never even got to Canada. I used to take three-hour walks on the beach every day and would dance every night. Now, I'm lucky if I take a couple of short walks per week, and those are exhausting and take a lot of effort. If, once in a blue moon I go out to see a band, I dance for maybe two or

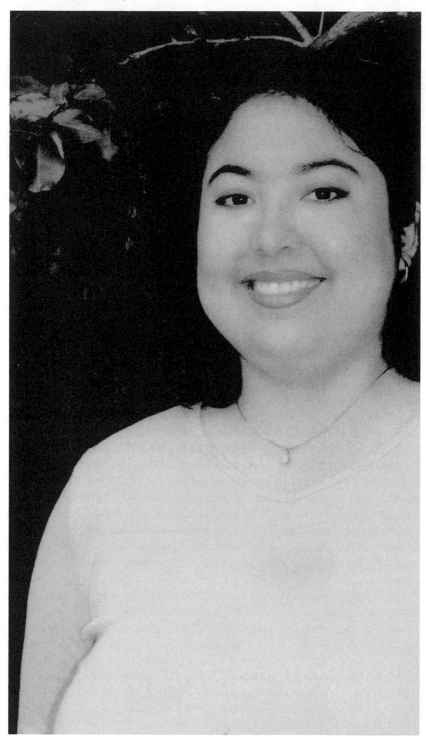

three songs the entire night and feel exhausted and out of breath afterwards.

I've had to live with my parents for the last four years because I have been too sick to work and was denied Social Security insurance and disability benefits. I have not pursued that further as of yet because it takes energy, effort, motivation, and a clear head—all things that I rarely have anymore. I do not date and cannot make new friends because I'm always too tired to go out. I have to avoid the sun. I have to be very picky about my sleeping arrangements because I need quiet, dark, and comfortable sleeping space and about ten hours of uninterrupted sleep or I will become more symptomatic. Therefore, I can no longer be spontaneous and just sleep anywhere. I can't just crash on someone's couch or go camping at the drop of a hat.

Strangers have questioned my symptoms. My friends have not. The others wonder why I can engage in a few fun activities, and yet I am unable to work. They think that I must not be really sick. The reason I can do this is because, with a fun activity, I am the one who makes all the rules. I can do it every day, or once a year. I can do it for one minute, or five hours. Work is not the same. Who would hire me and allow me to work only when I was up to it? No one. There are days when I feel great amidst months of feeling horrible; and yes, I take full advantage of those days. Sometimes, there are months in a row where I feel good amidst years of feeling horrible. People do not understand this inconsistency, and I lose my credibility because of it.

I wish some people could live my life for a week, just so that they could understand what this is like on a daily basis.

On occasion, I feel very envious of others. They're going jogging, dancing, traveling, and are dating, working, and sunbathing. They are financially independent. My friends don't live with their parents. They don't have to go to medical appointments all the time, or take medications and experience the side effects. Some people don't understand the problem of not knowing when they are going to feel good or feel ill, and not being able to make plans for fear they will have to be canceled. They can wake up every morning with a to-do list and actually get things done instead of having the same list sitting around for months. They can think clearly. They can have conversations with people and sound smart, not spacey. Sometimes I feel like that is so unfair. On the other hand, sometimes I feel like I have so much patience. I have been sitting in my room for months calmly accepting that all I can do is watch TV or just vegetate while others are living a real life. I wonder how they would react if suddenly they were put in my circumstances. Would they be as cheery and patient as I am? I try to hold onto hope and still live my dreams in spite of this. What also helps me is meditation, tai chi, being at the ocean, reading books, listening to music, being with friends and family, utilizing good doctors, indulging in fantasies, and day-dreams.

I wish some people could live my life for a week, or even five minutes, just so that they could truly understand what this illness is like on a day-to-day basis. Every emotional, mental, and physical symptom would be theirs for that time, and only then would they truly understand what this is like. I try to do what I can, but I also take it easy when I know I have to. I watch good movies and read books. I treat myself to good food and imagine my perfect future. I philosophize about exactly why this is the best thing that could have happened to me. Because of this illness, I am growing spiritually in ways that I couldn't have done otherwise.

The advantage of having a concealed illness, as opposed to one that is visible to others, is that as long as I can pull it off, I can easily blend in with everyone and not feel like an outsider. The disadvantage is that people need visual signs to offer credibility and to give them an explanation about me. Without that, it can be hard to deal with strangers, acquaintances, and especially difficult to begin new relationships.

For me, having lupus is everything you can imagine it to be. Not only has it been very depressing, but it has also caused me to feel angry, hopeless, frustrated, annoyed, isolated, bored, sad, disillusioned, unmotivated, unattractive, exhausted, groggy, and filled with pain. On the other hand, it also has caused me to feel relief and inspiration, and to feel that I am special and lucky. I know that I was given this challenge because I have the strength to deal with it. Not everyone has that inner strength. I feel like this is really an opportunity for growth and that the whole point of our existence is to evolve spiritually. Therefore, the disease can be experienced as a very spiritual thing.

My feelings about living with lupus cover the extreme ends of the spectrum and everything in-between. I have good days, I have very bad days, and I have days where thinking of my lupus affects me about as much as thinking about the beauty mark on my left elbow. In other words, it doesn't always have a significant effect on me. Sometimes, it feels like no big deal. I have brown hair, I wear contact lenses, I'm half Mexican, I have an ingrown toenail, and I have lupus. That is all there is to it. There are other days when it feels like a tragedy and my entire destiny has been completely altered because of this disease. I feel like a failure in life. On those bad days, I think of the potential I was born with and what I was supposed to become, and I realize that this will not happen now. This realization can feel like a nightmare.

As much as people complain about their lot in life, the majority of people, if given the choice, would not trade their problems, disease, or circumstances for anyone else's. I think that says a lot. Whatever is wrong with me, there's something familiar about it, something telling me that it was meant to be, for whatever reason. The bottom line is, no matter what I must experience, I view it as a challenge towards a deeper understanding of myself, and of life.

Nancy G., Social Worker

Fibromyalgia

I sometimes wish that my illness were visible so that people would be more likely to believe me. When they cannot see my symptoms or my illness, they question if it is real. They are less compassionate because they have never experienced such pain themselves.

People question this illness all of the time and assume it isn't really that bad. I have had to quit my business and go on disability insurance. I am always thinking of what physical price I will pay for any given activity I may want to do. I am always thinking of ways to minimize the consequences of an activity, such as how to do the dishes or laundry. I am no longer a planner; I always have to be flexible when I take part in activities.

I feel envious of healthy people all of the time. They remind me of the life I used to have before my car accident, which brings up feelings of loss and grief. My spiritual beliefs, spiritual community, meditation, friends, and family have helped me to cope. There are times when I wish I appeared handicapped, especially when I use my handicap parking permit and someone confronts me about it. I wish the public would become more educated and aware about concealed illnesses. This book will surely help.

I try to remind myself of my previous inner strength and try to learn the benefits and lessons of this new experience of being in pain. Talking with others who have fibromyalgia has helped me to gain information on new treatments and support. I also receive great healing and comfort from my animals.

I try to appear perfectly fine when I go out, especially when meeting new people. Usually, I go beyond my limits and then suffer more pain and sleep problems that night and the next day. This leads to feeling more discouraged and depressed, because I am not like I used to be. I think about self-care a great deal, but I don't seem to practice it often enough.

People expect more of me than is realistic because I look healthy, even if I am not. They don't always believe me and are not sympathetic to my pain, or they forget that I am in pain even within hours of my telling them.

Having this illness has been the biggest challenge I have ever had. It has turned my life upside down and sideways. After nine years, I still am grieving for my old self. I cope by not giving up hope, practicing my spiritual principles, constantly trying things that might help, slowing down, lowering my expectations of myself, crying, laughing, exercising, and watching my diet. I have found the most helpful approach to my symptoms has been eating raw foods, fasting with juice, and a regular exercise program of swimming.

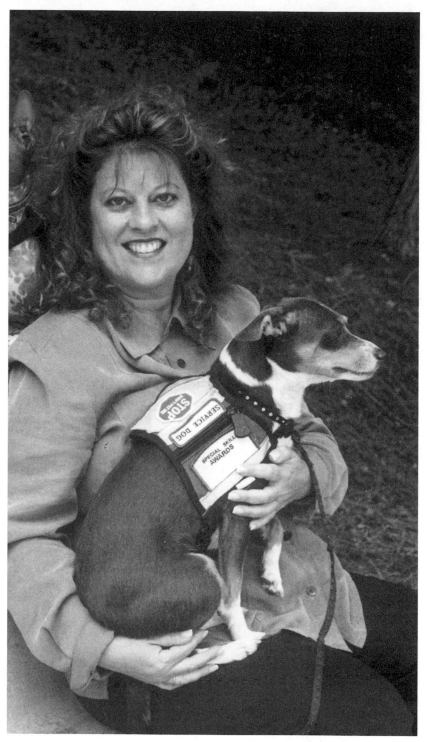

Prior to my car accident, my health team was almost exclusively alternative medical care. Initially, alternative care did not cure my symptoms, and I resorted to traditional Western medicine and medications. Over the past eleven years, I have alternated between alternative approaches and conventional medicine. I prefer alternative approaches, especially after I experienced more and more side effects with the medications. I dislike the toxicity of medications, especially with long-term use.

Biofeedback was initially very helpful to me in overcoming the post-traumatic stress syndrome from a devastating car accident. Gentle yoga is always helpful, though I need the structure of classes to do it consistently. Sometimes my symptoms interfere with my plans to attend class, and I lose ground in my progress. Meditation is helpful, but difficult for me to do, especially when I have not slept well due to the fibromyalgia pain. Swimming regularly affords great benefits, especially for my emotional and mental sense of well-being and productivity. Psychotherapy has helped me adjust to the changes and limitations in my new life, and nutritional supplements help when I can be consistent about taking them. My spirituality is what sustains me above all else.

People with chronic pain know that the search for relief is often unending and discouraging.

People with chronic pain know that the search for relief is often unending and discouraging. A couple of years ago, I discovered a very unique and pleasurable pain management resource: a dog! Toaster is a Xolos, a rare breed that generates a great deal of heat to keep itself warm. In fact, Xolos are literally hot dogs, and my dog, Toaster, is like a heating pad, without having to be microwaved. I named her Toaster because she is quite toasty on my neck.

Toaster has helped me in so many more ways than just being my hot neck wrap. Many people with chronic pain suffer from secondary conditions, such as depression, and I am no exception. Xolos are extremely intelligent and sensitive to their owner's needs and moods. I believe that animals are angels for us, healing us in more ways than we can imagine. They provide us with compassion and unconditional love. Animals enable us to feel connected to life, despite the challenge of pain and poor health.

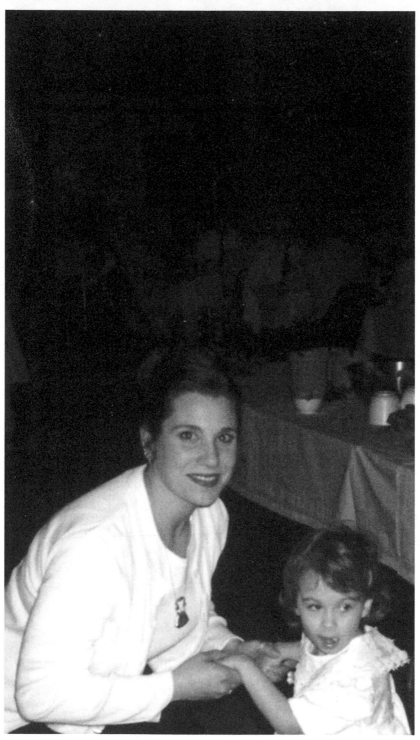

Shawna F., Allied Health Worker

Endometriosis

Society validates a visible illness more than a concealed one such as endometriosis. Being in the emergency room in the middle of the night is both disheartening and frustrating. Here I am doubled over in pain and trying to hang on, while the guy next to me with a bad knee is called in first. If his knee appears swollen and discolored, his complaints are listened to. For those of us who have endometriosis and other concealed conditions, medical professionals are less likely to be as understanding, since the source of our pain is not visually obvious.

The biggest adjustment that I have had to make is in learning to accept my limitations in spite of my highly competitive personality and my love of sports. I was an all-state, tri-sport athlete and had to turn down three scholarships when I left high school. My body simply could not keep up with my mind anymore. I have great frustration, because I was raised in a very active environment and have talent in many sports, but I am no longer able to participate in the activities that I love.

I always used to wish to appear disabled, not to gain sympathy, but because it would give my illness validation. . .

People have constantly questioned the existence of my illness, unfortunately, even some doctors. I have never been one to let anything stop me. Before I was diagnosed and was feeling so bad, I heard the word hypochondriac whispered behind my back rather frequently. Even though that was years ago, I still feel as though I lead a double life at times. I still feel safer and more accepted if I go to great lengths to hide how bad my symptoms are.

I often feel envious of the good health and vigor of others and wish that I could be the old me once again. It's my competitive nature. I see Olympic softball players with just as much talent as I had, and they are doing what I want to be doing, what I could be doing if things had somehow been different. Sometimes it bothers me when I meet a woman who has not only had children already, but who doesn't even take asprin because she has never had a headache. I suddenly get a case of the why me's.

I always used to wish that I appeared disabled—not because I would gain sympathy, but because it would give my illness validation, and people would understand my challenges. I used to secretly wish that I had cancer or something like that, and I have always felt guilty about those feelings. I am sure there are many with concealed illnesses such as mine who periodically have to go to the emergency room or be hospitalized when the pain is out of hand and the normal medication regime loses its effectiveness. We look just fine. It is frustrating and humiliating because even our blood tests come back with normal results.

My stubbornness and tenacity has helped pull me through the rough times. There have been times when I have desperately wanted out of this pain and suffering. Fortunately, I was unable to simply give up the fight. No matter how many times I have heard, "There is nothing more that we can do for you; you've exhausted all treatment options," that just is not good enough. I have empowered myself with education and knowledge and have made it my life's goal to find the answers needed to heal.

I have always felt the need to appear normal and healthy, to blend in with other people around me, especially if they are people I have just met. Sometimes, I think that if I just went into acting I would make a great actress. I'm already well trained enough to win an award for some of the roles I've had to play. When I am feeling particularly bad, the act is too much work. I will make up an excuse as to why I can't join my friends. Then I'll hide out somewhere and lie around, watch movies, read books, and get upset about the fun I am missing.

The only true advantage to not looking as ill as I feel is that strangers don't pity me. The downside to those scenarios is exactly the same. When my condition becomes acute, I rarely get taken seriously because I look healthy and just fine.

Even though I have had this concealed condition for over a decade, it is still very difficult to deal with. As I said before, I am very competitive; I love sports and being active. Even if there is a backyard or beach volleyball game taking place, I will still jump in. Not only do I pay the price later, but I also get frustrated because my mind is trying to do one thing and my body cannot follow through at the same pace.

I once coped with my condition by self-medicating with street drugs and alcohol. Now that I'm older and a little wiser, I'm trying to make cognitive changes in how I feel about my physical condition. I used to hate it, fight it, resent it, curse it, and get angry at it. There came a time when I had to accept that these concealed symptoms are a part of me; however, they don't have to define or consume me. I am learning to accept my limitations and realize that I am being put through these tests for some reason. I need to take advantage of what this illness is teaching me about myself. I am learning to cope with my symptoms, and my situation, one moment at a time.

Bill H., CEO, Inventor

Fibromyalgia, Chronic Fatigue Immune Dysfunction Syndrome

After receiving my diagnosis, I felt a great deal of relief that someone had finally put a name to what was going on. I was not crazy after all. I also thought to myself, now that I know what it is, I can fix it. Ha! Little did I know that would not be the case.

Having concealed and chronic symptoms is different than contending with disorders that are more noticeable to others, especially if one is not able to work for oneself. When I worked for others it was tough. I had to hide the way I felt. I had to hide the pain medicine I lived on for fear that I would lose my job and have no way of supporting my family.

Guilt is the most challenging thing about living with my chronic health problems. I am constantly feeling like a burden to my wife and children. Not being able to exercise and go places is difficult on me and my family, and it feeds into the guilt. Counting the minutes until I can take a hot bath and climb into bed is not a fun way to live. Once I reach home, I stay in bed.

I have finally forgiven myself for being sick. (Not really. I just try to fool myself into thinking that I have forgiven myself.) I try to rest a least one day on the weekend, and I take a nap when the pain is too severe to cope with. I try to focus on my business. I find that when my mind is engaged in solving problems, my pain is not as noticeable. However, as soon as I drop my guard, the pain rushes in and overwhelms me.

What has helped me secure periods of peace and what has helped me to adjust to these chronic disorders is simply having a wife and children that understand this illness and look out for me. They try to protect me. Looking back on what I have been able to accomplish, and how it has helped others cope with their illness, has given me some peace of mind as well.

I find that in my professional life, it is sometimes tough to keep up the pace. For instance, tonight I have two business associates from the East Coast coming to town and we have to take them to dinner. I am already in so much pain I could cry, and yet I have to act like I am enjoying myself. Sometimes, I wonder if I will be able to make it home. Inside, I am just weeping.

I often try to appear pain-free, especially when the symptoms are severe. I am a master at this. I smile and drink my coffee or eat my dessert. Each morning when I get up at 5 A.M. to go to work, I tell everyone I feel fine, but I don't. Do I tell them how I really feel? No. "How are you feeling?" they ask. "Great. I feel great." The line I use most often is "If I were any better I couldn't stand it." Well, part of that sentence is true. I can hardly stand it.

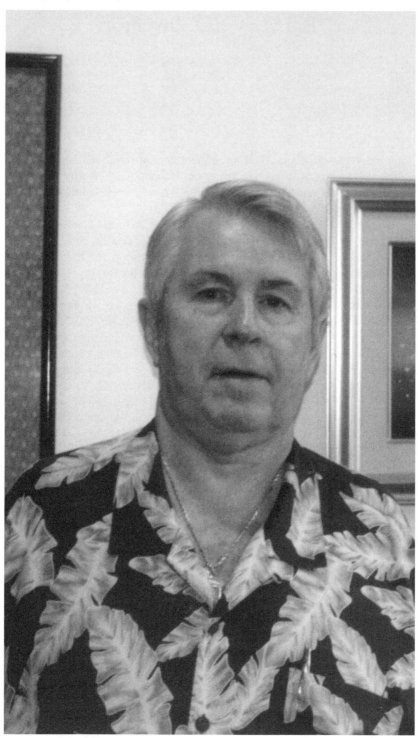

It is hard not to become irritable or frustrated when I am in constant pain. I handle it the best I can most of the time; however, sometimes I snap a little at my wife. Since we work together and are with one another day and night, she understands and is great about my little blowups. I do not know how I would survive without her.

I use my pain as a motivator. Just like hitting your thumb with a hammer, it feels so good when it stops. Each and every day when I wake up, I tell myself I will not be defeated by this illness. I will win in the end. I may even discover a cure. Maybe today will be the day.

People do not question my symptoms any longer. They did thirty years ago, but not anymore. I can still work any younger person under the table. Unfortunately, I pay a high price for it. I think most people who know me respect what I have been able to do, despite this illness.

I used to be a millionaire. I lost everything to this disease. Now I am fighting my way back. I may not enjoy the physical things success can bring, but it has made me a much stronger person, mentally. I am proud of what I have accomplished with such a handicap.

I lost everything to this disease. Now I am fighting my way back.

I would be here a year if I had to list all the things I have tried to help with my pain. Surgery, nerve blocks, biofeedback, enough pain medicine to fill a football stadium, and doctor after doctor until I hate most doctors and dread seeing the inside of each and every hospital. I have tried acupuncture, herbs, vitamins, and visited every medical center from coast to coast. Having to take so many medicines at one time had me looking and acting like a zombie for a while.

I am angry with my body. I hate feeling this way, and I hate the burden it places on loved ones. I feel certain that without this condition I could achieve anything I desired. Strangely enough, however, having this illness has actually strengthened my spirit. I will not be defeated by some unseen monster that is trying to steal my life away. I will defeat the monster and not allow it to control my life. Never!

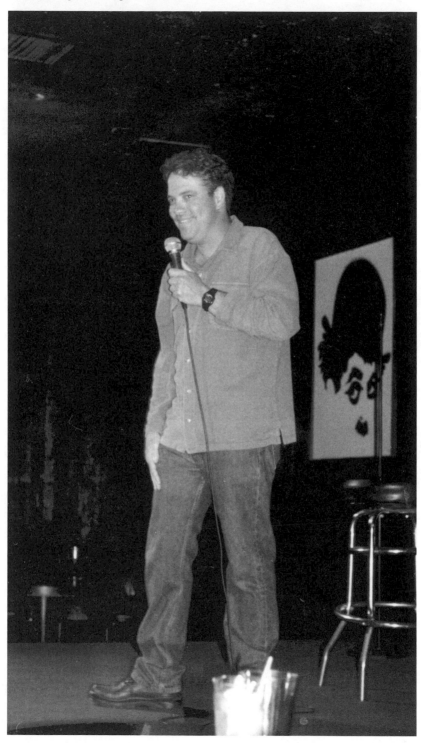

Mike E., Stand-up Comedian

Nephrotic Syndrome (Kidney Disorder), Ulcerative Colitis

Although no one comes right out and questions my illness, I often get the sense that certain people will never understand a concealed illness. If they cannot see it, it simply does not exist. . . at least, to them. When I was first diagnosed, there was a feeling of "Why me?" because I had always taken good care of myself. I had trouble accepting that while others smoked and drank and I didn't, I was the one who became ill. That seemed unfair, and I was envious of other people's freedom and active lives. Once I accepted that there would be some limitations in my daily life, I was able to secure some periods of peace.

I had trouble accepting that while others smoked and drank, I was the one who became ill.

I have sometimes wished that I appeared disabled or had a more acceptable or recognizable illness. It seems rather funny now, but I once told an employer that I had been diagnosed with diabetes. Although a person with diabetes may not appear disabled either, it is a familiar illness, and thus does not require a lot of explanation. It is also far less embarrassing then explaining the symptoms of ulcerative colitis. Although I often try to blend in with the people around me, I have learned that blending in is not as important as staying healthy. For instance, what I do to blend in is to resist the urge to use the bathroom for long periods of time.

Having these two illnesses has helped me appreciate life much more. Most people never realize how lucky they are to be healthy until they become ill. I have become so accustomed to living with kidney disease and ulcerative colitis that it now feels normal to me. Sometimes, however, I feel overwhelmed and want to crawl under a rock and hide. That usually doesn't last long because I remind myself that although things could be better, they could also be worse. These chronic physical challenges have been a learning experience. Having a concealed illness has humbled me and made me think twice before judging others. I often remind myself that just because someone looks healthy on the outside, their appearance does not always tell the entire story. One of the thought processes that I use is to think about people who are worse off than I am. In comparison, I have nothing to complain about. I feel grateful for who I am, illness and all.

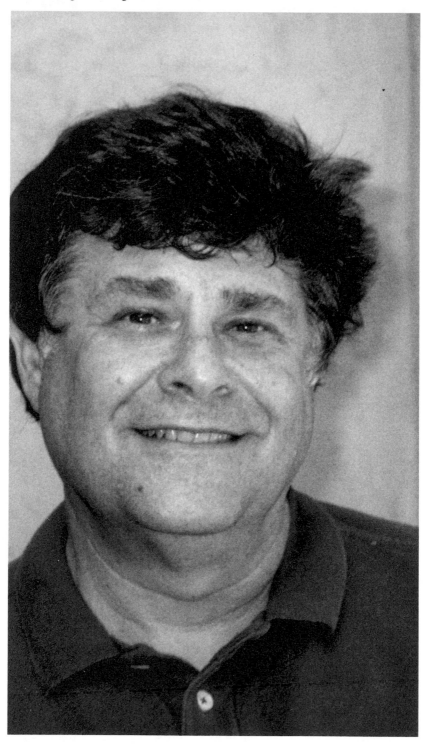

Marc H., Retired Attorney

Chronic Fatigue Immune Dysfunction Syndrome, Fibromyalgia,

Insulin Resistance, Depression, Sub-acute Celiac Disease

I've been ill for twenty-nine years, and for the past twelve years I have been disabled. Not totally bed-ridden disabled, mind you, just tired enough and with so little energy that I am exhausted most of the day. I have learned to adjust, cope, and live with a body that is just too sick to perform the daily tasks of life or work as an attorney. It's just too hard. On those days, I push myself beyond my limits of endurance; the extra effort only results in worsened conditions immediately or the next day. It's just not worth it. But, to see me on the street, you would not know I was sick. I look too healthy.

I can't let myself get rundown or I will become sicker. It is just part of my life.

For the first ten years, my symptoms were chronic fatigue (bordering on exhaustion), and a compulsion to overeat. As the fatigue worsened into chronic exhaustion, I ended up sleeping twenty hours per day. Going to the market was overwhelming.

Over time, despair replaced hope, and suicide seemed the only way out of the endless days and nights. I told God I was coming home unless he fixed me. And He did. In the next few months, He put the most unlikely medical doctors and dentists on my path.

Over the next few years, I began to recover. I have gained some strength and energy, but not enough to return to work. At most, I can work just a few hours every other day. But, I look and feel fairly well.

The realization that I had sub-acute Celiac disease (difficulty digesting wheat and other glutens) helped complete the puzzle of my symptoms. Finding out that there were real tests that showed I had a really sick body relieved a lot of my psychological stress.

I felt good that I had concrete reasons for my chronic exhaustion and thus my inability to work. Once I had labels for my illnesses, people could handle my disabilities. Until I had those tests, I was someone who was just too lazy or crazy to be employed. Until I had those tests, I was viewed as the eccentric hippie from the Sixties who just didn't want to work.

When I helped start an information and support group in my community, I met a lot of people like me. For many reasons, that turned out to be a good thing. I found I was not alone in my illnesses. It was reassuring to know there were many people like me in the world. I also discovered I was lucky because my wife did not leave me when she found out I was sick. That happens too many times to too many people when they become disabled.

Health issues define my life. It is a constant struggle to stay alive. I am always monitoring my level of vitality and my reserves. I cannot let myself become rundown or I will become sicker. It is just a part of my life, just as someone on oxygen is always monitoring the level in their tank.

I am lucky because I have many other interests, so when I first meet someone, I usually tell them I am a retired attorney who is interested in economics, financial planning, stock markets, and spirituality. If the occasion occurs, I share that I have CFIDS, that I spend a lot of time and money on doctors and medicines, and like to help others by sharing my knowledge and experiences.

I don't hide my illnesses; I just don't make it a point to say that I am chronically ill in the first sentence after I meet someone new. However, the topic often comes up casually enough in the conversation as we discuss health issues. Most find my knowledge, opinions, and experiences helpful because I try to remain constructive.

My joy comes from the love I have for God, my wife, my friends and family, and the abundance of nature. My humor comes from the ironic paradoxes in life.

My health issues take up a lot of time, which could be spent on other more productive forms of activity. But, that is not up to me to decide. That is up to the Universe. If it wants me to play a greater role in the world, it knows how to fix me. For now, I am limited in what I can do and when I can do it.

Diane J., Former Musical Theater Actor

Cerebellum Lymphoma, Central Nervous System

Lymphoma (including Eye Lymphoma)

One time, a salesman in my house noticed that I was moving a bit slowly and being careful when I sat down. "Bad back?" he asked. I responded, "No, brain cancer." Nothing wrong with having a little honest fun.

I have been in both places, having this illness as both visible and concealed. I know from experience that dealing with each one is very different. I have had brain cancer twice, twelve years apart, which was visible in the beginning because I was unable to walk, stand, feed myself, or do any and all functions that most people take for granted. My condition is much more visibly concealed now. I look healthy and appear to be just like everyone else. I have chosen to work hard, to recover, and to regain the best quality of life that I can. My bout with cancer is barely noticeable now. People are shocked to hear that I have had brain cancer, not once, but twice.

Those around me often get the impression that I am strong and independent, and not at all the way they think that I should be. In other people's eyes, a person who has had brain cancer twice is not supposed to look this good, be this strong, be this happy, or have such a positive attitude. I had to become more organized and more creative to compensate for my slowness in the beginning. For example, when I was first recovering from the cancer and trying to become more independent, part of my routine was getting my breakfast ready without any assistance. Because preparing and then eating breakfast was very tiring, I had to prepare breakfast the night before.

People make assumptions. If you cannot walk very well, you must not be able to dance. I can dance anyone under the table. I weaned myself from the walker to the four-pronged cane, to a regular cane, and then, no cane. The no-cane part was the hardest. Why? Well, when you have a crutch or assistance, other people realize that you are disabled. While you are training yourself to become more independent by walking without assistance, and look wobbly or off balance, people either ask if you are okay, or think you have been boozing like a drunken sailor.

I don't really envy others. Before my days of cancer, I was a single mother who worked full-time, performed singing and dancing in community theater, played tennis, and climbed steps two at a time. Even though I cannot do what I did before because of my limitations, I have had many successes and accomplishments.

What has helped me the most, in my recovery from surgery and in maintaining my good health, is doing mild aerobics. For two years, I've been using

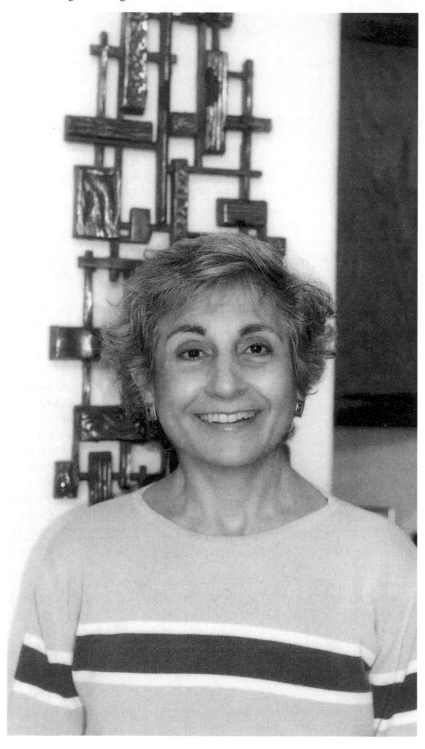

an upscale "soft bounce" mini-trampoline with a bar. I just take off my shoes and socks and dance or jump for joy. I started with small bounces, and even sat on it and gently bounced. Eventually I worked up to grander movements. I use it in conjunction with weights and yoga. This combination of activities has been my lifeline back to good health.

I know it is hard to believe, but having had cancer has been a gift and a continuing blessing for me. I am a successful human being because I have accomplished so much with my strong resolve and a determined step, literally and figuratively. I am a person who has faced seemingly impossible odds. I have always had peace because of my faith in God, which continues to grow every day. The battle is His and not mine. I just turn all of my burdens over to Him. Living with these challenges has strengthened my faith in God, to "lean unto him" and not my own understanding. Exercise, diet, helping others, and doing random acts of kindness all have helped me beat my illness, not once, but twice. I don't ask why this happened to me. I have no answer. I don't try to analyze or kick myself. I think of this as another chapter in my life. It can be a better and more exciting chapter than before. Birds fly; I cannot, so I don't even try. But I can strive to be the best person possible by maintaining a positive attitude.

A person who has had brain cancer twice is not supposed to look this good.

Having a concealed condition definitely impacted my social life. Participating in activities with partners is difficult. Dancing is fine, but things that require more coordination and movement are out. No tennis, volleyball, jogging, hiking in the woods or unsettled ground for me. It is difficult to go to baseball games or theater because there are no railings to hang onto for balance. Heck, going down steps without a railing requires that I go down on my butt! How sweet would that look on a first date? I am also unable to wear shoes with a heel of any height. Since getting sick, my friendships have increased in breadth and depth. However, few men want to be with a woman who has had brain cancer, especially twice— unless he is extraordinary or very lonely. Cancer is scary. "What if she gets it again?" they must think. On the other hand, there are men who might know my condition and admire and respect me for my courage and fortitude. If a man is concerned that I will become sick again, and he will have to take care of me, better think again, because I will probably be taking care of him.

My primary care doctor suggested I keep a journal to improve my fine motor coordination. My neuro-oncologist, even before diagnosis of the second cancer, reported that I was likely the longest survivor of brain lymphoma in the United States. I am hoping to be an inspiration, not only to cancer patients and their families, but also to those who feel they are facing seemingly impossible odds with any concealed illness or condition.

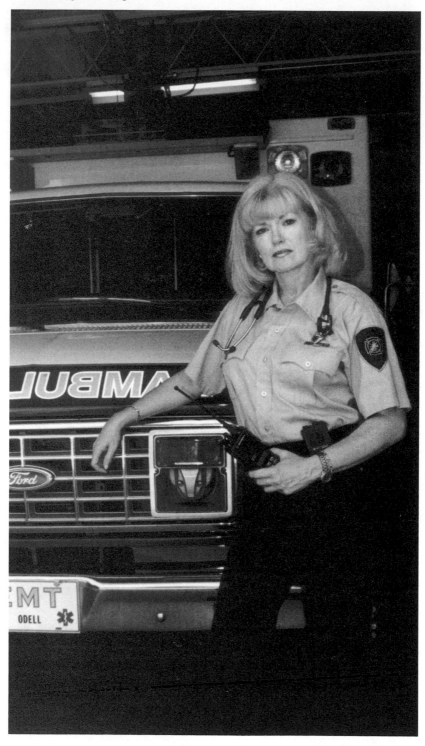

Jaye B., Nurse, Community Volunteer

Interstitial Cystitis, Crohn's Disease, Irritable Bowel Syndrome

It is difficult for me to remember how it was to be healthy. When someone tells me that they can work all day and then are able to go out in the evening, I marvel at how they can do all that. I forget for a moment that this is how healthy people live. Hearing about their successes and accomplishments is difficult, even though I am not a jealous person by nature.

I believe certain things happen to people for a reason; we have lessons to be learned. As a nurse, I saw the human condition from all sides. But the intensity of my compassion went way up after becoming sick with my own illness.

It is difficult for me to remember how it was to be healthy.

The adjustments I've had to make because of this illness are many. They include: gauging energy expenditures and deciding what is important and what can wait until later, deciding which places I can feel comfortable going to (such as those with bathroom facilities), deciding whom I feel comfortable riding in a car with, making work adjustments such as fewer hours or reduced duty, worrying about being in public and having a mind-altering pain session—the sort that doubles you over, limiting my traveling and, making wise food choices. I have to be very careful about each meal and what I ingest every day.

I do not want sympathy at all. If I looked disabled, I think that people would have a tendency to pity me. I prefer quiet understanding and acknowledgment. My true friends give me that. They know when I am putting on an act and when I really do not feel well.

I put on makeup every day, do my hair, get dressed nicely, and even do a small workout routine. This is the therapy I give to myself. It's my own form of positive thinking, because I approach the day with my personal best. I don't let myself lounge around in my pajamas on the couch, even though it is deliciously tempting.

Chronically ill people have enormous adaptive skills. I know I could be an award winning actress on many days. I'm playing the part of being just fine while inside I am reeling in pain, or mentally hunting down the next restroom. Looking normal has great social benefits, but doesn't tell the whole story.

The uncertainty of my life and the route it might take in the future bothers me a great deal at certain times. It is as though I am not in control, the disease is, and I do not want it to win. So, I try very hard to take care of myself. If some negative disease progression comes about, I can honestly say that I did nothing to cause it.

Food selections and restaurant choices have to be made with the disease in mind. The amount of energy I can expend has to be chosen with the disease in mind. Medications have to be taken for the disease. You can well imagine the effort it takes to manage this disease on a daily basis.

I can never forget this disease, even for a moment, which makes me sound as though I am obsessing and thinking negatively, but I am not. I just have to make choices every single day based on my symptoms.

Crohn's disease can be painful, and the medication I take can leave me fatigued. Since I am not able to work right now, I am a volunteer emergency medical technician in my community. There are so many people out there that need help. I am the first responder to the scene of car accidents, heart attacks, and other emergency calls.

I began volunteering after reading an article in the newspaper. The free clinic provides care and medicine to 600 patients and prescriptions to another 480 on Medicare. I feel there's a major need in this county for this type of agency. This place where I'm volunteering could grow like crazy if we had the ways and means to let it. If you have talent and training in a field, it's important to give something back to the community.

Jill V., Licensed Acupuncturist

Chronic Fatigue Immune Dysfunction Syndrome

The advantage of having an illness that is not easy to see is that people do not look at you differently. The disadvantage is that they do not look at you differently. They expect you to be able to do what they are doing. It is a double-edged sword.

Other people just don't understand, or they forget you are ill, because you look fine. People remember the old me, and that's who they see, even if I am challenged with an array of symptoms. In fact, I am still more active when I am sick than most well people are who are not sick at all. At one time, I went to a physician who told me that I didn't have chronic fatigue syndrome because I had too much energy!

The advantage of having a concealed illness is that I can work and socialize without having to answer questions from others. If it were apparent that something was wrong, I would have to deal with people's curiosity. This way, I am able to keep it private. The disadvantage is when I try to share my experience of being ill with others, they really do not understand. It is frustrating if I say to someone, "I am so tired," and they say back, "Yeah, I'm really tired, too." There is just no way to explain the depth of my fatigue.

This illness is like waves in the ocean, because it is always moving in a cycle. After six years, I have a good sense of the cycle. I start to feel better, get excited, feel that I should take advantage of feeling better and get things done, do too much, crash, get scared and panic that I'll never get better, let everything go and rest, start getting better, and the cycle begins all over again.

I've only recently learned the concept that, instead of trying to get a lot done while feeling well, I need to temper that phase so that I don't crash. This is so hard to do because it's so exciting to feel good. I have asked friends and family to let me know when they see me in my higher functioning phase where I am doing too much. Their feedback really helps. This is one reason I would really like to be in a support group. I have been through a lot of challenges in my life, like most people, and I'm a strong person. I have the confidence to know that I can handle a lot of different situations, but at times this illness has really brought me to my knees. I've had moments of total hopelessness and that is definitely the scariest experience of all.

Since becoming ill, I find that large groups of people, and being around all of that noise and energy, wears me out. Therefore, I make choices based these limitations. I avoid certain people and situations that I know will be too draining. I have had to give up most of my social life. I no longer go to crowded

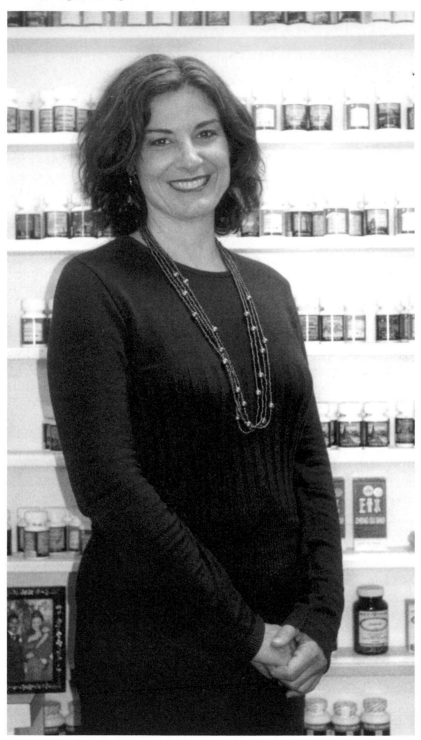

gatherings, such as street fairs, concerts, or malls, because the overstimulation wears me out. I don't drive very far anymore because freeway driving stresses me out so much that I get panic attacks. I cannot take all the classes I would like to, which is difficult since I love to learn new things. I haven't been able to read since this all began because I have trouble concentrating. I love all kinds of music, which has always been a refuge for me. However, for the past four years I have not been able to listen to music because it too is overstimulating. As I have gotten healthier, I am again able to listen to music.

It is so difficult when people invite me places and want to get together. Explaining the whole situation over and over again is very difficult. I've finally learned how to just say, no thank you, and not feel guilty. I still cannot believe that I can feel so ill, as if I am dying, but I look just fine. This has been the scariest time of my life, especially because of the few real answers I seem to have about this illness. What causes it? Why are there no effective treatments? How do I live with something that makes me feel so ill, but allows me to appear perfectly fit? I understand why so many people who have this disease give up hope.

Because I still keep on my happy mask, I get very tired around other people.

When I see people going to the gym, or to exercise on bicycles and treadmills, I often want to say to them, "You don't know how lucky you are!" Sometimes, when I see a jogger running along the coast, I just cry. Just having a normal social life, where I can go out for dinner after work, seems so far away from my current reality. I don't have difficulty hearing about other people's successes, but at times I can get into a pity place and feel sorry for myself.

What has helped me the most in dealing with this condition, is surrendering to it instead of fighting it. I plan my days carefully now. I don't return every phone call. I take naps. This is all new for me. I hate to say no to anybody or anything. I have had to learn all over again how to take care of myself, such as going to bed when tired and not running around all the time. Once upon a time, I hated to cancel planned activities for fear I'd appear flaky. All this has changed. I realize now that I have only a certain amount of energy and I have to be very picky about where I spend it. Like the waves in the ocean, I must continue to surrender to my illness again and again. Only when I surrender do I find peace. This realization is very important.

I have been able to turn the self-pity into appreciation of what my illness has brought to me. I am truly grateful for the lessons and opportunities I have gained from having this illness. It would be so much easier if my illness were visible, but I have been able to fake my way through my work-life because I appear fine. In that regard, I am glad that my illness doesn't show.

I have always been trained to be a good girl and to make sure that everyone around me is comfortable. I automatically put on a happy mask without even thinking about it. After awhile, this leads me to emotional and physical exhaustion. I still do this, but I try not to control every situation any longer. Because I still keep on my happy mask, I get very tired around other people. That, of course, is one of the reasons no one can believe I am sick, because I appear so happy all the time. I just can't seem to let myself be down or negative around most people. I wish I could be more genuine and stop taking care of everyone's feelings. This is something I am working on very hard, because it is just so exhausting and is hampering my recovery.

Many things have helped me throughout my healing process: journaling, doing gentle yoga, leaving open spaces in my schedule everyday, canceling things at the last minute if I am not up to doing them, surrendering to my illness and accepting the limitations it brings, embracing the chances I now have for creativity, and finding new skills and passions.

The only things I've done that have made a noticeable change in my symptoms are short yoga classes (so I don't become too tired). The yoga helps me feel balanced all over, and I feel I have better circulation and oxygenation. I am more peaceful and less stressed. I also used intravenous hydrogen peroxide (administered by a Western medical physician), which made a huge difference in my energy level. Eliminating all gluten from my diet has also made a positive difference as well.

I practice daily gratitude. I thank this crazy illness that has grabbed my attention and changed my life and my awareness in so many ways. This is not always easy, especially when I'm in a flare-up. Somewhere inside I am aware that there is meaning in this illness, as long as I am willing to uncover it.

David Y., Retired Teacher

Raynaud's Syndrome, Fibromyalgia, Prostatitis

I am a fifty-nine year-old retired teacher and coach who happens to live with fibromyalgia. I taught and coached for thirty-three years. I am an avid long-distance runner and have completed five marathons. My most pain-free times are on a natural endorphin high that can last as long as six to eight hours after running. I still run but not as much. My condition won't allow me to be as active as I was in the past. When I overdo, I have long periods of severe pain, periods of chronic fatigue, and sleepless nights, but I refuse to allow these symptoms to stop my enjoyment of running. I usually run with a group. This has become a social occasion that I feel is necessary. I have found interaction with others is essential. When I retired, my fibromyalgia pain and other symptoms increased and my socialization decreased. I know the guidelines for fibromyalgia say mild exercise and stretching, but my ego, and the sense of well being that I get from running are more important to me than following the guidelines. I suffer the consequences. On the positive side, I have the blood pressure and heart rate of a teenager. On the negative side, I have to take a number of medications.

I first knew something was not right in my life in my early thirties when I began to feel the symptoms of what I later learned was fibromyalgia. Around the same time, I also developed prostatitis, an inflammatory condition of the prostate gland, which also became chronic.

As a teacher in the classroom, I usually was so busy that I was able to block out almost all symptoms except when I sat for lengthy periods and then arose to move about. I would find myself having difficulty getting into motion because of stiffness and pain. Coaching became a more challenging matter. It hurt to stand for any period of time on the basketball court and I would have to warm up for each demonstration. I could run and play ball with my junior high athletes; the pain would come later. I coached basketball for twenty-five years, but when I started running, I became a cross-country and track coach and trained with my athletes. I lived with the pain and tendonitis. The pain in my forties was not as severe and I had periods when it waned.

Living with Raynaud's syndrome requires a few adjustments in my life. Whenever I run, I wear gloves. I dress warmly beyond what many would do for outdoor activities in the winter and spring. I am extremely sensitive to cold water. If I am sprayed by cold water or get into it, the water feels like an electrical shock! (I swear, if I ever have a heart attack, it will be due to the shock of cold water.) I try not to do activities that require standing or sitting

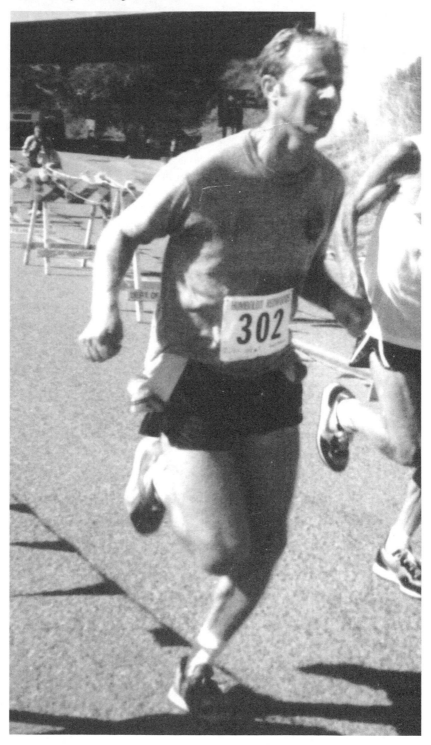

for long periods of time, although I do not let it stop me from going to football games two or three times a year.

Pain produces depression over time. I try to live without antidepressants but do better with ones that will let me sleep. Pain management is the key for me. Some mornings it takes me several hours to control the pain with medication so I can function. I often wake up in the night in pain. One fibromyalgia patient described it as having a bear on her back. I describe it as compression pain. I take a pain pill an hour before I run. I have one in the morning and one before bed at night. I find it best to control the pain before it controls me. Sometimes I take less medicine. Occasionally I need more. (Headaches, neck pain, backaches, and leg pain—no part of my body seems exempt from fibromyalgia pain.) I get involuntary spasms, and loud noises make me jump. A light touch can make me spasm. Sacral-cranial therapy has relieved some symptoms and offers me relaxation. I have a physical therapist that treats me, and I find it useful. I have a low tolerance to pain, and my pain is almost always present. I know others have felt self-conscious of this condition, but my doctors and family have understood and we talked about the nature of fibromyalgia. My extensive reading has also helped me understand the nature of these disorders that I live with. The condition has been discussed in the medical news, so my friends and associates are usually aware of it. I tell people who do not know or understand what fibromyalgia is, that I have a form of soft tissue arthritis that produces tendonitis and muscle pain that is not deforming.

When I overdo I have severe pain, fatigue, and sleepless nights, but I refuse to allow it to stop my joy of running!

Because I have stayed so active in my life, most people might not have even noticed that I have any disorders or physical challenges at all. My challenge has been to stay active. I even periodically lift weights to maintain muscle tone and strength. My theory is to stay as fit as possible so there is less pain from normal activities. Being strong makes dealing with the symptoms of fibromyalgia easier. Fibromyalgia has affected my life. I can't do what I would like because the energy is not present. Travel is painful. It has affected my married life. It affects intimacy. I do not see my grandchildren as often as I would like, nor do the things with them I would like to. I lack patience when I am hurting and dread certain household maintenance tasks. I am not angry about having this condition because being angry is wasted energy.

I am fortunate that I have an understanding wife and adult children who are supportive. I do not make an issue of my conditions with others. I explain when necessary. I listen to others and read extensively about fibromyalgia. Generally, I have always been an optimist and do not dwell on the past. The present and planning for the future are more important concerns.

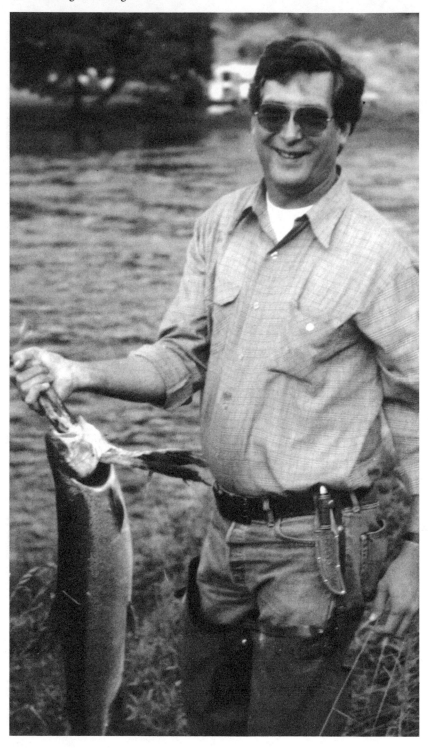

Don E., Sales Representative

Rheumatoid Arthritis, Diabetes

People I meet simply don't understand why I can't go fishing or hiking, or even stroll around with them. They can't seem to comprehend that I even have trouble crossing a street. If I have to hurry, I could easily fall down and do more damage. I sometimes use a cane at home but can't seem to be able to use it in public yet. I happen to love classical piano music. And when I am playing, I seem to be in a different world. No problems; no worries; no thoughts of symptoms or illness or anything other than beautiful sounds. And for many years, I loved getting out on some river and fishing for steelhead trout. All of these things calmed me, even if they didn't calm my symptoms.

I am frustrated when my symptoms worsen. It is difficult to make people understand these challenges.

My chronic conditions hit me very hard. Maybe not so much now, as I have learned to live with them, but when I was first diagnosed and began having severe episodes of pain and weakness. I thought all was lost. When first diagnosed, I lived in the country. There was certainly a lot to do. I had been very athletic all my life and had no problem keeping up with all that had to be done. All that caretaking and working the land was actually fun for me. But, all of a sudden, I couldn't do some of the things that I had to do because the symptoms came on so quickly. At one time I was told that I might be in a wheelchair by the time I was forty-five. But, thanks to good medical care, that never happened. I beat the odds.

I become more irritable and frustrated when my symptoms worsen. It is very difficult to make others understand these challenges, and strangers don't believe my pain is real because I appear to be quite healthy. We all have our limitations, and even though we know, other people just don't get it. I would certainly love to be able to do some of the things that I used to do, like going fishing on beautiful streams. But, I simply can't trust my legs to get me through this activity. I would certainly not be able to ask a dedicated fisherman to take me along. That would not be fair to him, as I might not be able to keep up.

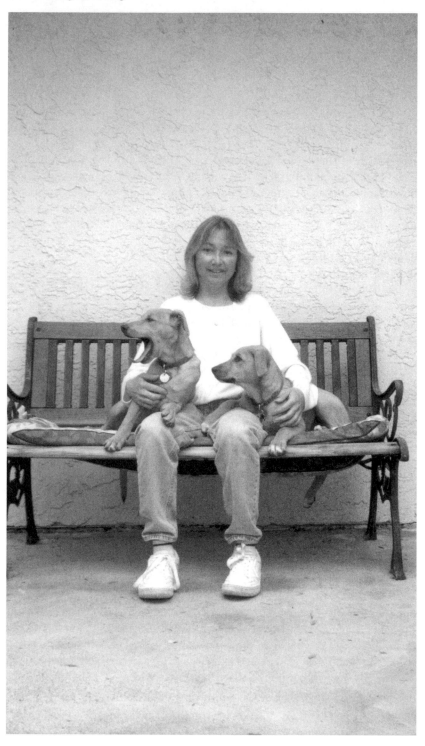

Sue T., Medical Worker

Nephropathy, Ulcerative Colitis

I have lived with these diseases a long time and will not allow them to stop me from feeling confident about my capabilities. Five years ago, I felt as though I couldn't be who I wanted to be because I had this disease. I had only one child. About the time I thought about having another child, I was already on many medications. I didn't feel I should expose an unborn child to my regime of serious medications.

I have had to slow down the pace of my life. I have to conserve energy for the times when I need it rather than do many of the things I would like to do. I also changed my career path. I was diagnosed with ulcerative colitis about the time I wanted to go back to school. I needed time to get this disease under control. At that juncture of my life, the medical field intrigued me, so I went into the field of medical administration. Working in an office suits my energy level, but mentally I am extremely bored. After three years of watching my disease progress and trying every medication available for treatment, I am doing okay again, at least for the time being.

If someone can't understand this illness or doesn't want to, that's their problem, not mine. I'm not ashamed anymore.

People tend to help out more when they can visibly see that a person needs help or is at a disadvantage. With my particular concealed illness, no one can tell or see that something is wrong. I'm treated as normal no matter what my circumstances may be, even if I'm grimacing from the pain. No one has ever questioned my illness. My family has been very supportive. Other people tend to change the subject very quickly. They do not ask questions, nor do they really want to hear much about it.

I don't envy the achievements of other people. I am always happy when I hear someone is doing well for themselves. I do feel a bit sad inside, however, and even a little sorry for myself, because my path and life has been difficult. Had I been healthy, I would have gone further in life a little sooner, and with greater confidence. I am not envious, just sad. I secure most periods of peace by always finding the positive aspect in things. For example, working with doctors has gotten me over my fear of them. After working in a hospital setting, my fear of medications and procedures has faded quite a bit. There are so many people, even children, who are so sick and much worse than I am.

We recently adopted a couple of collie dogs. They need so much attention, care, and love, that my mind is preoccupied with thoughts about them. I don't think about my disease half as much now that I have them wrapped around my ankles. My energy level is up because of this. Happy thoughts make me go on longer and much further than depressing thoughts.

I do not want sympathy from anyone, nor do I want people to feel sorry for me. Sometimes I just need a little understanding from those close to me when my system is down. I want to be normal and appear normal in every way that I can.

What has helped me is planning and looking forward to fun events, such as going to school again or going on a vacation. Anything that makes me look forward to the future is a diversion from my symptoms. Sometimes when I am sick and taking all kinds of medications, the end always seems near, and that can be very depressing. But, I refuse to give up.

I try to stay as healthy as possible. I eat properly and am very conscious of my weight, being the steroid-user-for-life that I am. I would probably be healthier than most people around me who take their health for granted, if it weren't for all the medications I am on. The only scary part of this concealed illness is that some of the medications have a negative impact on my overall health. I appear healthy and can blend in rather well. I do tend to go to bed early, but I do not hide this new routine from anyone. I do not hide or pretend in front of anyone any longer. If someone cannot understand this illness or doesn't want to, that's their problem, not mine. I needed nine years to get to this point. I am not ashamed anymore. Life is too short to be living it for others.

The biggest disadvantage and the hardest thing I have trouble coping with is health insurance. What if I lose my job? Getting insurance privately would cost me an arm and a leg. I cannot work any place I want to or for anyone I want. I must work for a large business that will insure me with my preexisting condition. I cannot hop around in jobs or try things out that I might enjoy because of my issue with insurance. I often feel stuck in a rut because of this. This is the one thing that can bring my mood down the most. It is truly discouraging. Having a concealed illness has been the biggest challenge I have had to face in my life. In some ways, it has made me stronger, but in many ways it has left me sad. If given a choice of being in the world this way or not at all, I would choose to stay and make the best of things, which is what I do. It does not seem fair, but I will not give up. I am not a quitter, never have been, and never will be. Knowing that I am not alone helps. There are so many people out there having hard times, too. I suppose overcoming obstacles is what life is all about.

Hope M., Office Manager

Chronic Back Pain, Scoliosis

People tend to have less compassion for people who have an illness where the symptoms are less visible or obvious. It is harder for people to conceptualize your pain when they cannot see it. Out of sight, out of mind. However, pain is still pain.

Throughout my life, I have made many compromises and adjustments to compensate for my chronic pain. For instance, although my personality tends to be more adventurous, daring and carefree, I will often take extra precautions and be concerned and protective about the way I approach certain activities. I have to always be aware of my energy level. It fluctuates so much that I must honor the times that I just cannot keep up the same pace.

The most common comment people make to me is, "Wow! You look so happy and your body looks so strong and healthy that I would never have imagined you are in chronic pain." I maintain my life by keeping a positive outlook on life and trying not to let the little things bring me down. I do not allow myself to become a victim, and I always make time to be aware of my limits and honor the way my body is feeling. This is not always easy to do, however. It takes a lot of attention and focus on my part.

This is my body, my life, and my karma. For some reason that I don't fully understand yet, this is what I have been given to deal with. I must learn some difficult lessons in this life. What is behind these lessons has not yet been revealed, but I truly believe that we all have the ability to heal ourselves. The more aware I become of my body, the more I am capable of trusting in this process.

The only time envy rears its head is when I go through periods where I am trying so hard to get better or to shift my pain level. If the results of my efforts are too subtle, or things don't shift at all, I become discouraged and resentful.

When people share their success stories with me during those times, and as much as I want to be happy for them, I find myself feeling discouraged. I do not feel like or want to be a victim, but I do think to myself, "Why can't that be me?"

Since others do not easily detect my condition, people don't have to feel sorry for me or be burdened with catering to my special needs. That's a good thing. I don't have to deal with people continually asking me about my condition, since it is not apparent. I like to have the freedom to choose whom I share it with.

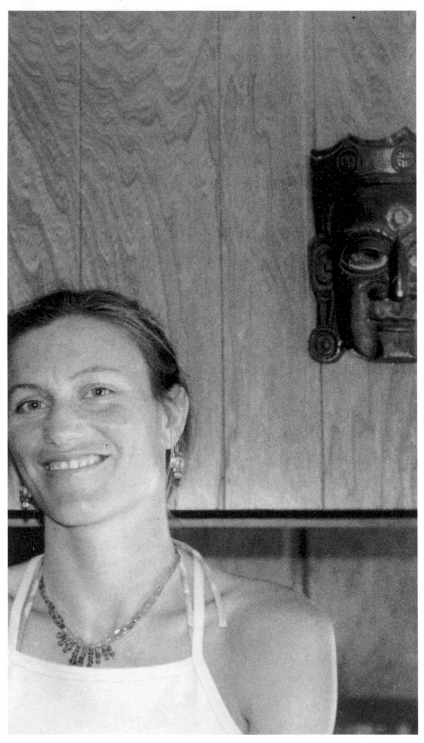

I think that it would be extremely challenging for me if my condition were more obvious, because I would often feel self-conscious and concerned about being judged or talked about.

At times, I become frustrated with people because they tend to forget my limitations and expect me to be this superwoman that they see. They perceive a physically strong person in front of them and think I am perfectly capable of doing anything they can do, even though this is not true.

I have benefited from practices such as tai chi, which is a form of moving meditation. Chiropractors have often been able to help relieve acute pain from my spine, and acupuncture has also been useful for relieving acute pain on a short-term basis.

Massage therapy allows me to be present in my body, which is not often easy when you are in chronic pain. It also allows me to truly feel my emotions and not be as afraid of them.

Chronic pain leaves me restricted in all aspects of my life. I might have been a totally different person than I am if I did not have this condition. My natural personality tends to be optimistic, outspoken, open-minded, positive, caring, loyal and loving towards all types of people. However, I am not sure that I would still have those same qualities if I had not had this physical condition. A large part of who I am has been influenced by my pain.

Part of who I am has been influenced by my pain.

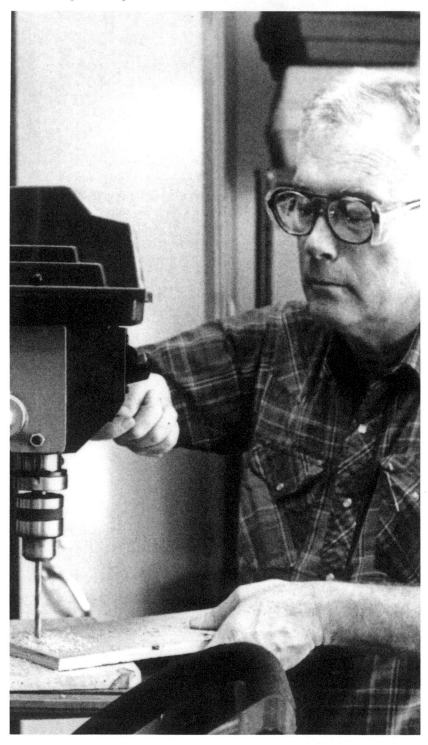

Dave K., School Teacher, Engineer

Crohn's Disease

Living with a concealed illness is definitely different than having a physical problem that others can actually see. Most people assume that if I look normal, then I am. Many people cannot accept an illness that they cannot see. One of the ways that I have coped with this is to make friends with people who understand the problems of having a concealed illness.

I have learned about my own physical limitations and have learned to live within them. I plan what I will do around those limitations. For instance, I need more sleep than most people, so I just go to bed earlier. I also do not plan strenuous physical activities or too many different activities for any one day.

No matter how sick I have been, I have accomplished the goals that meant the most to me.

My disease can be extremely painful at times, with severe cramping that may last for several hours. Several doctors diagnosed my disease as "all in my head" early on, and told me that I had too much stress in my life. "You have to learn to calm down and relax," they said. In order to help me relax, they prescribed various tranquilizers (which are really depressants).

I took these tranquilizes for a long period of time—not because I wanted to, but because I believed they would help me relax and be free of the constant and severe pain I was in. What I didn't realize was that I was already depressed and the tranquilizers were making me even more depressed.

After experiencing constant pain for ten years and becoming tired of fighting with the doctors on this issue, I stopped seeking medical treatment. A psychologist friend told me about the good results some of his patients had received from a hypnotherapist. He explained that the hypnotherapy would be a palliative, not a cure, for my pain.

After my first hypnotherapy session, I felt much more relaxed and much happier. By the sixth session, I had learned to control the spasm in my intestines. Whenever the pain became severe, I would hypnotize myself and cause my intestines to relax, significantly decreasing the pain.

I now use the art of self-hypnosis for many different problems. It can help me fall asleep faster, stop worrying, relax, and generally feel better. I have since met many people who successfully use self-hypnosis.

I do not envy others who have good health. For one thing, I know that many of the supposedly great and successful people have problems that are much worse than mine. I have had much success in the endeavors that are important to me, such as taking good care of my family. Many of the most successful people have had to neglect their families, which can adversely affect children. Seeing my children happy means more to me than job success, power, or material goods.

No matter how sick I have been, I have accomplished the goals that meant the most to me. In addition, I have learned to live each day for that day alone, and to live life to the fullest. I let tomorrow take care of itself.

I concentrate on my accomplishments, rather than on what might have been, or "if only. . ." thoughts. I have never worried about what others might think. I am myself. Others have to accept me as I am or they can find another friend.

The major advantage of having a concealed chronic illness is that people do not give me a lot of sympathy or ask questions because they do not know about, and cannot detect, the illness. I am very lucky in that my job and my friends have allowed me to be myself.

I was able to take early retirement from my former job as an engineer and take up a totally different field (teaching), so I am getting a whole new set of experiences at this time in my life.

Perhaps I would not have taken a more fulfilling road if it had not been for this concealed chronic illness. I truly appreciate and enjoy my life now.

Diane P., Prison Facility Social Worker

Type I Diabetes

Having and living with this concealed illness is like living with anything that one feels the need to hide. It can be emotionally draining to have to keep something secret and not be able to share it with others. I used more energy to hide my illness than to bring it out into the open. Of course, this process of coming out with my illness has taken many years. The process has been gradual, but in the end, quite rewarding. Why some of us should take so long to accept our disease is a mystery, but some of the less brave souls just need more time to feel comfortable with being different. I have found that the more comfortable I am with my disease, the more comfortable others become.

I would like to live without diabetes, but the sad fact is that I do live with it. Consequently, I have been forced into living an extremely healthy lifestyle or suffer the consequences. I have always wanted to be part of the group and to be as strong and sure of my health as the next person. What I do to reconcile not being as healthy as they are, is to overcompensate. I out-walk, out-run, out-play, out-life everyone.

All my life I have felt ashamed of having this disease. Yes, I realize that this disease is not my fault and is nothing I should be ashamed of. I know that intellectually, but emotionally I have trouble accepting that I have limitations. I know that I could always be worse off, but I still have challenges to meet in living with this particular disease, even if it is hidden from view. My struggles may be silent and invisible to the world around me, but they are still very real and, at times, quite challenging.

In some ways, having a hidden disorder is more difficult than living with one that is obvious. For example, I can pass as "normal" with Type I diabetes until a problem surfaces. The worst of these problems is an insulin reaction. During one of those episodes I appear drunk and demented, which blows the lid off any semblance of normalcy that I'm trying to present. The difficulty and embarrassment are compounded because those around me don't know why I'm acting in this manner. If I looked diabetic, that is, like someone who could have a reaction at any time, then the public would be prepared to deal with this bizarre behavior from someone who looks normal.

I have lived with Type I diabetes most of my life. When first diagnosed, adjustments ran contrary to my lifestyle as an eight-year-old tomboy, wanting to play dodge ball, hide-and-seek, and baseball without having to stop the game, go into the house to test my urine, and eat a snack if my blood sugar was low. This was torturous, especially if my team was winning.

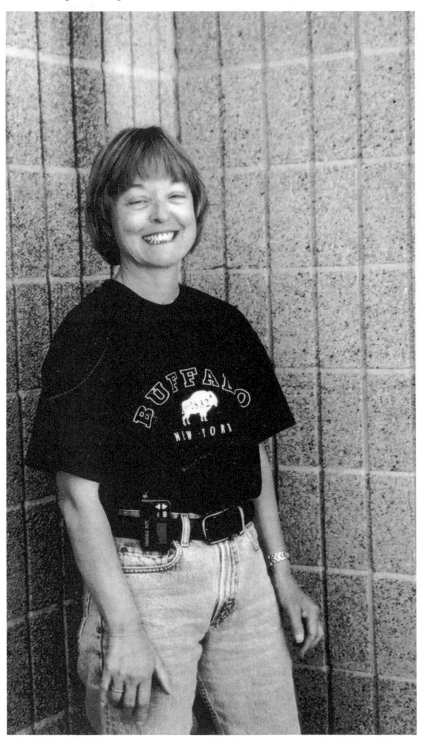

Most of the people in my life are familiar with diabetes and its symptoms. After five, ten, even twenty years, diabetics experience what is called hypoglycemia unawareness, which to me is a cruel joke. Not only are you having a reaction, but you also don't know you're having a reaction and can't do anything to stop it. After the profuse sweating, comes the confusion, and the inability to string even two sentences together that make sense. In the past, when someone would try to pull me out of a reaction, I'd come out fighting. People personalize it, but it is truly part of the disease and the blood sugar level. This can be quite alarming for casual onlookers and quite embarrassing for me. This has happened more often than I care to remember. People will generally be supportive and not ask questions. I'm sure they must wonder what's happening and what they can do to help. I prefer that they ask me about this than not ask.

I envy people who don't have to worry on a daily basis about their mortality, whether they will wake up the next morning, or whether they will die in their sleep from a hypoglycemic episode. What helps me stay afloat is supportive friends who understand the illness and what to do in case of hypoglycemia. I am also helped by my sidekick, an insulin pump, which does its best to keep my blood sugars stable. I keep my blood sugars in check by eating at regular times and testing my blood sugar often to ward off the demon attacks.

I have found that the more comfortable I am with my disease, the more comfortable others become.

The advantage of a concealed disease is that I can blend in with the crowd. The only disadvantage I can see is the element of surprise for onlookers if something should go wrong, such as having an insulin reaction. You've heard that song, "I can do anything you can do. . . " I've always lived my life as if I could do anything anyone else could do, and I have. I refuse to let a disease get in the way of my doing anything I want to do. In all honesty, diabetes has not held me back from living my life to the best of my ability. I am active, still healthy, and so far I have not developed any life threatening complications. I plan to stay that way.

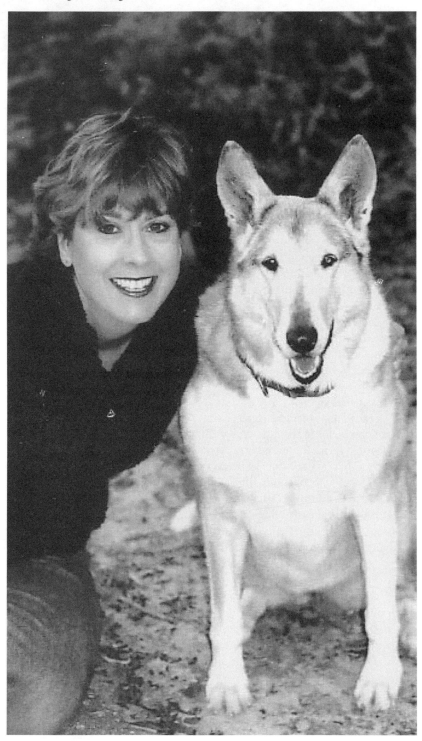

Marianne R., Legal Office Administrator

Crohn's Disease

People have questioned some aspects of my disease, because they do not understand how it can be so debilitating. Since I appear so healthy, diarrhea doesn't seem to be such an awful thing to them. They don't understand the constant urgency and frequency concerns I have with my bowels. They don't understand the mental anguish of knowing I will be on medication for the rest of my life.

I envy everyone who can eat whatever they want. I hear my fellow coworkers chatting away about what they have for lunch (onion rings!), and it is only a distant memory for me. I know better than to eat those kinds of foods with my diseased colon. I envy them their youth, health, and vitality, and their sheer joy in eating whatever they want to.

If necessary, I can live with this condition for the rest of my life utilizing the coping measures I've learned along the way.

I always need to know beforehand exactly where each and every bathroom is, as well as how long it will take to get to a destination while traveling. I need to plan what to eat or not eat before taking a trip. I need to pack my own food, stock up on enough medications, and make sure my insurance is accessible wherever I may be going.

I've also learned to not throw away any clothing. I discovered a while ago that my weight could seesaw a good twenty pounds in each direction with this illness. During a flare-up, I have to wear my big clothes! Then, when I'm losing weight after coming off of steroids, I wear my "small clothes." I always try to wear a bit of make-up during my sick days, if only to have some color on my face.

I started going to a support group with great trepidation at first, but quickly realized what a great source of knowledge, comfort, and friendship it provided. Others were going through, or had already been through, what I was experiencing with this illness. We not only shared information on the illness, but more importantly, we shared our feelings surrounding the illness. What were our daily obstacles? How did we cope with them? We laughed about it, and sometimes we cried about it.

I was so grateful to be able to talk with those who have lived with this disease longer than I had, and could tell me how to make peace with it. They didn't just tell me how to cope, but they showed me how to cope by merely being a living example of strength and determination. I learned that passing along my good spirits and positive attitude to others could help, especially those who were newly diagnosed.

I wish I didn't have this illness. I know that Crohn's disease is 15%-30% genetic, but so far, I'm the only one in my family of four siblings to be diagnosed. I wish someone else had it so I could talk to him or her about it. Just having this condition is one thing, but then there are all the secondary symptoms of which I have to be cognizant. I recently had the skin eruption called pyroderma gangranosum, which was just another reminder that there is something wrong with me and that there is a flaw within my body. I think I'm coming along, doing fine, dealing with my life and then, BAM! Something happens to remind me that I'm not really whole.

I try to remember that I have a life-altering illness, but not a life-threatening one. If necessary, I can live with this condition for the rest of my life using the coping measures I've learned along the way.

I'm the sort of person who can continue to cope as long as there's hope on the horizon. I follow all the medical research and breakthroughs with great interest because therein lies the cure, and the sooner I can get it, the sooner I can get back to onion rings.

Lynda P., Mixed-Media Artist

Obstructed Airway, Chronic Enteritis

Since I have had to deal with both evident and concealed health challenges in my life, I feel extremely qualified to comment on the differences of living with one over the other. The two situations carry wide variance in how I am perceived. My evident condition has always been part of my life. My voice is always soft, and my speech is quite raspy at all times, because of damage caused to my vocal chords. The damage was caused at an early age, so I cannot recall a time without it. Luckily, I was raised in such a way that I just tried harder in everything that I tried to do. People would stare at me when they noticed the vocal problem. That is dreadful for anyone, but particularly tough on a youngster. Luckily, my parents had given me the message that I should just keep on keeping on no matter what, so that's what I did. I loved school, but was often absent due to illness, so I spent a lot of time making up schoolwork. Yet I look back and perceive myself as being very fortunate. I always felt extremely loved and valued by my parents, and that can get a young person through a lot of very tough situations.

The multiple damaging surgeries on my vocal chords are my worst memory associated with childhood. They left me with scars and additional problems, such as difficulty with speech, that made my situation more evident to others. In spite of this, I graduated from high school with honors and from my college's honorary society. I also found gainful employment and became self-supporting. My health remained quite challenging, so my work record had gaps, but I still kept moving forward. Then in midlife, I faced the challenge of a concealed chronic illness. The diagnosis of chronic enteritis took a couple of years to confirm and I suffered a great deal in the meantime. I have never been a complainer. Family and friends were very supportive. But since the medical profession wasn't being helpful, it was very difficult. I still managed to keep working by taking short periods of disability.

I cannot quite figure out what caused the long delays in obtaining a proper diagnosis from the medical process. But I know this happens quite often with diseases of the colon, as they are a bit tricky to diagnose. I just had to find the right doctor, and when I did, he was able to diagnose me moments after meeting me. I kept trying to work, but I finally went part-time, and am now on total and permanent medical disability. In looking back, I realize that I tried too hard for too long. Maybe that is because our society doesn't want us to give up or acknowledge our limitations if we have them.

When my secondary illness came along, it forced me to go on a very

249

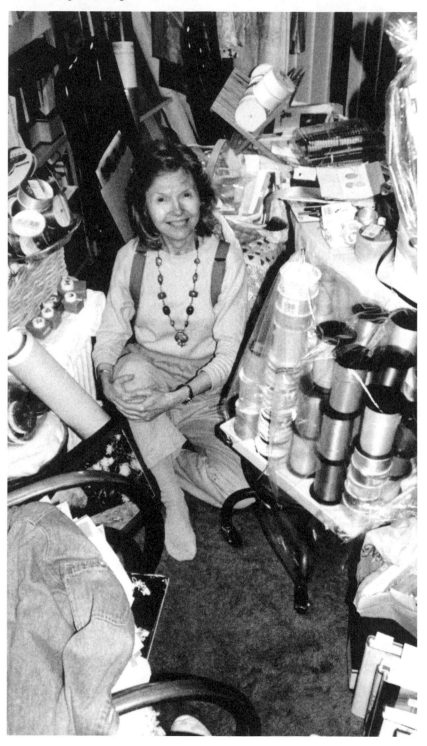

restricted diet. That was quite a challenge in this food-is-fun society. I had people wonder if I was eating correctly after the chronic illness appeared. I suspect we are all guilty to some degree of wondering if a person is doing all that they possibly can to rectify their situation. I certainly have turned into an expert on self-help measures. I wish I could eat like other people. Someone once asked me, "If you could have a day without your chronic illness what you would do?" That's easy. Eat. I would have a pork tenderloin sandwich, malted milk, and a piece of cake. Yeah!

I turned to alternative medicine when Western medicine was so slow in diagnosing and treating my chronic illness. I was at a crisis level with fissures, extreme weight loss, and severe pain. In desperation, I sought out an acupuncturist for the first time in my life. I'm so glad I did. The acupuncturist made an immediate and accurate diagnosis. I was told that I might need ten to twelve treatments to control the ghastly pain, but within three treatments, my comfort level had improved dramatically. He also prescribed herbs and eventually recommended a carefully tailored macrobiotic diet. After awhile, I did locate a medical doctor who also diagnosed my illness (using invasive tests, as opposed to the acupuncturist's noninvasive diagnostic methods), and he put me on medication for a one-year period. Several years have passed since that time. I remain on the diet, and by doing so, I am able to control my symptoms. I no longer require medication, herbs, or treatments

I may have five challenges, but I have five billion blessings, and isn't that a great ratio?

of any sort. I studied and practice the Alexander Technique for its known help with chronic pain. I recently began a serious study of qigong, which is a form of moving meditation. I continue with my Transcendental Meditation practice, which I have been doing for thirty years.

Staying connected with my loved ones has helped me. I am blessed with great family and friends. I give most of my limited energy to them and of course, get it back tenfold. I have kept very current on self-help approaches to better health. If something doesn't work, I'll try something else. I do believe we can help ourselves a great deal. Exploring my creativity is also a source of healing and joy. Since I cannot totally disguise my challenges, I do have to deal with some reactions to my situation. I present a happy exterior, so I believe people are sometimes perplexed and taken aback when they realize the depth of my challenges. The bottom-line is, I try to gauge my energy output, but I often fail. My illness is part of my life. I deal with it one day at a time, one hour at a time, and one minute at a time.

I have kept a gratitude journal for over five years. I can always easily think of at least five things that I'm grateful for to write about at the end of the day. I may have five challenges, but I have five billion blessings, and isn't that a great ratio?

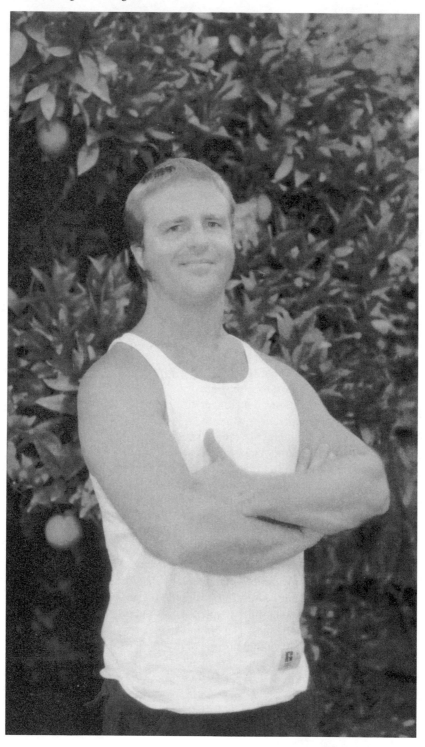

Ken L., Musician

Narcolepsy, Chronic Pain

Most people have questioned the existence of my pain. The doctors swear they can help me when I first come to see them, but quickly become frustrated if I don't respond to their treatments, or if they can't seem to make the pain vanish. Then they suggest that it is all in my head or that I am holding onto my pain. Doctors do not take their patients with hidden illnesses seriously, or believe there is a problem at all. Also, people with a concealed chronic illness are not able to obtain Social Security disability insurance or other financial assistance very easily. You have to do battle, but who has the strength when you're in pain or feeling ill?

I accept that I cannot keep up with my peers, and I don't try to any longer.

I had to give up a lot of things in my life because of this illness and its symptoms. I had to quit my last job, and I still cannot work. I can't sit for extended periods of time, or drive for very long. I can't lift weights, mountain bike, do karate, or even surf the Internet. I cannot read for more than twenty minutes at a time because downward positioning of my neck causes great pain. I cannot type or use a computer. I even had to move back in with my parents at the age of twenty-nine in order to survive financially. I wish I could be financially successful. I accept that I cannot keep up with my peers and I don't try to any longer.

They only reason I would want to appear disabled and not have a concealed illness would be to finally gain some financial assistance for my medical problems, and to achieve some independence. The things that have helped me to cope with my symptoms and pain include the Buddhist teachings. The belief that this is not forever has helped me hold on to hope for the future. Maybe someday I will find some relief.

There are no advantages to having this illness except for the fact that I look okay. There are many disadvantages, but the main one for me is feeling like a baby and a burden. Having this illness has made me realize how good I used to have it. I just try to cope day-by-day. I can honestly say that if my mother were not alive now, I would have it much tougher and would most likely have suicidal thoughts. Heck, I didn't go to college for a decade to be in this position of helplessness and pain.

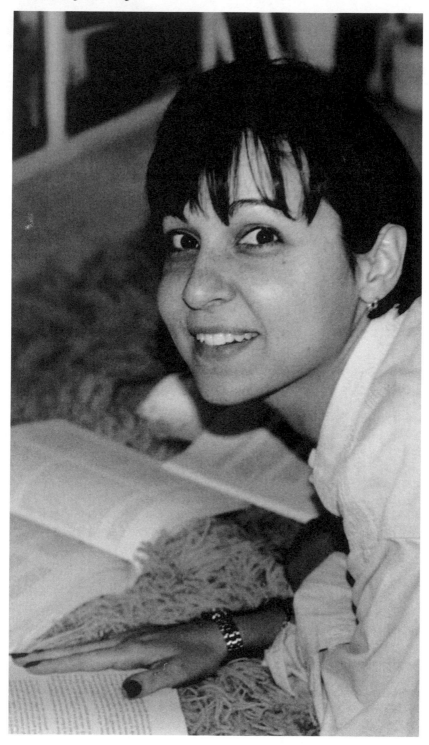

Nancy T., Clinical Psychologist

Crohn's Disease

Other people have always minimized my symptoms. For example, they might say, "You just need to watch your stress level." They do not appreciate the impact this illness can have on my daily life.

Having a concealed illness certainly requires more explanation to others. I am likely to be questioned or scrutinized when asking for special accommodations, or turning down invitations. My own adjustments have included reduced work hours and income, dietary changes, travel limitations, and increased expenditures for doctors and prescriptions.

The danger is in going beyond my limits and feeling worse as a result.

I envy others who are well, and I envy their boundless energy, although perhaps they are faking it, just like me. I envy their health and the apparent ease with which they can do things. I always want to remind them to be grateful for their health and to take good care of it. Good health is such a gift. Unfortunately, many of us learn that lesson only after we become ill. I have always been an extraordinarily healthy person. Having a concealed chronic illness is a new challenge for me.

My spirituality, my faith, and my husband have helped me the most in dealing with this illness. I'm glad this illness is concealed and not visible. People make hasty decisions based on physical appearance. I wouldn't want to be labeled or stereotyped because of my looks. A concealed illness affords a certain level of privacy. The illness is not out there for all to see. Not everyone has to know, only the people I choose to tell.

I have used acupuncture to help me deal with some of my pain, which helped a lot. My night sweats and fatigue from the blood loss went away after such treatments. I've also done amma therapy, a non-needle way of stimulating acupuncture points through the use of massage instead of needles. However, when I get a bad flare-up, the only thing that seems to put a stop to it is medication.

What has helped me to cope is keeping a journal, attending support groups, prayer, relaxation, and hobbies. I have discovered that I'm stronger than I ever thought. Sometimes, I try to appear better than I feel. The motto: fake-it-until-you-make-it has been useful to me. The danger is in going beyond my limits and feeling worse as a result of overextending myself.

There are ups and downs with this illness. Not knowing from one day to the next how I will feel is very frustrating. Many of my routine activities require extra planning and effort. Some things are just not as easy as they used to be. Having this illness has been limiting and often makes me feel out of control. It has been my greatest challenge. Never a day passes that I do not think about it on some level.

Many times, the mental aspects of coping with the illness are harder than the physical aspects. Most days, I cope just by putting one foot in front of the other, thinking positively, and honoring my limits. What is the alternative?

I'm still the same person I was prior to my diagnosis. I still have a life to live and contributions to make to society, to my family, and to my own career. I still have a child to raise and a household to run. I have my career and so much more to be thankful for.

I could easily turn sour because of these new challenges my illness has put in my path. But, I will do everything in my power to remain optimistic and as strong as I can possibly be.

Pete M., Retail Store Manager

Rheumatoid Arthritis

I do not want friends, employees, or associates to know about my illness. The fact that my family knows I have it is enough. I am forty-years-old, and I see many people getting overweight, out of shape, becoming less active, and giving up on their bodies.

It makes me angry to see them doing harm to themselves, but I say nothing. If they knew what a gift a healthy body is they wouldn't take it for granted, as so many people do.

Because of my illness, I never know if today will be the last day I am able to walk, swim, or ride a bike, so I am in a hurry to live each day the best I can.

I want to walk, swim, ride, and be active every day. I do not want to look back and find I wasted my last chance to take a walk. I cannot rest today for I may not get a tomorrow.

As much as I desire to be a consistently positive person, I find my illness wears me down. I refuse to give in to the pain, I refuse to give in to the illness, but there are days when I am exhausted and in excruciating pain. I try not to show it. I find strength in my commitment to be a father to my two sons, ages eleven and fourteen.

I push myself to be a positive example for them. I was told several years ago I could take a disability retirement, but how can I teach my sons to be proud workers, strong men and leaders if their father doesn't work?

The desire to be a good father helps me overcome my symptoms. My love for them helps me ignore any level of pain. I sometimes wonder what reason I will find to push myself past the pain when my sons are grown men.

As my sons grow up and move from elementary school to middle and high school, they develop new circles of friends. As we connect with many of the parents and develop new friendships, I find myself in the dilemma of what to tell and how honest to be. I find that waiting is best. I do not want to reveal, even to the closest of my new friends, the illness that I have.

People's responses have ranged from shock, dismay, and disbelief to sympathy and feeling sorry for me. I don't want any of these. I would rather they do not know, so I fake it even when I feel terrible. Otherwise, the conversation becomes an hour-long talk about how I got this as a youth, what caused it, how bad is it now, when did I get my hip replacement,

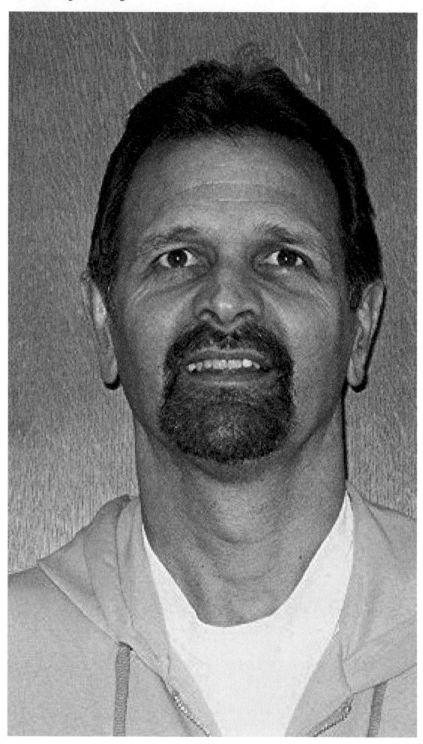

when did I get my shoulder replacement, and on and on. I know they mean well but I don't like to relive it, so I would rather not talk about it.

I find it very frustrating to not have control over my own body. No matter how well I take care of myself, or how disciplined I am, this illness just isn't going away.

Worse than that, I sometimes get angry at my body and my God for this sickness. I have found my faith in God to ebb and flow over the years as my illness flares up or goes into a remission.

I chose to disconnect from my battered and broken body. I chose to feel nothing. It is the only way I can go on.

I can work, I can live, I can exercise, I can hide, I can conceal, but I cannot admit my pain.

This is my cross, but I will bear it.

How can I teach my sons to be strong men if their father doesn't work?

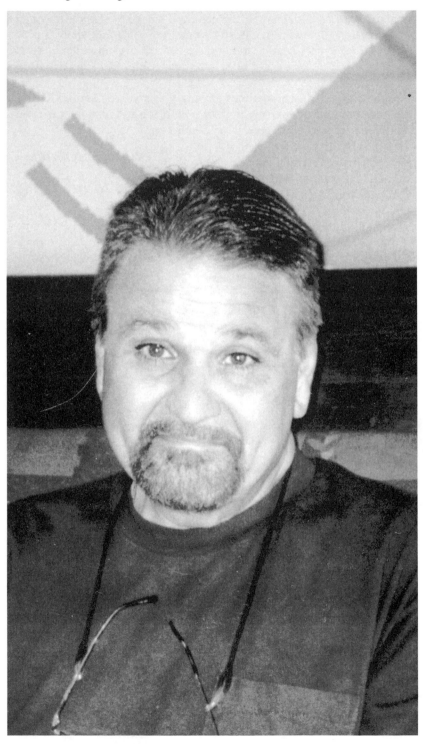

Gene C., Former Boat Dealership Manager

Chronic Atypical Pain, Depression

When I pull into a handicapped parking space, hang my placard and exit the car, it's not unusual to get some rude stares from the people around me. I can tell they are trying to figure out what's wrong with me because I appear as healthy as they do. Some of them seem angry at me, as if I owe them an explanation. Little do they know that I have fallen six times since the initial accident that caused my injury, and that I've been hospitalized twice for this injury. I find myself getting angry in response to their rude stares, and then I feel upset for the rest of the day. Sometimes I give them what they want—a good limp. If you park in a handicapped parking spot, you are expected to appear handicapped. To appear healthy is offensive to some.

If you park in a handicapped parking spot, you are expected to appear handicapped.

I believe that at birth, each of us is given a basic set of tools to help us deal with what life presents us. As we grow, we master the tools we have, we establish favorite tools, and we acquire more. Just like a master technician, the more tools one has, the more one can accomplish. However, sometimes we are confronted with new situations that cause us to use every tool in our tool box to no avail. We are forced to give up or find a new tool to use in our struggle to survive.

In my case, that new situation happened to be severe pain resulting from a work-related injury. As a high school and college athlete engaged in football, wrestling, and boxing, I learned to deal with pain. I played these games in an injured condition more often than not. I grew up in a rough neighborhood where physical strength and a few good punches were the name of the game. I thought I had developed a high threshold for pain, but at age fifty-one, I faced pain more powerful and debilitating than I had previously experienced. It was a pain so constant and unbearable that I felt hopelessly defeated, even after using every tool I had. Medication certainly helped, but not enough. Acupuncture was useful, but not enough. The pain, now accompanied by emotional turmoil and depression, was simply too potent. I am now worried that my doctor has used every tool available to him as well.

I started to refer to my newfound friends as Mister P (for pain) and Mister D (for depression). Mister P found his way into my face, my arm, and hand. He's highly skilled at what he does. He can deliver pain in several areas simultaneously and he wasn't going to let me forget it. Mr. P knows I'm very vulnerable in the morning since that's about the time my pain medication is wearing off. He does some of his best work between 8 A.M. and 10 A.M.

As I started to sense I was at the end of my rope, my doctor informed me of a new program that he thought we should try. It was as if the tool truck had just pulled up to offer the latest that science and technology had to offer, but this wasn't the case. The new tool was a stress reduction program that had been used for thousands of years—meditation and yoga—but with an added dimension; a heavy emphasis on mindfulness or mindful living. Adding these tools to my tool box and learning how and when to use them has renewed my hopes that the pain I have may be manageable. Now, when the pain awakens me in the morning, I take my medication. Instead of leaving my powerful rival Mister P to have his way with me, I frequently meditate during this period. It sort of creates a smoke screen on the battlefield and takes the edge off Mister P's morning assault. As I master the use of these powerful methods, I have reason to believe my situation can only improve.

Living with chronic pain is a full-time job. All of the tools I learned in sports have served me well with this latest episode in my life. Some of the things that caused my pain so many years ago in my wrestling and football days have given me the tools I need to survive my pain today. I have learned to face my fears just as I faced my fears on the football field. Am I the guy who is going to be defeated in this game of life? No! Do I have fear about the future? Of course. What will I feel like two weeks from now? What about six months from now? Will I still be in pain?

I've had a lot of time to think. I had to recuperate from surgery to my spine and lay in the hospital in a cast for weeks. I had to learn to rely on other people. The nurses, and even my mother, had to take care of me. She changed my diapers when I was a baby, and here she was taking care of her fifty-one-year-old baby! I learned to be humble in a new and profound way. Anxiety, depression, and crying fits will leave any man humble. Luckily, mindfulness meditation tools have given me new confidence and comfort with my pain and depression.

Terry H., University Academic Counselor

Ulcerative Colitis

Having a hidden disability is so different from having one that is visible. Not better, not worse—just different.

People often do not know that I am dealing with any health issues until I choose to tell them. I am not faced with inaccurate assumptions that might accompany a more visible disability such as employers inaccurately assessing my ability to work, or even assumptions that people might make during the course of everyday life. On the other hand, people often assume that I am healthy and pain-free. They might not understand these health issues that are very real.

With inflammatory bowel disease, I never feel completely well and likely never will again. At the very least, I feel as though I have the flu because my immune system is constantly fighting. Most days I am in pain. I don't act sick, but I always feel sick. People don't really know what it's like for me, the limitations it has created in my life, how I have a hard time pulling myself away from fun activities, conversations, and intimacy. to get the rest I need, and how it affects my overall health. They don't see all the emotions that I feel about being ill. They don't know about my experiences with doctors, my expectations about life and my health issues, the essential pain of losing one's health and facing pain and limitations, and the conflict between what I need and what my body needs. There are times when this causes me to be less cheerful and patient with others. Though I do not let pain and fatigue stop me from getting out and doing many things, it does send me to bed earlier. I stay well rested so that I do not get run down. No more burning the candle at both ends.

Drinking alcohol is very much out of the picture, not that I would overindulge anyway, but I don't have the choice anymore. Since I almost starved to death when I was seriously ill, I decided to put on forty extra pounds of "insurance fat" once I got well. As a result, I now have to deal with other people's issues with weight. People make a lot of assumptions about weight, health, and heavy people. Often they are incorrect.

Another adjustment that I've had to make is to increase the planning of activities and to decide whether or not I'm up to certain actions. For example, I really want to take a six-day saddle-pack trip to Yosemite National Park this summer. In the past, I would have just made the reservation and set out on an adventure. Now I have to make sure I can make the trip without risks to my health, and I have to put some special arrangements in place. Will I be able to

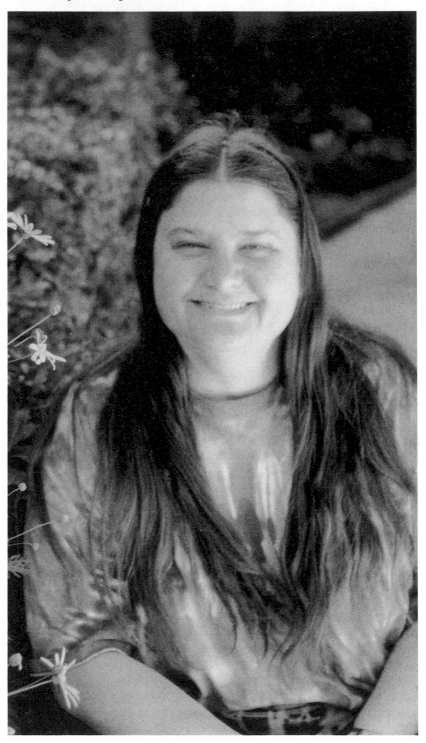

stop as often as I need to? What will I do if I'm miles from the comforts of the nearest restroom? How can I provide for the possibility that I might have an accident?

I also have to make sure that I drink plenty of water, as I get dehydrated very easily. Strenuous physical activity on a hot day could be potentially dangerous. I have to be careful. Will I get the extra water that I need? Will it be too hot for me to be out in the sun all day? Who wants to deal with this sort of anxiety and worry on a trip? Not me.

I seem to have less believability with doctors now because I have a big fat medical file. Before getting this illness, I was an exceedingly healthy person. I had hardly been sick a day in my life. Therefore, my doctors seemed to believe what I said. Now that I have a thick medical chart and an impressive group of symptoms, doctors seem more likely to scrutinize what I say. They seem to think I'm making these symptoms up. I do not know if some doctor somewhere put a note in my file, or if just the sheer size of my file makes doctors doubt me more now, but I have seen a definite change. I have even thought of finding new doctors and not giving them my medical history, just so that I can start from scratch again without prejudgment or prejudice. However, with my belly full of scars, doctors always want to see my records. Some doctors who are not experts in inflammatory bowel disease do not understand that there are symptoms that go beyond the bowels. Joint pain, skin problems, and other extra manifestations are all part of this illness. Still, my doctors sometimes question these additional symptoms.

I may not have 100% of the life I once had, but I live with passion and enjoy 100% of what I have left.

I remember one incident when I was very ill and only able to do a couple of hours of activity each day. I stayed in bed all day so that I could attend and help at a group meeting. After helping for only an hour, I was so exhausted that I could hardly stand. I excused myself early. On the way out, I walked into the restroom feeling drained and ill. I caught sight of myself in the mirror. I looked positively robust, healthy, and full of energy. I couldn't believe that I could look so vigorous and yet be unable to support my own weight. I thought to myself, "How can I expect anyone to believe me when I look this healthy? Can't I at least look a little tired?"

I am more apt to envy the healthy person that I once was rather than the good health of others. Even after years of being less healthy than I once was, I still compare my current stamina with what I used to have. My previous healthy self is like a dear friend that I have lost and still grieve for. I envy the people who live pain-free with normal bowel habits. They truly do not know how lucky they are.

Life is awesomely good and I have learned to float. You see, life is like a river. Swimming upstream does not work; I've tried it. I get knocked down if I try to stand still in the current. I become bruised if I try to cling to the rocks. Even swimming downstream is too much work. Lifting up my feet, letting go and floating is easy, fun, and gets me to where I'm going.

Most importantly, I have called upon the physical and emotional support of people that I love when I am feeling ill or depressed. I asked for help when I needed it. I use natural childbirth breathing, as well as a self-hypnosis relaxation technique, to float through periods of pain.

I won't pretend any differently—I hate being sick. I hate being in pain. I hate being tired. But I am. It is not going to change much. I may not have 100% of the life I once had, but I live with passion and enjoy 100% of what I have left.

Marie Z., Registered Nurse, Gourmet Cook

Multiple Sclerosis, Lupus

Most people in our society seem to feel more comfortable with visible evidence of an illness or disability. They have a problem envisioning what they cannot readily see. There is a trust component to accept what they are hearing, rather than what they are seeing. A visible illness is easier to accept simply because visible evidence is harder to doubt.

I have had to give up my professional nursing career of twenty-five years and modify my activities to meet my decreased energy level. I had to learn to reset priorities. Housecleaning is now proportional to my energy level. I do not like to see the messy result of letting things go but that has become a reality for me. I used to maintain everything at home and at work so effortlessly. Now, I am learning to let go of the need for cleanliness and control.

The biggest adjustment I've had to make took place three years ago. I lost my driver's license privileges because of seizure activity, and that resulted in a complete loss of independence. I have regained my license at the present time, but live in constant fear that I may deteriorate neurologically and be unable to drive in the future. I now allow my husband to shop for me and perform the tasks I was easily able to manage prior to my illness.

I have to write down important messages and communications, as I routinely forget details and cannot recall conversations I have had. This has resulted in appointment glitches on many occasions. Many financial adjustments have had to be made since I lost my ability to work and earn a salary.

I try to appear normal and in good health to blend in with others. I try very hard to apply makeup when I go out in public and try not to show fatigue. I try not to sit down at times, even when I feel I need to, so as not to draw attention to my symptoms and myself. I will sometimes try to lift or move things just to show I can, but I usually end up paying later. I feel the need to always prove that I can still do it. I have not found an effective way of eliminating the need to prove myself all the time, but I wish that I could.

I have many friends who still enjoy nursing careers, and I wish I could return to my career; but, I am beginning to accept the loss of that part of my life. In my home care management position, I was involved in many quality control aspects of healthcare delivery. Ironically, I am now experiencing, first hand, the difficulties with unprofessional, poor quality healthcare.

I envy the friends who can take vacations to Europe and other destinations, as I cannot tolerate long plane rides and cannot be too far away from my healthcare support system. I constantly remind myself that there are many

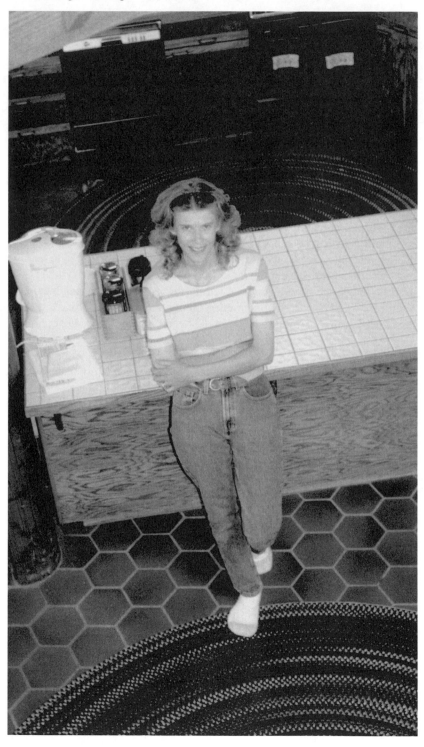

people in the world in much worse condition than I am. I try to remember all of the supportive friends I have. I know someone who is severely disabled and endures her own disability with such grace and determination that she is a constant inspiration to me. I also try to remember that even though my priorities have changed, I can still experience great joy by spending time with my cats, sitting quietly on my deck, and having time to keep in touch with my friends. These become all the more important since I am faced with a lifestyle loss and adjustments.

I wish people would believe me when I tell them about this illness. I wish they would be open to educating themselves about my illness process. Instead of worrying about others and their opinions, I try to focus on what I can accomplish versus what I cannot. I've always enjoyed cooking and baking. Instead of trying to prepare and present a large dinner party now, I occasionally bake something for my husband's coworkers. I've learned to scale down my hobbies, but I still enjoy them.

My close friends are very understanding, so I try hard to nurture those relationships. I also try to ignore the ignorant attitudes and remarks of those who do not choose to understand or accept my illness. My true friends take into account my limitations and sometimes are more realistic than I am. They make sure I am taking it easy.

I was devastated when originally diagnosed, but also relieved.

The advantage of having my illness concealed is that I can deny the illness to people to whom I do not want to disclose it. The disadvantages are receiving reactions from people who think I am lazy, attention seeking, or complaining; feeling guilty about having my illness in the wake of negative reactions from others; and my own difficulty with accepting the limitations caused by my illness.

I was devastated when originally diagnosed, but also relieved. I had experienced vague collagen vascular symptoms for seventeen years prior to my lupus diagnosis. I experienced unexplained infections, meningitis, and fatigue without a proper diagnosis. I was in denial about any possibility of serious illness. Approximately ten years ago, I came home from making home health visits and was experiencing numbness in my feet. I quickly discounted this sensation as just being on my feet too much. The next day the numbness had ascended to my ankles and I surmised, "I must be looking for a psychosomatic way to get out of seeing so many patients." After getting out of bed on the third morning, I fell, and the numbness was up to my waist level. I finally admitted to myself that what I passed off as being psychosomatic, was neurological in nature. By the time I could get to a doctor and was admitted to the hospital, I could not walk. I was terrified that the paralysis would become permanent; but, at the same time, I felt vindicated in a sense that now I knew what had been developing for seventeen years. My rheumatologist verified that the lupus had probably developed years earlier. I will always wonder if I had gone to astute healthcare practitioners when my symptoms started years ago, would my symptoms have been recognized instead of being discounted as just "female problems."

My lupus has destroyed or severely limited many aspects of my life, but has also clarified important priorities such as family, friends, and letting go of things over which I have no control. My neurological symptoms are the most devastating symptoms I have now. My neuroleptic medication suppresses neuropathic pain, but in turn it suppresses all nerve response. My sensory status has been severely decreased since 1993, and I have found that very difficult to deal with. At present, I have not found an effective way to improve this, but I do continue to look for ways to deal with the problem.

I try to contain my frustration as much as possible and try to focus on others. This gives me more pleasure and gives me back the feeling of fulfillment that I lost when I left my career. I am constantly looking for other ways to feel like I am a worthwhile person once again.

Marsha S., Quilter, Image Consultant

Hepatitis C, Migraines, Ocular Rosacea, Fibromyalgia

I often try to appear as if I have the energy of my old self, as if I am dealing with no health or fatigue problems. Sometimes my symptoms worsen when I try to do this, and other times I stretch myself a little too far. I end up being worse off by trying to do what everyone else is doing.

People tend to not take a concealed illness seriously. They think a migraine is just a headache, so what is the big deal? They think that fibromyalgia is just the "disease du jour" even though I was diagnosed about fifteen years ago.

People do not understand that because of my illness, being in the sun is something I cannot do. Sometimes I cannot go places if I have to be in the sun for any length of time.

I have had to move into my own bedroom so that I can get more sleep. I also have to rest more often during the day. I always have to be sure to carry migraine medication with me in case of a headache. I feel so fortunate that there are effective migraine medications on the market today. Sometimes, I think about my poor grandmother who did not have these medications for her migraines, and I feel bad complaining about mine.

People tend not to believe that these are real illnesses. Sometimes they act like I am being a wimp or party pooper when I say I cannot do something.

While I do envy the energy of some people, in no way do I mind hearing about their successes or accomplishments. I'm truly happy for them. I just wish I could do some of the things they are able to do.

I have a friend with fibromyalgia and one who has migraines. Being able to talk to them and share information helps me. Just knowing that there is someone out there who understands is a big help.

I simply wish that other people would not judge me and would be more understanding. Being sympathetic is difficult for people who have not experienced anything like this. In this case, the walk-a-mile-in-my-shoes adage is true.

Going to a fibromyalgia support group helps to validate what I am going through. I feel that I am better off than those with serious illnesses or life-threatening ones. I think to myself, this too shall pass, when I get a bad migraine or have some difficult fibromyalgia symptoms.

I have so many different symptoms that every day it seems there is something else wrong. I have very few days when I am symptom free. If I

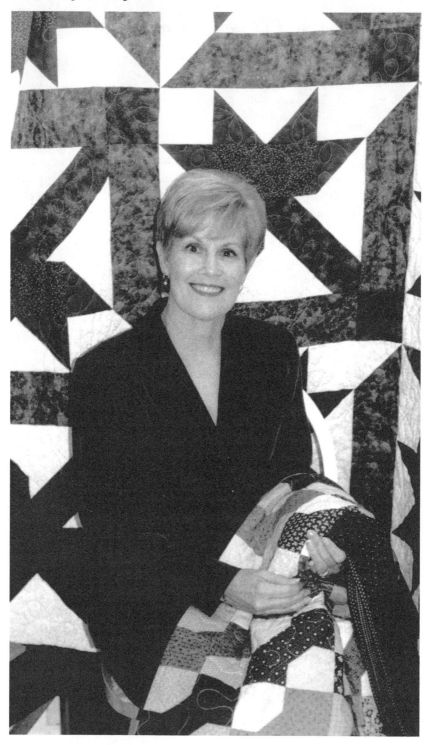

don't have a migraine, then my fibromyalgia is making me hurt, or I am simply fatigued, or my ocular rosacea is acting up and my eye is driving me crazy.

If I'm outside in the sun for any length of time, I burn and swell up and become fatigued. I feel like such a burden sometimes, because I have so many things going on simultaneously.

Sometimes I cope pretty well, and other times I get very upset. Recently, our little four-year-old grandson was visiting us, and my husband had to take him hiking by himself because I was simply too tired to go with them.

While I love having him visit, there are times when I don't feel I can cope with the visit. These sorts of limitations bother me the most.

When friends invite us out, sometimes I have to decline because of all my problems. This is difficult. I'm afraid they will think we do not want to go and we're making up an excuse to get out of it.

I try to cope with my illness on a day-by-day basis.

Sometimes I cope well and other times, I'm sorry to say, I do not.

I stretch myself too far and end up being worse off.

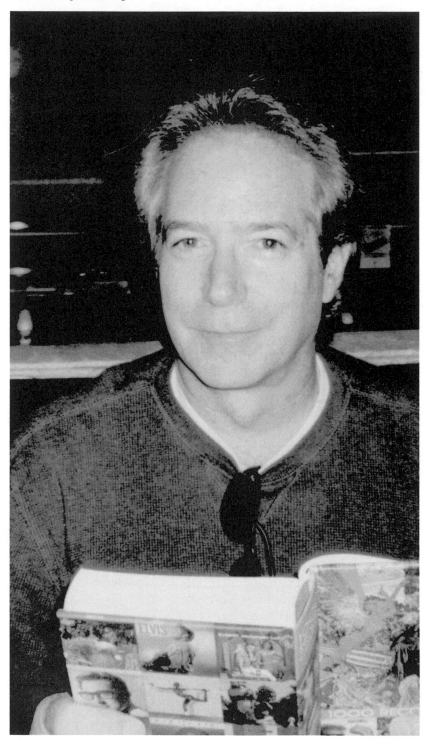

Michael N., Product Developer, Musician

Cluster Headaches, Migraines, Epstein-Barr Syndrome

I often try to appear healthy and problem free, even when I'm experiencing a migraine or other symptoms. This has been an issue, both consciously and subconsciously, throughout my life.

I've had serious migraines since I was a child. At that time, doctors attributed it to allergies, but I discovered later that was not the case. My cluster headaches have been with me for decades. I never know when they will strike or how long they will last. It's the unpredictable nature of these headaches that makes them so difficult to deal with.

I constantly felt off-balance and vulnerable in my life. I was like a boxer waiting for a punch, but not knowing when it would hit.

My life goes on, but I try hard not to let anyone see my pain or weakness. That's getting harder and harder to do. For example, a couple of years ago I was under extreme pressure and stress at work. I started having intense migraines on a daily basis. This continued for twenty days straight, but I continued to go to work and accomplish my daily tasks and job responsibilities. Finally, after nearly three weeks of intense daily pain, I couldn't hold up the facade of feeling fine any longer. After seeing the state I was in, my doctor sent me directly to the hospital and insisted that I be admitted.

In the past, some people have questioned the severity of my symptoms. That has always been an issue for me, but it happens less frequently now because the general public seems more informed and aware of this malady and how incapacitating these headaches can be.

At times, I envy other people's good health. They are not suffering from debilitating migraines that can strike at any time with extreme severity. They don't know what this is truly like. This leaves me hyper-aware of other people's freedom from such ongoing pain. I have to admit, I feel a little jealous of that freedom. In the beginning, and because of not knowing when it would strike or what was setting it off, I constantly felt off balance and vulnerable in my life. I was like a boxer waiting for a punch but not knowing when it would hit.

I recently was diagnosed with Epstein-Barr syndrome, which helped to explain why I'm constantly battling fatigue. I'm a very intense and active person by nature, and have a hyper-personality. Therefore, for the past ten years, I could not understand why I was experiencing this unwanted sluggishness that seemed so unlike me and the way I used to be. Not knowing what it was made me feel my spiritual and emotional life was to blame for this weariness.

I was very depressed for a long time because of this listlessness in my body. Once my doctor diagnosed me with Epstein-Barr, I had a name for what ailed me, and this helped me cope a little better. There's no remedy or cure for Epstein-Barr, and very little is known about it, but at least I now have a name for what has been dragging me down and making me feel so low in energy.

Mark E., Sales Manager

Crohn's Disease, Ileostomy

Although my disease and symptoms have been relatively quiet for many years, scars from surgeries and an ileostomy serve as a reminder of the challenges I faced.

The scars are a reminder of the pain, and the ileostomy serves as a milestone of when things started to turn positive for me. For it was only after the ileostomy that the pain started to subside.

My scars and ileostomy are visible, but I don't see them or think of them anymore. I think of myself as a normal healthy human. I have never asked my wife of twenty-five years if my body, that was once so perfect, is a turnoff to her. I can't change it and I don't want to know. Still, I've had to make, and continue to make, adjustments because of the ileostomy.

Activities that are normally associated with not wearing a shirt cause me to think about and see my ostomy. I don't want people to know about my prosthesis. So, if urged to go swimming, I wear a dark tee shirt and claim I want to limit the amount of sun my body receives.

I love massages, but wear gym shorts I can pull up to cover my pouch. Working out at a gym and then using the public showers is something I can't bring myself to do. Other adjustments have also been made. When sleeping in a strange bed, controlling what and when I eat becomes a priority, as I don't want to have an accident from a full bag during the night.

When making a presentation to a group, or sitting on a long flight, I may not be able to get to a bathroom at a specific time. So once again, I limit my intake to help limit the output. I also request aisle seating so as not to impose on those around me.

I have to make a lot of small adjustments, and I often think about how great it would be not to worry about all those things. Still, without the ostomy, I was in pain and couldn't lead a normal life. The trade-off was, and is, well worth it.

I don't associate the disease with who I am. A disease is like a job; a job isn't who I am, but what I do. Similarly, a disease is not who I am, but a challenge in my life.

When my disease was very active and the doctors couldn't seem to help ease the symptoms, I tried self-hypnosis. It was an interesting experience. At first I was hopeful. I was so desperate; I would have tried most anything. I normally would not have tried hypnosis if it had not been for my disease.

277

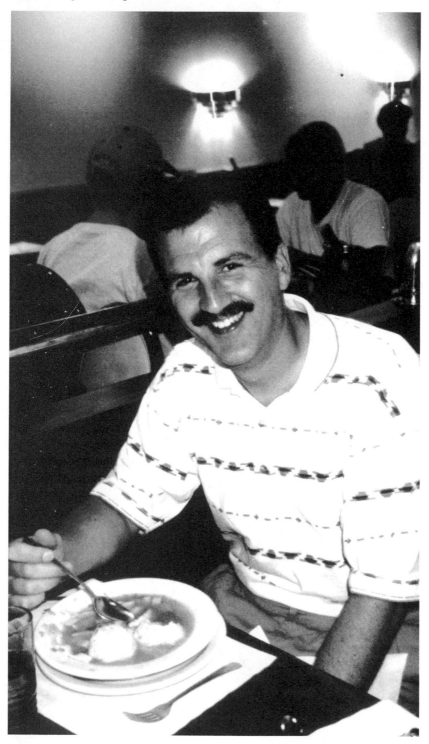

I had always wondered how people could be pulled into certain scams or off-the-wall treatments for getting better (not that this was one of them). There I was, grasping for anything that might cure me. It was something I could try with little risk.

I don't think I envy other people. That's not the right word. I think everyone wants to be disease-free and live a life that doesn't require adjustments.

During some of the adjustment times, such as the ones I already mentioned, I sometimes think about those who are fortunate enough to lead normal lives. Wouldn't it be great?

But there is so much I don't know about their lives. Plus, what does the future hold for them? And are these thoughts of being in their shoes even possible? No.

So, thoughts of changing places are replaced with a comfort of where I am today and an optimism for the good things that may be heading my way.

A disease is not who I am.

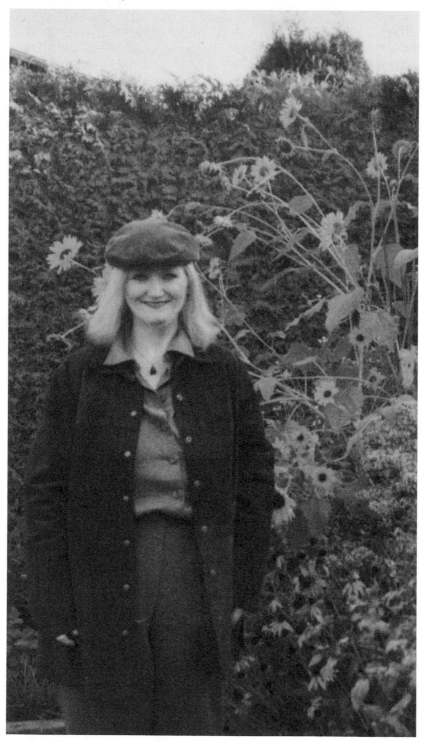

Donna L., Teacher, Writer

Ménière's Disease, Sjogren's Syndrome, Raynaud's Disease,

Polymyalgia, Interstitial Cystitis, Asthma

Living with a hidden illness is a double-edged sword. On the good side, at least I do not appear to be different from other people, so I am not treated as an invalid or given unwanted pity. On the other hand, I do not feel normal. It is as if no one is truly seeing the real me. I may want to feel well, and I certainly look healthy and normal, but I know that I am not. I am actually quite pleased that I look normal. I am glad people don't look at me and know what is inside. I can choose who will know the truth and who will not. I feel in control because of this. I now find this is a gift—this invisibility of my illness.

I was mourning for the death of a life I had once enjoyed, and for the person I had always been.

I was tired and in pain all of the time, but people's expectations of me remained high. I looked healthy, so they assumed I should be as productive, active, and sociable as I had always been. As a result, people did not believe that I was really ill. I was considered to be lazy, or burned-out, or depressed, or whatever label they chose for me to explain what they perceived as my change in behavior. They saw no visible proof of my claims of pain and my inability to work or function. Therefore I was seen as a malingerer. They assumed I did not want to work or I did not like my job. I was seen as an attention seeker and as one who was bilking the insurance company for money by using false claims. I even heard this from doctors who did not as yet understand these illnesses, and who were supposed to be helping me. I looked normal, even glowingly healthy at times. It was confusing to them as well as to me.

My whole life was irrevocably altered by these illnesses that seemed to pile on, one on top of the other. In the beginning, I missed a lot of time at work. I ended up losing a career I loved, which threw me into a deep depression that lasted a year. A psychologist helped me over this hurdle, but I never fully recovered. I don't know why I identified myself by my job, rather than by my person, but I did.

This was actually a period of mourning. I was mourning for the death of the life I had once enjoyed, and for the person I had always been. I was changed in both good and bad ways. It took me a long time to realize the positive impact my illness had on my life. I clearly became more empathetic to others'

281

physical or emotional pain. I appreciated much more the kindness of a stranger and the love of family. Unfortunately, I lost many friends. On the other hand, I also found friends I would not have known otherwise. Illness is a double-edged sword. Not everyone has this chance to find out who really loves them, so that was a blessing in disguise. However, it took me a long time to appreciate this blessing.

I had to accept that I would not have the life I had envisioned. I could not do the activities I enjoyed most, such as dancing, skiing, and skating. I also lost interest in dating. I became discouraged when men got turned off after finding out I was not very healthy. It eventually came out, even if I looked perfectly fine. I realized I might never find that right person for me. The things I envied most in others were their opportunities and abilities to find a loving mate, which I felt had been taken from me, and the opportunity to have a family, which I had always craved. I had to find new reasons for liking myself. I had to decide who I was now and my reason for being in this situation. One of the hardest things I had to adjust to was the enormous weight gain due to the medications. Steroids were the obvious culprit, but many other medications also caused weight gain. Society judges us by appearance, so now I was deemed both unhealthy and unattractive. I had to learn to accept myself all over again and believe in myself in the face of other people's opinions and reactions. All I thought about, night and day, was finding deep sleep and pain relief. These were my only two goals.

My love of books saved my life and sanity. At times, I would read four books a day. I was lucky at that time to have a phenomenal memory and ability to concentrate. I don't understand why I retained it. As my body weakened, my mind seemed to expand. It was a bit of nature's grace, I suppose. I did crossword puzzles like a fiend. I soaked up knowledge on anything and everything like a sponge. A huge thing that saved my sanity, gave me a purpose, and helped me to find new interests in life was the Internet. I did not discover this until I had started feeling better. I resisted until then, as I was always too tired to bother. I rediscovered teaching on the Internet. There I met a number of people from Third World countries who were very motivated to learn to speak English. Teaching English as a second language had been my career, and now it was again. I had a purpose, a role to fulfill again. By word of mouth, I amassed over fifty students. These people were friends as well as students. It was a delight to know them. I even learned to speak Spanish from the Spanish-speaking people that I met online.

Trying and doing new things again is like emerging from a coma or a time warp. I have had moments of complete despair; however, at the root of who I am is an optimist. I never entirely lost hope. I am a terribly curious individual. I sought knowledge from books, other people, and myself about my diseases. Hope is sometimes the only fuel to keep our bodies and souls running.

Harry K., Piano and Organ Tuner

Crohn's Disease

I would have liked to have completed schooling in telecommunications and gone into television production, but this illness changed my mind and my career. I now run my own piano and organ repair business. Having my own business has its good points and bad points. Flexible hours are helpful, but the lack of a pension is a problem. Therefore, I will need to work through what would have otherwise been my retirement years, simply to make ends meet. Having a chronic illness can definitely determine your financial security, or lack of it. I feel fortunate, however, as companies I've done business for have been understanding and very patient with me when I've gotten sick or had to go in the hospital.

Presently, my family and my faith help me cope. My wife keeps me on a positive plane. My parents planted some great early tools and strength in me at a young age to help me fight though the hard times. I've moved closer to my Catholic religion over the years. In the beginning of my illness, I felt angry. I kept asking, "Why me, God?" Of course, the answer came back loud and clear. "Why not?" At that tough time in my life, my priest and the good friends I spoke with helped me through.

I feel as though I can help people by disclosing that I have this disease. If I can help someone else by sharing what I've been through in my thirty-five years with this illness, why not? When I was first diagnosed with Crohn's disease, the doctors weren't sure what I had. I was losing weight week by week and quickly went from 165 pounds to 140 pounds. I was quickly put in the hospital where I was given high dosages of steroids. My weight kept dropping because I was not absorbing or digesting anything, and my weight dropped to 100 pounds. They had to stabilize me before they could operate. Without the medication, I would have died.

At the time, I had to leave my job as an electronic technician for four to five months. Once I gained back some weight, I returned to work. Within a year, I had relapsed and had to permanently leave my job. For the next three years, I was on serious medication and had to have surgery again. I had a hard time getting or keeping a job in consumer electronic repair, in which I had a background. I was not physically able to maintain a full-time job, which was a very difficult and humiliating experience.

I went back to college and began working part-time in a music store doing electronic repairs on organs. This part-time job went to full-time, and I eventually started my own business repairing electric organs, pi-

283

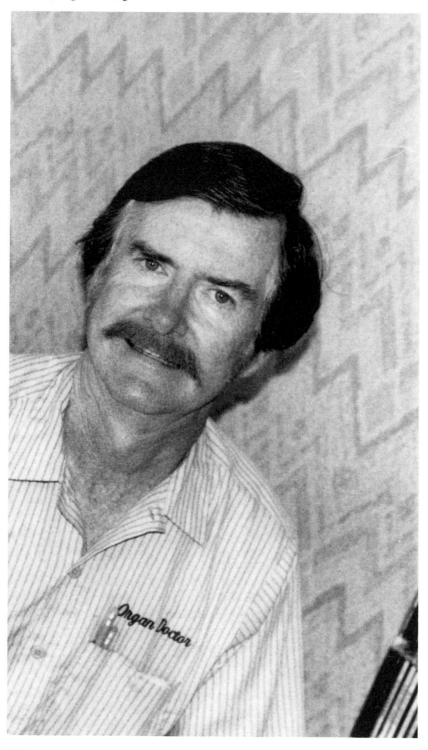

anos, and keyboards. I've had relapses and major surgeries many times over the past thirty years, but I am still working. Having my own business is easier on me as I can take time off without having it impact my job. I've met some great customers, technicians, and engineers during my career and I feel honored to know them. I feel fortunate for the way my career has turned out, even though it was not the path I had initially chosen. I've met many great people I wouldn't have met if I hadn't developed this disease. Many have become very good and dear friends.

Since I am so thin, some people say to me, "You are either a long-distance runner or you have Crohn's disease!" They say it as a joke, but it is so true. Other people want to know how I can stay so thin, as if that's a good thing. In their eyes, I look healthy because I am thin. The reality is, I'm thin and my bones are damaged because of this chronic disease of the intestine.

I have had this disease for over thirty years and have undergone a great number of surgeries. I've lost half my stomach due to Crohn's disease. Also, part of my small intestine has been removed. I need to watch what I eat, how much stress I put myself through, and how much rest I get. But then again, who doesn't?

I kept asking, "Why me, God?" Of course, the answer came back, "Why not?"

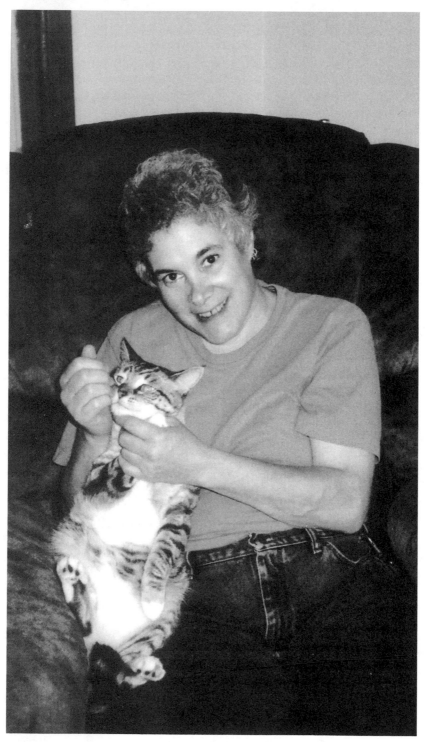

Margie K., Disability Retirement

Bipolar Affective Disorder, Chronic Fatigue Immune

Dysfunction Syndrome, Crohn's Disease

Living with a concealed illness is very different than living with an apparent one. This is especially true on those days and weeks when I feel just awful, and someone says to me, "You look so good." I know this sounds odd, but I just want to scream. Being told how I appear to them puts me on the defensive. I feel the need to point out the truth of the matter and how I actually feel, rather than how I look. That is not a position I enjoy, or one that I take with ease.

I don't go out much, and if I do, I have to scout out the bathrooms. For the past year, I have been unable to eat a normal diet so I never go out to eat, even to a friend's house. Many times, I have wished I could trade in this body for one that works better. I often envy other people's vitality. If only I could feel as healthy as I look.

I'm stubborn and determined. These traits have helped me recover what I thought was lost.

I'm stubborn and determined. These traits have helped me recover what I thought was lost. I spent five years depending on a motorized scooter to get around. For some time, I didn't believe I would ever be able to work or drive again, but I never gave up. I had to accept not one, but several health disorders. I have a dear friend who is quadriplegic, and she helps me feel okay with my physical condition and accept the state of my health, without giving up. She is a real inspiration to me.

I am always being questioned and scrutinized about my health problems. I run into this many times when parking the car with my disabled placard. If I appeared disabled, I wouldn't be questioned so often about why I have to use the disabled designated parking spaces. People seem to assume that if they can't see my pain or condition, it must not exist. I don't enjoy being scrutinized in this way. The more pain I'm in, the less tolerance I have for the ignorance of others.

If I looked the part of someone disabled, I wouldn't have had to deal with the hassles I received from the state government about financial assistance, which is based on my disabilities. I feel that I have to continually prove the existence of these concealed disorders in order to receive assistance. I would rather not have these illnesses that I don't look like I have. But, if I have to have them, I wish I didn't have to feel so much doubt from others, or feel the need to prove my case simply because my symptoms are not visually apparent.

I don't have to try to appear normal. I just do, even when I have low-grade fevers, as they give me my rosy cheeks. Sometimes, I do not want to explain that I do not feel as good as I look, so I suffer in silence. It is very hard to get a healthy person to understand what living in this sort of body is like. I am slowly learning that when the pain is bad, asking for help is okay. If someone doesn't understand why I am asking because I look so good, that's their problem, not mine.

I rely upon certain principles to help me through my health challenges. I have learned to trust in a power greater than myself to take me through the challenges and obstacles my illnesses present. One thing that I know will help, but that I have not done lately, is to go to a support group for people with chronic illness. The difficult question is, which illness do I select?

The advantage of not looking ill is that I do not have to deal with unsolicited sympathy from others. The disadvantage is I have to ask for sympathy, because no one can see my symptoms. Being chronically ill is very difficult and is made more difficult because it is not readily apparent to strangers. Because of the hidden nature of all that ails me, I feel a great deal of stress, because I continually need to explain myself to others. I find that sharing my feelings with someone who also has hidden illnesses helps me to cope better with my own.

Judy R., Computer Consultant, Student

Crohn's Disease with Multiple Intestinal Resections

Living with a concealed disability forces me to be more open and verbal about my disease. I look rather healthy. Therefore, people do not understand how I can become so ill in a matter of an hour or two, or how I cannot do things unless it is on the spur of the moment. So, I am forced to explain a disease that I would prefer to have stay in the shadows.

I always have to know where the restroom is and to carry a change of clothing and a purse filled with different types of medications, depending on my needs that day. I avoid social situations so that I don't have to constantly explain the disease. Initially, doctors said that I was exaggerating my symptoms. They looked for all kinds of other causes, physical and mental. It took two years to receive a proper diagnosis. Even with ten surgeries under my belt, literally and figuratively, and two near fatal bouts of peritonitis, some people continue to tell me that this illness is in my imagination.

My stamina level does not allow me to be a superwoman. I no longer participate in many activities when I know I will pay with several days or weeks of recovering. I'm working more and more on my faith, in not asking, "Why me?" but instead asking, "What can I do to help someone else who has just been diagnosed?" One of my gastroenterologists has been instrumental in more than physical healing. He has been there to listen, to guide, and to challenge me. And, of course, my friends have helped, compliments of the support groups I have located in my community.

I have certainly been in denial in the past. First, I felt anger, but then my good ol' sense of humor began to come back. It's difficult to maintain a sense of humor sometimes, when my life feels so out of control. I try to calm down and keep life as normal as possible, unless it becomes too exhausting. Then I take special care of myself and just accomplish what's necessary to survive at that particular time. Appearing normal takes a lot of work. I become stressed if I am somewhere and might have to leave because I do not feel well. As a result, I push myself, which in turn causes me more stress. I am starting to listen to my body more and not do what tears me up inside and aggravates my symptoms.

This has been a particularly rough year for me, and my feelings of hopelessness surrounding this illness have resurfaced. I'm usually an upbeat person, but after my eighth resection surgery a few months ago, I felt pushed to the edge of what I could tolerate. Surgery is usually no big deal for us veterans of surgery; however, this last one was difficult, not only on my body, but

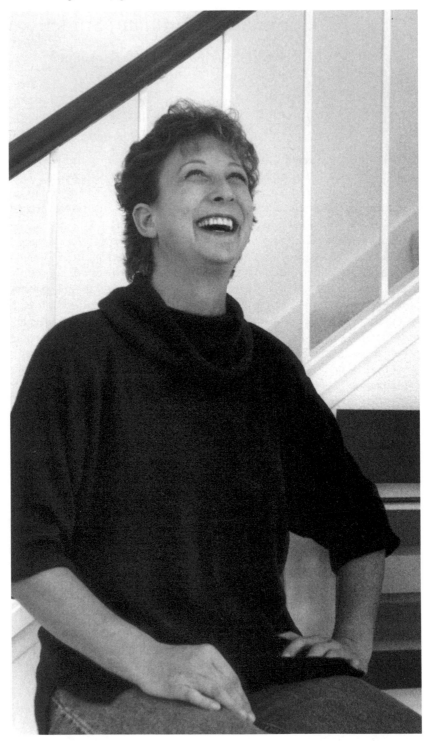

on my spirit. I am still here, so I won the battle, but I feel as though I'm losing the war. I have not come through unchanged. I almost died on the operating table and was left with an ileostomy pouch that I'm still not accustomed to. I now have three months before my next surgery (number ten, for those who are counting) to reverse the ileostomy; I'm terrified. When people look at me, they are unable to see the illness. They cannot see the fear, anger, frustration, pain, and isolation that accompany my chronic symptoms. All they see is my confident, sometimes aloof exterior and the ever-present smile plastered on my face.

This illness leaves me feeling like I'm defective—not just physically, but emotionally. When I am doing this badly, I have difficulty remembering what good times are like. When things are good, I often forget these very frightening and depressing moments. This time I came through the emergency without hope. My ability to cope got lost in the surgery, lost in the medications, lost in feeling so utterly alone. I had several weeks of feeling totally helpless and miserable before returning to my spirituality and the Catholic faith of my upbringing. Over the last few months of spiritual counseling, I am finding my sense of humor beginning to return. My wry, dry wit is my saving grace. I cope with these more challenging times by going for short drives, being out in the sunshine, or talking to my best friend on the phone and charging up large long distance bills. I also love to garden and put my hands in the dirt. I play with my two cats and only enjoy being around the people I truly trust.

I will forever have this disease, but as long as I can inject it with an overdose of humor and good friends, it will not have me.

After fourteen years of dealing with this illness, I am most grateful that I do not have to contend with something else in addition to this disease. There can always be something different and much worse than Crohn's disease. I needed several years to work through the anger, grief, and loss stages of living with this illness, but I did. I am going to college and working again after fifteen years of not being able to, and am going out dancing on the weekend when I am able to do so. I need to feel productive and alive. I need to move forward in my life, wherever that might lead. I don't know if I will be working tomorrow, or if I will get to class this week, but I am happier than I have ever been, because I am trying. I will forever have this disease, but as long as I can inject it with an overdose of humor and good friends, it will not have me.

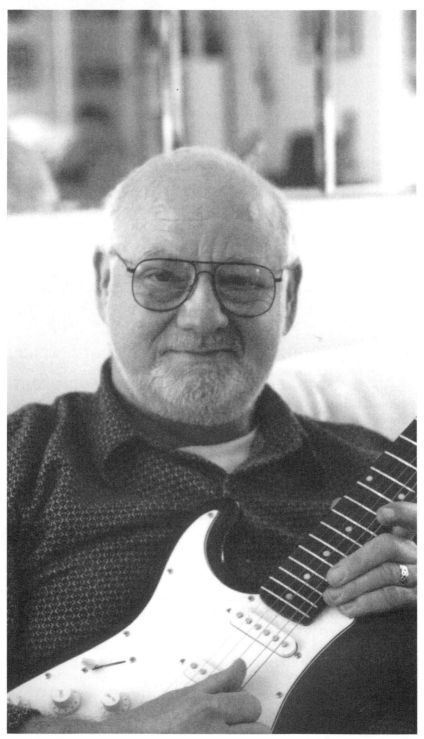

Steve B., Former DJ, Traffic News Reporter

Diabetes, Neuropathy, Heart Bypass

Complications from my diabetes have caused me to spend several months in a highly visible wheelchair. And while people may offer common courtesies, the biggest impact is that you are aware that they are aware of your disability. The concealed aspect of my diabetes now offers a degree of anonymity, which I find comforting. I have had to make considerable lifestyle adjustments, mostly in dietary habits, because of my concealed illness. Diabetes is a disease that reveals its complications microscopically over a very long period of time, attacking the cells of every component of the body. Adjustments have to be made for physical, as well as emotional, stability.

This disease tests all the human emotions.

Exercise is a major factor in the control of diabetes, but exercise is difficult for me because of some aspects of the disease, like a few missing toes. Other adjustments include eating my meals on a specific schedule each day, testing my blood glucose levels, and injecting insulin, or taking oral medications depending on the severity of my condition. Unfortunately, self-discipline is the best virtue that can control this disease, and I lack self-discipline. Periods of making peace with this illness are few and far between. I tried hypnosis as a last resort to control my eating, as food choices and weight management can have an impact on this form of diabetes. I had always had a fascination with hypnosis, and I truly believe it can work. The trouble is finding someone reputable who does it for medicinal purposes and not a stage act. The hypnotist I worked with was quite good and helped me stick with a good eating plan where I didn't cheat.

In most cases, outward appearances won't identify this disease. About the only thing that would identify me as a diabetic is if others witness me injecting insulin. This disease tests all of the human emotions. Even though I did nothing to cause my diabetes, I am the only one who can control it. Therefore, guilt has become my constant companion. I feel sorrow for the normal life I might have led otherwise. I feel jealous of the people who don't have to cope with my illness. I try to live my life as normally as possible. Sometimes that means ignoring my condition, which is the worst thing I can do. Coping with diabetes, for me, requires a momentary denial of the condition. One advantage of having my diabetes concealed is anonymity. Sometimes I just want to be left alone. Other times you cannot shut me up. The low visibility of my disease helps me to choose which way I want to be at any given moment.

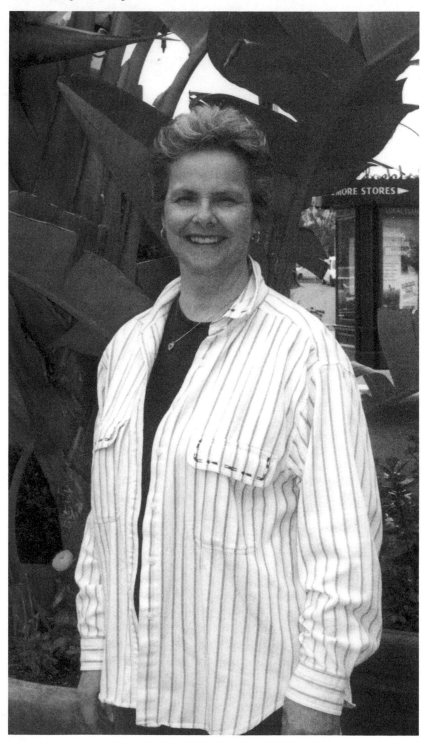

Maria D., Homemaker

Hepatitis C, Chronic Back Pain

I don't do well with pity, so I'm glad my illness doesn't show. I have always been on my own and able to handle life. Now I feel very vulnerable, as if I am not able to take care of myself financially, or without some help. I have tried to learn everything I can about my disease, and I am trying to take the appropriate actions to help myself. I like to read inspirational stories. I have read great books that give me insights about my situation and remind me that life could always be worse. That helps me deal with my disease a little bit better.

I have shifted my entire life around my disease. When we go out, we cannot be out for an entire day. The sun really tires me out as does too much walking. I avoid most of the things I used to do. Walking with my husband or going to arts and crafts shows in the summer is no longer an option. I have to clean my house in shifts, a little at a time. By the time I finish, I have to start again.

People don't question my condition to my face, but I always feel like they think I'm fooling.

I have to make sure that I don't overplan my day. I no longer work, which is a big adjustment. I have worked since a very early age, so this is new and unwelcome territory for me. When I exercise in the morning, I make sure that I have time for rest before and after my exertion. If I have appointments, I don't make plans to go to the gym. I can't seem to do both.

People do not question my condition to my face, but I always feel like they think I'm fooling or am not really that sick. This is very hard, as I have always been a pretty strong person. Sometimes people say to me, "Just live for today." Uh, it is very hard not to think of hepatitis C every day, especially when your liver causes your body to hurt and tire easily.

I envy every person I see running or playing sports. I love to play and have fun, but since my diagnosis, I have been running downhill. I have been through two treatments; the first one almost killed me, and the second one, I had no response to. They left me feeling weak and very discouraged.

I don't try to blend in with others as much as I used to. I used to plan a big day and then be miserable. I don't feel normal, so I have trouble acting like I am. I plan my activities for the day. For instance, today I have a yoga class, and I need to pick up my medications and some vegetables. I am worrying about how I will do everything. I get so frustrated living my life this way. It is so hard when you cannot just shop and clean your house on the same day.

The advantage of having a concealed illness is that I do not have to tell people there's anything wrong, and I can act like a normal person. The disadvantages are that I need a lot of rest and a special diet, because I can no longer tolerate fats. I must make sure I eat before I go out. We rarely eat out any longer, which used to give me a break from cooking. Aches and pains are a problem, because I have to keep shifting positions if I sit too long. I don't want people to think that I am bored. Most people probably assume I am just lazy. But laziness is not a part of who I am. I was always on the go. My mom is eighty-five this year, and she is still on the go.

Having this condition is a nightmare. I pray all the time for this illness to be gone and to just have my energy back. Sometimes I feel like God is punishing me for my past.

I try to cope with this chronic illness in a multitude of ways. I have a counselor and a psychiatrist that I see regularly. I am on antidepressants. I belong to Alcoholics Anonymous, and the meetings help a lot. In fact, a lot of my support comes from these group meetings. I don't know where I would be without them.

I guess I am a survivor. I have been all the way to the bottom with drugs, drinking, and physical problems, but I have never given up. I guess I'm just a stubborn person who refuses to give up until I can no longer do anything at all anymore. I meditate, do yoga, and go to Alcoholics Anonymous meetings about five to six times a week. That is my salvation.

Steve G., Accountant

Ulcerative Colitis with J-Pouch

I try to appear problem- and pain-free around other people when I'm experiencing symptoms of my illness. After a while, I get tired of people asking me how I'm feeling, or if I'm doing okay. People don't understand the difference between discomfort and pain. Many times, I simply respond that I'm fine just to avoid having to go into detail and to get people to stop worrying about me.

When I'm in pain, it is very hard to describe. Most people don't, and can't, understand the pain. I'm very fortunate to be working for such a great company; otherwise, my recovery and illness would be difficult. When I do have a flare-up, my employers take my word on it. I don't give them the details, I just call in sick and let my boss know that I'm having a flare-up. I could see where some bosses might not be so understanding, since nothing looks wrong.

I wanted to go to a football game just four days after my surgery. Looking back on that now, it probably was not the smartest thing, but I wanted to be normal and didn't want another surgery to get in the way of my life. It's difficult to rediscover a workable balance in my life. When I originally returned to work after my surgery, my wife, kids, and boss wanted me to work half-days the first few weeks, but I was going to show them. So, the first week I worked half-days, then the next week I went back to full-time. I didn't look too good, but I wanted to be back at work and functioning normally after being out of the office for three months.

Just last night, I had a flare-up and could not go to a much-anticipated baseball game. So, not only was I in pain, but I was missing out on something I wanted to do. When I do have my pain, or discomfort, I just want to be left alone. There is nothing anyone can do, and no one can understand what I'm going though. My wife does a good job of knowing what I need. If I want to be left alone, she will just check on me every hour or so.

I feel angry toward my body and this whole situation. When I experience pain, I cannot seem to identify what causes it to come on. The medication the doctors originally gave me for my illness caused damage to my hips/bones. I seemed to fall into every category of "If it could happen, it will happen." Blockages occur in about 15% of the people with ulcerative colitis, and I've experienced blockages. Following that surgery, I got an infection. And now I'm suffering from side effects of the medications. With all this history, it is hard not to feel angry.

On most days the thought, "This is better than the alternative" works, but

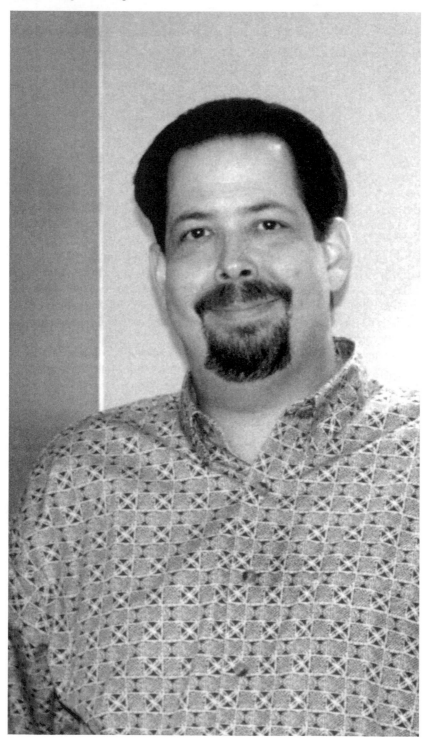

not always. After all the stuff I have been through, I don't want to lose the battle now. Therefore, I will not give up. I don't have a real clear memory of what life was before all this happened. For instance, I just assume everyone goes to the bathroom ten or more times a day. Don't they? Maybe I'm the normal one, and all the other people are the different ones. When I'm talking about myself, my illness often seems to come up. I don't do it because I want people to feel sorry for me; it is just a part of who I am.

Planning ahead is very important in my life. I have been able to figure out some of the foods that work best for me, and I try to eat them before I go out because it may not be convenient for me to go to the bathroom. Additionally, taking medication prior to an activity helps reduce the pain.

I do envy other people at times. I would be lying if I said otherwise. We joke at our house when someone says they haven't gone to the bathroom in a couple of days. I wonder what that must be like.

Before I had this illness, I traveled extensively for business. However, once my condition accelerated, it became very difficult, if not impossible, to hop a plane and travel from city to city. My illness impacted where I went, and I always had to be concerned with finding a bathroom. I started getting an aisle seat on all planes and started planning trips to the bathroom depending on the length of the flight.

After all the stuff I've been through, I don't want to lose the battle now. So, I will not give up.

The situation with my hips has forced me to give up something I loved. For the past thirteen years, I had worked as a high school basketball referee. After my illness, I was able to return for one year. It was great! In the past, I took all this for granted, but not anymore. I thoroughly enjoyed each game.

In one way, my illness has brought my twenty-one-year-old daughter and me closer together. My illness taught us both that life is not guaranteed. It is important to treasure every moment we have together. This realization was one of the benefits of my illness.

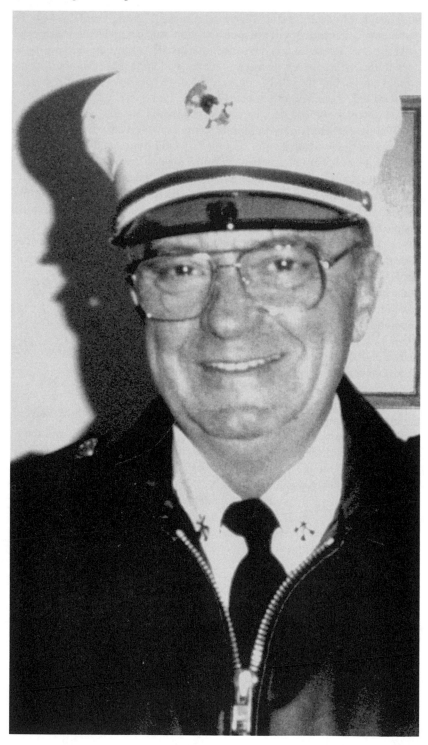

Robert B., Retired Deputy Fire Chief

Lung Cancer, Ulcerative Colitis

I never thought of myself as being disabled. One of my illnesses, ulcerative colitis, came on in a rather subtle manner at first. I dealt with the problem privately for years. People in my age group did not discuss bathroom problems. The subject was not exactly talked about at cocktail parties or with friends. We referred to my lung cancer as the "Big C," never admitting to anyone that a person in our family had such a disease. The only one who was truly aware of my condition was my wife. I did not discuss it with my children or my parents.

I am a retired deputy chief officer of a local fire department. As I rose through the ranks from firefighter to lieutenant to captain and finally to deputy chief, the job became more stressful. It was at this time that my condition became a problem. For some twenty-five years, I had not used many sick days, but the sick days were becoming more frequent.

I was not looking for sympathy. I was looking for understanding.

My job required that I be at a certain place at a certain time, and there was no middle ground. This became a real problem. When I was flaring, I took sick time. I could not command a fire scene when I might find it necessary to find a bathroom at any moment. The stress was taking its toll.

I am not a smoker. My lung cancer was caused by my occupation as a firefighter. When I discovered I had lung cancer, I was quite upset. Then my wife and I sat down and discussed this latest development and decided that it would do no good to worry about something that had not happened as yet. I was assured that the cancer was operable and so we went on the assumption that everything was going to be all right. The operation was successful. I am cancer-free coming up on five years.

The operation for lung cancer brought on some rather unusual symptoms. I suffer from almost constant pain in my ribs. The surgeon had to cut one rib to get at the diseased part of the lung. I also have difficulty breathing in times of weather extremes (either very hot or very cold). Here in the Northeast where I live, the temperature range is from below zero in the winter to above 100 degrees in the summer.

As a retiree, I don't have to go outside in extreme weather. I could never have afforded that luxury had I been still working as a firefighter. I also obtained a handicap license plate. I use it only during extreme weather, and frankly I get strange looks, because I do appear to be healthy. But I use it in those times when I have difficulty breathing and have to walk long distances.

I am now retired from the fire department. My condition has eased somewhat, although I am having some difficulties at this time. I have regular colonoscopies and make sure I know the location of every bathroom in every mall and along regularly traveled routes. When working, I drove to work on a route where I knew I could find a bathroom. I was aware of every bathroom in every department store, grocery store, and gas station wherever I went.

My wife and I love to travel. When traveling by airplane we request seats near the lavatories. I recently did some traveling, and the excursions were well planned. I noted rest areas, and I was always on the lookout for gas stations and restaurants. Thankfully, the interstate system is overflowing with gas stations and restaurants. I also carry a portable toilet with me in the event I cannot reach any facilities.

All in all, I consider myself a very lucky man. I deal with my situation, as I know I must. I do not envy anyone else for I know that there are many problems in this world. I have learned, and continue to learn, to deal with mine.

Laura H., Retired Art Teacher and Dancer

Post-Polio Syndrome, Diabetes

I recovered from polio in 1946 at the age of thirteen. My left side was para-lyzed (face, throat, arm, leg) before I recovered movement. Physical therapy helped me regain control of my body, except in my throat and with the pro-cess of swallowing. No one can see that part of my illness, but I do have great difficulty swallowing. I have also lost my ability to sing more than three or four notes. I can no longer make the sound of laughing or crying, and I cough and sneeze in a funny way. I cannot drink at a fountain, because the water would come out of my nose, since I lost the ability to close off my throat. I have to be very careful to chew my food thoroughly. I choke quite often, if I am not careful, and I have difficulty catching my breath. I cannot talk and eat at the same time or I risk choking. I do not eat steak because it does not break up enough when I chew. I almost choked to death twice before I got smart and switched to chicken and fish. No one has questioned me about my illness. I just explain that I have to eat slowly, and all my friends seem to understand.

The thing that really bugs me is not being able to sing. I have perfect pitch and know almost every standard musical tune. In my pre-polio days, I was quite the entertainer. All through high school and college, I was active in modern dance groups. My physical education credits were mostly in dance or swimming. I decided that if I couldn't be a musical comedy star, I would become a teacher (the next best way to have a captive audience). Girls could only be teachers or nurses in those days. I became an art teacher because I didn't have to lecture too long. I don't have a very loud voice, and in class I could give individual instruction after introducing a lesson.

I graduated from the University of Minnesota with a bachelors of science degree in art education and a minor in speech and theater arts. My voice would not project across the footlights so I learned about costuming, lighting, sound, directing, and all things backstage. Later, I earned a master's degree and bought my own house. I had a near death experience with meningococeal meningitis about ten years ago. I survived, taught one more year, and then retired. This life of mine has been quite an exciting roller-coaster ride.

I am very proud of what I've accomplished on my own, despite my ill-ness. I do not really envy other people's good health and energy because I am quite lively. At my age, I'm in better shape than most of my contemporaries. All I can complain about now is an arthritic thumb.

I always had my parents' love and support. So many children were af-fected by the polio epidemic in 1946 that I never felt ostracized or isolated.

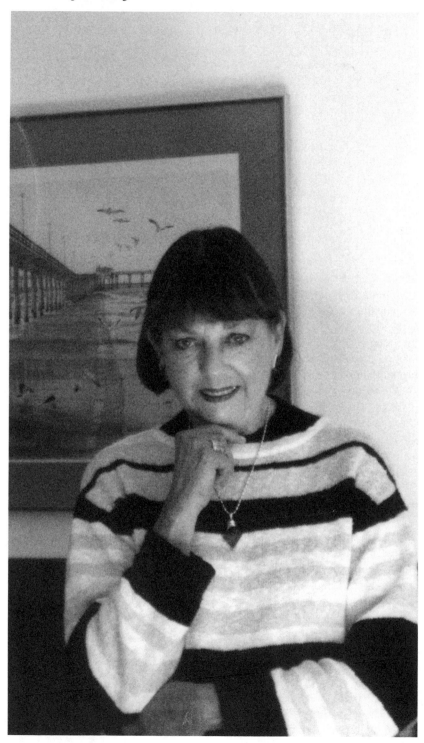

There were many of us in the same boat. We were not shunned. We were respected, because we were survivors. All people with chronic illness or conditions are survivors. It is something to be proud of.

I maintain a positive attitude and I don't let the little things in life, of which there are plenty, get me down. A sense of humor helps. When I attended my first post-polio survivors meeting, I was amazed at the number of people with braces, crutches, and wheelchairs. I felt out of place with my concealed symptoms.

I was recently diagnosed with diabetes, which really threw me for a loop. For years I have eaten right, exercised regularly (swimming three times a week), and I am not overweight. I had no symptoms and knew of no one in my family with diabetes. So, there you go. You never know what life is going to dish up for you.

I've accomplished a lot and feel I have led a full and satisfying life. I have had more than my share of adventures, here and in Europe. I have seen what I wanted to see and accomplished what I set out to do. My kids are fine now, I have many good friends, and I made it to my fiftieth high school reunion. I don't let things get me down. I don't worry about things I have no control over. I can laugh at myself, and do just that all the time. My saving grace is my sense of humor.

My saving grace is my sense of humor.

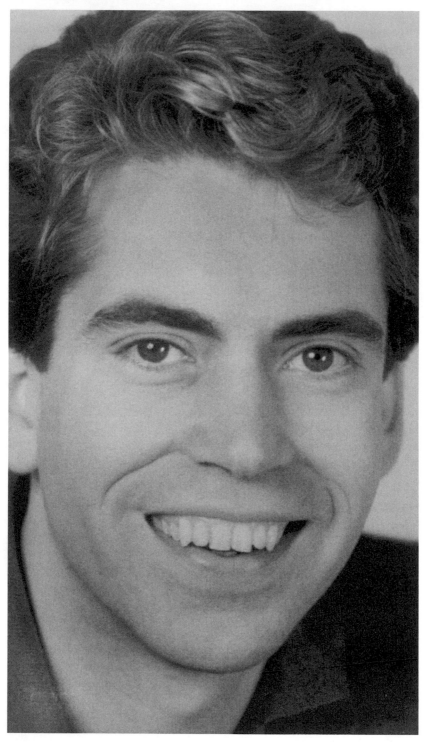

Tim C., Volunteer Peer Support Counselor

Crohn's Disease

I've been thinking a lot lately about how other people think of my disease, and ultimately, how they think of me as a person. As much as I try to convince myself otherwise, the part of me that is about my disease, and the rest of me that is not, are no longer distinguishable.

For twenty-five years, I have been living with Crohn's disease, a chronic inflammatory bowel disease. I'm okay with that, I really am. But it seems that no one else I know can quite grasp the concept of its chronic nature.

Having a chronic disorder is a problem for people because of their own expectations. People expect a sick person to either get better and be well, or get worse and die. Those of us with chronic conditions deal with something that is ongoing. Chronic is not good or bad, or right or wrong. It just is.

You really get stuck with a credibility problem, trying to prove yourself all the time.

If you add to that the fact that your chronic condition is concealed from view, then you really get stuck with a credibility problem, trying to prove yourself all the time. People who look sick get sympathy and understanding; those who don't, don't. It reminds me of when I was about to leave work on disability status (itself a huge and totally life-changing decision). The experience was so difficult that, if I could have, I would have brought poster size blow-ups of the films from my latest colonoscopy to prove I wasn't someone trying to fool the system.

It's not sympathy I want. Oh sure, sometimes when I'm feeling really sick and my illness is symptomatic, I'd like someone to stroke the back of my head and whisper softly, "You poor dear. . ." But usually, that's not the case. Understanding would be nice, but I don't even need that most of the time. But not being believed really makes me nutty.

Sympathy and understanding are nice, but belief in my honesty and belief in who I am as a person, including my disease, is something I'm just going to have to insist upon.

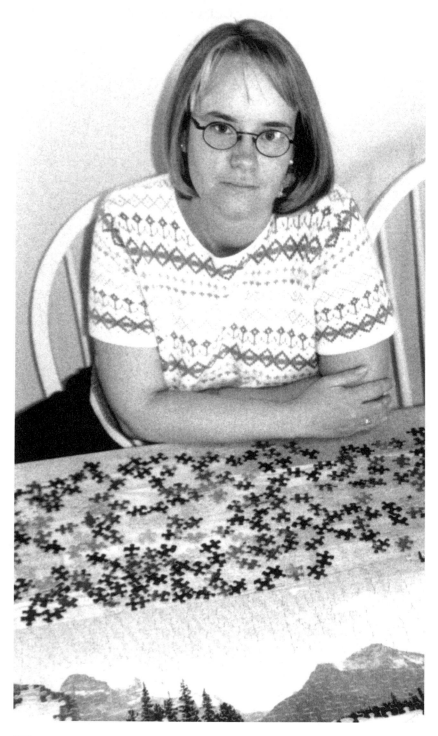

Kristen B., Mother and Homemaker

Crohn's Disease

An advantage to having my illness concealed is that people do not treat me differently because I have an illness. The disadvantage is just that. People think that I should be able to do everything, since I do not look sick.

Because my disability is hidden, many times people will comment, "But you don't look sick," as if to say that I am lying and making an excuse. I often have to justify the fact that I am sick. Those individuals with visible and noticeable conditions may get unwanted sympathy, but every once in awhile, a little unsolicited sympathy would be great.

Once in awhile a little unsolicited sympathy would be great!

Having a child has forced me to take better care of myself and to control this disease to the best of my ability. The hardest thing for me has been to learn how to ask for help taking care of my young son. I feel helpless when I have to acknowledge that my flare-up is to the point where I need assistance providing my son with the care he needs. That's a feeling I don't like to experience. However, asking for help, as difficult as it is, provides blessings that I could never have imagined. I'm learning how to ask for help when I need it and not just give help to others. That's quite an accomplishment for me.

I always have to know where all the bathrooms are in every store and restaurant I visit. This is a must. Another adjustment I have had to make is planning on when I am going to eat my meals so that I won't get caught out somewhere and have an accident.

I try to be positive and focus on the many wonderful aspects of my life, including my husband and son (although I would by lying if I said I was never envious of others). I always try to keep a positive attitude and stay focused on the good times. I also try to give my problems up to God. Through prayer, I get the power and faith I need to sustain me through the rough times.

I rely heavily on those close to me, particularly my husband. I remind myself that seeing me ill is not easy for family members either. If I can make light of the situation, their troubles will be lifted as well.

I just live the life that I have been given. It is frustrating when I am so tired and don't have the energy I need or want to have, or when I need to change my pants, time and time again during a given week, due to bathroom accidents. But I always say to myself, things could be much worse.

Living with Crohn's disease is a challenge, but having it makes me a better person. Dealing with the bathroom accidents, not having energy, and other associated factors forces me to appreciate the times when these things do not rear their ugly head. As I said before, I have many blessings in my life. They help and encourage me to cope with this disease. Thinking of those less fortunate than myself and remembering my blessings helps me live a life full of faith and hope, despite my illness.

Barbara M., Volunteer Caretaker

Lupus, Fibromyalgia, Sciatica

Having a concealed chronic illness is certainly different from one that is visible. People don't understand how I can be so sick, yet look so good. My career was not doable any longer because it was too physically demanding. I also had to cut back to part-time instead of continuing to work full-time.

During flare-ups, I have lost acquaintances and jobs. I cannot be outside because the sun is damaging to my condition. Maintaining friendships is hard because of the unpredictability of my illness. Often plans need to be canceled at the last minute. I've learned to change my priorities in order to keep the little social life that I have. I cannot make commitments because of the uncertainty of the disease. Medical professionals and others have often questioned the existence of my illness. At times, I wish I appeared disabled. My illness would not be questioned as much. I watch others living a normal life doing many things throughout the day and I envy them. I've always been a high-energy person and now have to limit myself to one activity per day. I envy my friends who have good health.

What has helped me the most is to reach out and help others. By educating myself, I can become more proactive and work as a team with my doctors. Having a best friend with the same condition as myself is a comfort and a bond. Having role models who do not behave as victims teaches me how to live with this illness. I use positive thinking and affirmations as much as I can. I listen to music that makes me feel good. My cat is a great comfort and companion. I find examples around me of those who have things to deal with that are much worse than my own. I enjoy reading medical books and learning that I am not alone. I surround myself with an environment that is soothing by using candles and aromatherapy oils.

People might be surprised to learn this, but I consider aromatherapy to be the one thing that has had the most positive impact on my lupus. I was introduced to it by a friend and read a couple of books about it. I now use it on a daily basis. Nausea often accompanies lupus, so I use peppermint oil in an oil/candle burner lamp, or put two drops of this oil on a tissue and inhale it. The nausea stops at once. It truly offers instant relief and is quite amazing. Peppermint and grapefruit used together help calm my nausea and stimulate my appetite. I also use these oils when I am having a lot of sciatica and joint pain. Blue chamomile oil can be put right where it hurts. The relief is fast acting, but is temporary. Chamomile oil is also a good aid for sleep. I mix it with carrier oils or sweet almond oil, and it really helps me drift off to sleep

311

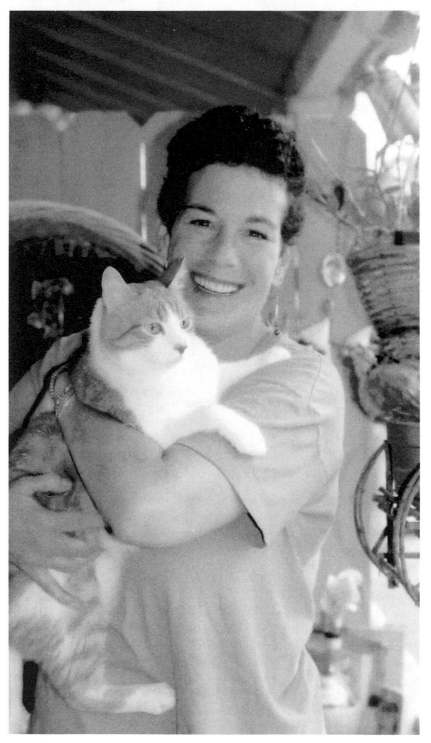

quickly. (Chamomile and lavender oils may be used without carrier oil, but other oils have to be mixed with them.) If I have trouble breathing, I use eucalyptus and rosemary oils. These oils are effective and people should really read more about their uses. My symptoms are severe, yet the results from these oils have been positive and dramatic.

I used acupuncture for three years and found it very useful for my joint pains. Now that my skin sensations are so intense from the fibromyalgia condition, I can no longer use acupuncture, but I highly recommend it to others. Another thing that has helped me tremendously is treating myself to a healing massage once a week. Yes, it is expensive, but I can't think of anything that has helped my circulation more. My particular massage therapist only sees clients with chronic conditions and pain. I also drink ten glasses of water daily and that seems to help as well.

Since I moved from an old and damp city apartment to acting as caretaker to an elderly man who lives in a close-knit and lovely community, my symptoms and energy level have improved dramatically. My walking has increased from forty five minutes a day to two-and-a-half hours a day. Sometimes a change of scenery and focusing attention on helping others can do wonders for mind, body, and soul.

I cannot make commitments because of the uncertain nature of this disease.

I often think of people who are much worse off than I am. I count my blessings. I distract myself, and if people ask me how I feel, I say, "fine," so I don't stand out. I can pretend that I am healthy and normal. The effect of this on my symptoms is that they seem less bothersome and are temporarily numbed.

The advantage to having a concealed illness is that I do not look sick. I can go out among others and appear normal. The disadvantage is that acquaintances question my disease. I have had several negative experiences with doctors who minimized my illness or sent me to other doctors because they were mystified about what to do. When an individual has an obvious physical ailment, people act kinder and offer help. People seem to believe that when something is not visible, it is not there. They have to see something in order to believe it.

I question my illness all the time. "Is it in my head or is it real?" It is alternately frustrating, depressing, lonely, and isolating. I cope by falling into denial, or distracting myself with art, music, or talking with friends. Humor is an essential part of my coping mechanisms. I joke about my condition and myself. I seek out opportunities to help others. It feels good to feel needed and productive. I also try to create an atmosphere at home that is peaceful, warm, and comforting.

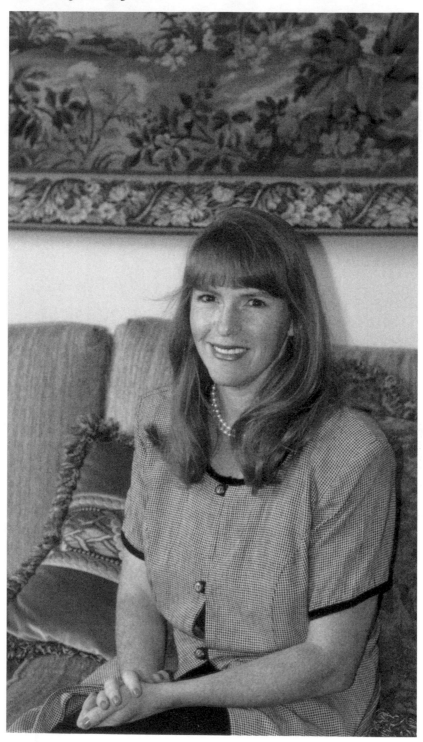

Cindy V., Mother, Administrative Assistant

Crohn's Disease

I have had Crohn's disease since I was three months old, and as a young child I had several surgeries. The medical doctors told my parents that I'd never be able to have children, and my parents relayed this information to me at a very early age. However, they did not explain about how fertile I'd still be. In fact, I sometimes joke that my sex organs are just about the only part of my body that works right. Despite having this disease, I've never had trouble getting pregnant. I have three wonderful children, and they were all born very healthy.

When I was younger and in my dating phase, I avoided telling any of my dates about my disease or the symptoms of my disease. I truly felt that no partner could accept me with the disease. I was so afraid of rejection that I would do everything I could to hide the symptoms. When I would start getting too close to someone, I would break off the relationship. At that time, I felt I couldn't risk having anyone find out about it. This went on for many years.

I was so afraid of rejection that I would do everything I could to hide the illness.

When I met the man who is now my husband, my first response to him was the same, even though I was in love with him. I did everything to hide my disease from him. I certainly did not want him to know I had diarrhea, so I would purposely not eat before our dates. Sometimes I would go five days with only water and bananas just to avoid having a problem around him. At the time, eating very little reduced my chances of having symptoms. If I was in his apartment and needed to go to the bathroom, I'd jump in the car and drive home, which was thirty miles away, without an explanation. However, I didn't want to break off the relationship like I had with the other men. It was scary, but fortunately he truly loved me and accepted me, disease and all. We've been married now for fourteen years.

I had a wonderful job and a great boss at a financial institution, and I really wanted to keep working, but my illness was just too severe at that time. I tried applying for disability benefits but was rejected. I appealed time after time, and eventually came to the point where I was to appear in court before a judge. I knew if I could explain my situation to a fair judge, I would be believed. I explained from my heart about everything I have been through

315

with the disease. It is not an easy disease to discuss, but I told him all about it in a way that was clear, accurate, and personal, but not crude. Usually after one of the hearings, one has to wait up to sixty days to hear the decision from the judge. But right after my testimony, the judge said he would accept my appeal and wished me happiness.

Sometimes others say things like, "I wish I could be as skinny as you." They don't realize that keeping weight on is one of the challenges of this disease. I always appear to be slim, and others think I am able to eat whatever I want, but in reality, I have to eat all of the time just to get through the day. My choices in relationships, careers, and friendships have all been impacted to some extent.

Because I have had this chronic disease all of my life, it's difficult to know what life would be like without it. On the other hand, I've often imagined, especially when I was a child, what life would have been like to be free of my many symptoms and the pain that goes with my concealed illness. In many ways, it was like a beautiful dream. A normal life has always been just out of reach for me, but I've learned over the years how to cope and make allowances for the things I could not easily accomplish.

Holding down jobs and working towards a career was challenging. I always had to miss days here and there due to flare-ups of the illness. School was also quite difficult because of my illness. I now try to make jokes about my illness and myself, but the truth of the matter is I have sacrificed a number of important academic and personal goals throughout my life just to remain stable enough to simply function on a physical level. I've had to give up many things, and this leaves me sad and mournful for the life never lived.

I always envy people who are high achievers. My biggest achievement is just getting through the week. Sometimes I need to lie down, but if I look okay, if I look just fine, other people think that I shouldn't be allowed to rest. They simply cannot, and do not, understand this level of fatigue.

Daryl W., Sr. Manufacturing Consultant

Diabetes, Glaucoma

The primary symptom of my illness is fatigue caused by the ups and downs of sugar levels. The tragic thing about type II diabetes is that the symptoms aren't obvious. A routine physical exam that I had a few years ago pinpointed my blood sugar; otherwise I wouldn't have known.

When I become symptomatic, I get very quiet. Most people don't know what's occurring, but since I'm not normally a quiet guy, some people will ask me if I'm okay. I don't get real highs and lows much anymore because I control the sugar pretty well. The frustrating thing is that I will occasionally get a sugar spike for basically no reason, i.e., I have not eaten anything that would spike it up, but the body does what it does sometimes without any help from us. Type II diabetes is like that: sometimes the liver hiccups.

This illness makes a significant impact in some areas of my life. I have to watch my carbohydrate intake which can impact the glucose level in my blood. Consequently, my diet is constantly under scrutiny. My wife has a tendency to have low blood sugar, so this is an interesting conundrum and challenge. Fortunately, type II diabetes is not uncommon, so there are far more food choices today than a few years ago. Our friends have to be aware of this as well, because we must consider food choices at social functions or restaurants when we go out. Restaurants aren't always prepared for sugar-free or low carbohydrate choices, so this can be a challenge. In addition, because diabetes has an effect on blood clotting, I have to be more careful about cuts and such. Last year, I had an accident trimming bushes and had to go to the emergency room for stitches. If I did not have diabetes, I could have used bandages at home and that would have been that. These are some of the lifestyle changes that I have to adapt to. For someone in his fifties who refused to conform to a senior lifestyle, these adjustments were particularly challenging.

With this disease, the major issue for me is recognizing that it is a factor of aging. That bugs me. I mean, it's bad enough I have to deal with aches and pains and the other issues involved with getting older. The addition of diabetes is just a huge annoyance. I refused for a year to take the medication and tried controlling the disease with diet and exercise, but it caught up with me. Basically, I hated taking the pills more than anything else. Plus, I also have to deal with glaucoma. Anyway, I have adjusted by just dealing with it. I still refuse to think of myself as a senior. I have always associated with people younger than myself, because my chronological age has always been older than my mind.

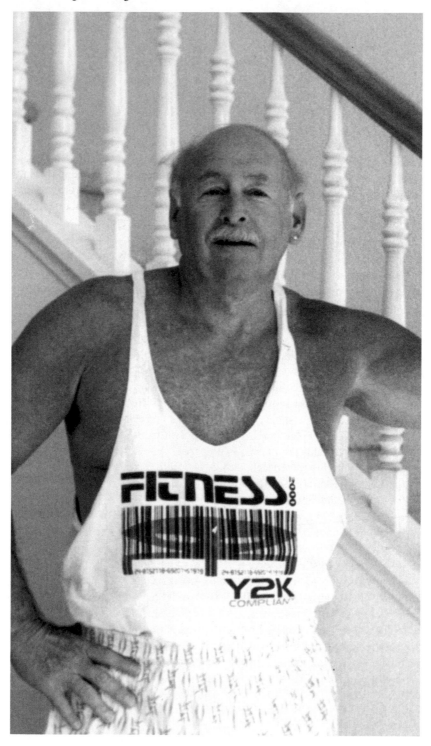

I decided to get educated about my disease. I found out all I could about the condition and began testing my blood throughout the day in order to determine the effects of different food. Now, I don't have to do the testing except when I feel tired and want to see if the sugar is up. I can control the symptoms pretty well. I see the doctor every six months for a blood hemoglobin test that averages your blood sugar level over three months. I guess the main thing I have to do is take care of my body. I plan on living awhile yet, and I want the time to be good. That motivates me to take good care of myself.

I'm in a lot better shape than a lot of people my age or younger. I'm thankful that I live now, when there are medicines and treatments for my conditions. Fifty years ago, I would have been blind with cataracts and glaucoma, struggling to deal with diabetes, and perhaps facing a premature death. Today, they take out the cataracts, put in lens implants, give me drops for the glaucoma, and I take pills twice a day for the diabetes. Such a deal!

Diabetes can affect potency because of its effect on blood flow, but I have not seen any effects, so far. My doctor has told me that there is a medication that would help with this, but I don't envision this to be a problem. I think that regular exercise helps offset any other issues.

The problems encountered in travel or social engagements involve the food choices. It can be a major hassle trying to find a place that has sugar-free syrup for my pancakes, will substitute veggies for baked potatoes, has low- or sugar-free desserts, and things like that. I can't have rice or bread, except sourdough, no corn or other white vegetables, and no cold cereals. I have to limit fruit and watch alcohol consumption. In dealing with this type of disease, I found out how much sugar is in everything.

I plan on living a while yet, and I want the time to be good. That motivates me to take good care of myself.

I am thankful this is all I have to cope with, and I am always cognizant of the fact that there are a lot of people worse off than me. My mother died of breast cancer at age fifty-three, and my Dad died of cancer at sixty-three. I intend to live a long time by taking care of myself.

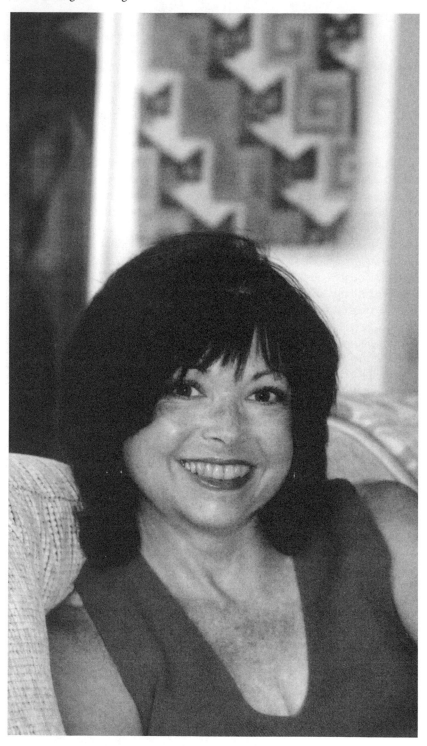

Kim H., Photographer

Short-Gut Syndrome, Crohn's Disease

I was diagnosed with Crohn's disease in 1970 when very little was known about treatments or helping patients maintain a decent quality of life. Treatments consisted of steroids or surgery. Living with this disease for many years has shown me how necessary it is to be an active participant in my own care. I have had numerous flare-ups, a few nice remissions, and multiple surgeries. Most of the drugs on the market have been tried with varying degrees of success. I have had four bowel resections leaving me with twenty-one inches of small intestine, and short-bowel syndrome, which carries its own assortment of problems.

My days, weeks, future plans, are all tentatively based on how I am feeling. There is always a 'Plan B' just in case.

Over the course of my life, the adjustments I had to make became greater and greater. I was forced to leave my career behind and go on permanent medical disability. My days, weeks, future plans are all tentatively based on how I am feeling at the last minute. There is always a Plan B just in case. This has affected the financial health of our household as well, and put added pressure on my husband to not only provide more money, but also provide good benefits such as health insurance.

Our friends have had to learn to be flexible since we may need to cancel plans or make some changes depending on how I feel at the last minute. I also eat frequently to keep calories going in throughout the day. This helps me to maintain my weight, but also takes a lot of time. If we are out or traveling, I have to stop to eat many times along the way. Those who travel with me usually gain a lot of weight.

There are several sides to living with a concealed illness. You're able to blend in with the crowd. No one stares at you or moves aside to let you through. This is the upside most of the time. However, there are times where more obvious symptoms might be useful. For example, when a bathroom is needed quickly and the lines are long, like at a ballgame, a wheelchair would get through very quickly. Generally, I'm glad to be able to keep some degree of privacy and to have my illness hidden from sight.

I get a little sad that I cannot do the traveling I have always wanted to do. However, I know that if I were healthy, I would be caught up in the hectic pace of today's society, which is so full of stress. I wouldn't have time for the things that bring great joy to my life now, such as photography and ferocious reading. It is a trade-off.

I developed my illness when I was fourteen years old. In some ways, having to contend with this disease most of my life has been easier than going from a full-blown healthy life to becoming ill in middle age and having to make that adjustment. For me, it is how I have always lived as an adult. Granted, I was able to work up to this point in my life, but I always had to deal with fatigue and the on-and-off symptoms of my illness. I guess I feel I have two choices: to enjoy life and make the best of what I have, or be miserable. I choose to enjoy what I can.

Having a full life is much more difficult when people treat you as if you are fragile. There are times I need help, and I am getting better about asking for it. I am also better about saying no. People who know me well can tell when I am having a bad day and they are very supportive.

I have always had a lot of interests. In the past seven years since my illness has worsened, I have moved into areas of interest that take less energy, or can be ongoing to accommodate the shift in good/bad day fluctuations. I indulge my creative side now through various forms of photography. Taking pictures when I am confined to the house is challenging. When I'm doing well, I am able to do the more traditional outdoor photography.

I keep in touch with friends and family through e-mail, phone, and personal visits. The support and energy that people pass on to me, even if they are not aware of it, makes a huge difference in how I feel. It's important for me not to isolate myself. I also try to learn new things. Whenever I am healthy enough, I take classes at a community college, just one class each semester, but it challenges my mind and gives me goals to reach.

I have cats at home. I find that pets are great companions and help with healing and depression. Some of the day-to-day things that need to be done I now do through the Internet. Using computer sites for shopping saves me a trip to the store, which can save me energy. I do as much of my shopping online as I can. All of these things combined help me maintain a good outlook, conserve my energy, enhance my spirit, and basically allow me to live a good life in spite of my illness.

I always make sure I am put together before I go out, even when I'm feeling poorly. I feel better when I look my best. I also gain energy when I am around others. I am usually exhausted by the time I go home, but I also feel better emotionally for having gone out and mingled with the crowds. If the day is especially full, I spend the following day doing as little as possible, or sometimes I spend it in bed.

The advantage of having a concealed illness is that I am able to live a fairly normal life. I am the one setting the limitations. The disadvantage of having a concealed chronic illness is in having to offer an explanation to others when I need help or cannot follow through with a commitment. For example, I had to drop classes due to health issues. I also need to find out beforehand what a class will involve to determine if my physical stamina can handle it.

I cannot say, "No, I am too busy," when people ask me to do something since I do not work. It requires a health explanation, and that can change a person's perception or treatment of me.

What has made the biggest difference throughout my life has been my attitude. I have always pushed myself to live as normal a life as possible. If that means taking prescription medicines, I do. If it means giving up certain foods, I do that too. For me it has meant long term, low dose steriods, giving up dairy foods, salads, most roughage, limiting sugar and, believe it or not, making sure I do not drink too much water. When I follow all this, it works beautifully. Yet, I am like everyone else on any sort of diet. If I cheat, I pay the price.

I have to take each day as it comes. This is a constant lesson in patience and flexibility. I have had to accept that I will always have a long to-do list and an unorganized house. I live my life within a detailed schedule of medications, eating patterns, and doctor appointments.

Over many years of searching for a cure, I have been to many clinics claiming to have the answers. They rarely do. I have tried supplements, teas, chiropractic therapy, allergy treatment, meditation, and many alternative approaches to treatment, all with varying degrees of improvement, but ultimately, very little change. This is not to say they do not work, but they did not work in my case. Crohn's disease is as individual as the people who suffer from it.

One important thing to note, I never stopped taking my prescription medication, even when I was trying something else that was considered more holistic. If I decide to try a new alternative treatment, I do so while still taking my prescriptions. If I start to improve, then the medication is altered with my doctor's assistance.

In my experience, many people searching for alternative healthcare are also searching spiritually. They are trying to figure out more about their inner selves and their place in the world. They are asking big questions and getting some worthy answers. A stroll down this path has led to the one thing that has made the biggest difference in my health.

I recently traveled to be part of a support system for a close friend who was undergoing leukemia treatment at her local hospital. At the same time, my own health was not doing well. I was rundown from the stress of travel and worry about my friend and was suffering some flare-ups of my disease.

My host, who was concerned about my fragile health during this stressful time, and being a practicing Buddhist, started chanting for my health to improve. She introduced me to Nichiren Buddhism and taught me to chant. I chanted while driving into the city each day to visit my friend in the hospital. I noticed a change in my health almost at once. This practice teaches happiness and taking control of your own life. As I practiced chanting, I noticed my energy increasing, weight increasing (which is good for me), and my overall symptoms starting to become more normal. That was incredible, especially for a skeptic like me.

I have been practicing chanting for over a year now and continue to experience greatly improved health. This is not magic. This practice promotes living responsibly. I take my medication and follow my diet along with chanting to improve my health. I have faith in the balance I am creating between myself and the energy in the universe. This balance leads to my improved health and happiness. I feel as if I have more control over my life and my health naturally improves in this condition.

We all have a connection to everything in this world, and this Buddhist practice also promotes peace throughout the world and absolute equality among all. By following this belief system, my life force has become stronger; I feel more connected to the world and my health has improved. When you can get outside of yourself and work for a greater cause—helping others—there is a direct benefit to your life. As long as I am a happy, well-rounded person with an illness, I can cope. As long as I do not become my illness, I will be fine. There's so much beauty and wonder in this world. As long as I can continue to see that first, I will remain happy, despite my illness.

Resources

Those who live with chronic disorders often seek relief using complementary as well as conventional methods. Therefore, many forms of symptom management were researched for this book. A comprehensive list of practitioners are located below.

Acupuncturists

Elissa V. Blesch, L.Ac. D.O.M. Bioset Practitioner. Fort Collins CO, (970) 484-8602

Julie Chang, L.Ac. www.sdhealthylife.com, San Diego CA, (858) 495-0771, info@sdhealthylife.com

Richard M. Gold, Ph.D., L.Ac. Pacific Center of Health. www.pacificcenterofhealth.com, San Diego CA, (619) 542-0884

Jill Van Meter, L.Ac. Acupuncturist, Massage Practitioner, Biofeedback, Herbologist. Encinitas CA, (760) 634-6990

Chiropractors

Susan Cameron, D.C., Director: Cameron Family Chiropractic. San Diego CA, (858) 627-9646

H. Ginakes, D.C. Integrated Medical Centers. www.imcdoctors.com, La Jolla CA, (858) 622-9266

Dan Kalish, D.C. www.drkalish.com, Del Mar CA, (858) 720-8380

Cynthia Leeder, D.C., N.D., C.C.N. Carlsbad CA, (760) 434-4615

Massage Therapists

Karen Jolley, C.M.T., Cranial Sacral Therapist. Bayside CA, karenmjolley@aol.com

Kevin Klatt, H.H.P., Integrated Medical Centers. www.imcdoctors.com, La Jolla CA, (858) 622-9266

Debra Kaye Peterson, C.M.T. Springfield OR, (541) 543-9495

Medical Physicians

Sidney Cassell, M.D. Eugene OR, (541) 687-0816

Roopa Chari, M.D. www.charicenter.com, Del Mar CA

Douglas Drossman, Professor of Medicine and Psychiatry, University of North Carolina, Chapel Hill. www.med.unc.edu/wrkunits/2depts/medicine/fgidc/welcome.htm, Chapel Hill NC

Margaret Elizondo, M.D., F.A.A.F.P., Practice in Family Medicine. San Diego CA, margaret.elizondo@cox.net

Bill McCarberg, M.D., Kaiser Permanente/Director: Chronic Pain Program. San Diego CA, (858) 581-8255

Artemio Pagdan, M.D., L.Ac., Board Certified Neurologist with special interest in headache and pain management. Chair of Pain Management Committee, Scripps Memorial Hospital. www.istopsandiego.com, La Jolla CA

Vijaya S.V. Pratha, M.D., Gastroenterologist. San Diego CA, (858) 455-7520

Malcolm Robinson, M.D., Clinical Professor of Medicine, University of Oklahoma College of Medicine. Oklahoma Foundation for Digestive Research. www.ofdr.org, Oklahoma City OK

Psychologists

Steven Hickman, Psy.D., Director, UCSD Center for Mindfulness Neuropsychiatry and Behavioral Medicine. University of California San Diego Medical Center, Department of Psychiatry. San Diego CA, shickman@ucsd.edu

Geneé Jackson, Ph.D., Licensed Clinical Psychologist, Brain Behavior Education and Resource Center. Gendeja Center for Growth and Healing. www.growthandhealing.org, San Francisco CA, (415) 860-6860, growthandhealing@att.net

Michael Wrobel, Psy.D., Clinical and Medical Psychologist. Qualified Medical Examiner, Medical Hypnosis. www.counselingsandiego.com, La Jolla CA, drwrobel@simplyweb.net

Reflexologists

Christine Issel, National Legislative Consultant. www.quantumreflexology.com, Sacramento CA quantumreflexology@earthlink.net

Cheri Reeder, R.N. C.H.T., Reflexologist; Registered Nurse. San Diego CA, (619) 269-1058 and (619) 743-3181, cheri@holisticreflexology.com

Therapists

Bejai Higgins, M.S., M.F.T., Chair of Social Services, University of Phoenix. San Diego CA, (619) 682-2150

Joanne Kezas Mason, M.F.T., R.N. www.sandiegotherapy.com, San Diego CA, (858) 974-6100

Jan Yaffe, M.F.T., CA Assoc. for Marriage and Family Therapy. Scripps Memorial Hospital. Del Mar CA, (858) 205-5269

Yoga Instructors

Lori Baker, CORporate Yoga. Vista CA, Lori@coryoga.com, (760) 644-3149

Diane Roberts, Foundation Yoga, CA Yoga Teacher's Association. www.foundationyoga.com, Solana Beach CA, (858) 616-8586, foundationyoga@cts.com

Nurses

Hollie Ketman, L.P.N. Springfield OR, Holliebuhn@cs.com

Cheri Reeder, R.N. C.H.T., Reflexologist, Registered Nurse. (619) 269-1058 and (619) 743-3181, cheri@holisticreflexology.com

Marie Zadravec, R.N. (Retired). Fallbrook CA, tomzad@prodigy.net, (760) 731-7455

Notes

Chapter One

1. Rollie McKenna, *Rollie McKenna: A Life in Photography* (New York: Alfred A. Knof, Inc. Publishing, 1991).
2. Malcolm Robinson, M.D. interview by the author. San Diego, CA, Sep 2002.
3. Jan Yaffe, M.F.T., interview by the author. San Diego, CA, Aug 2002.
4. Dianne Hales, "When The Body Attacks Itself," in *Parade/San Diego Union-Tribune,* Oct 12, 2003, 4–5.

Chapter Two

1. Geneé Jackson, Ph.D., interview with author. San Diego CA, Jul 2003.
2. Jackson, interview.
3. Michael Wrobel, Ph.D., interview by the author, San Diego, CA, Dec 2002.
4. Jan Yaffe, M.F.T., interview by the author, San Diego CA, Aug 2002.
5. Yaffe, interview.
6. Bejai Higgins M.F.T., interview by the author, San Diego, CA, Jun 2002.
7. Higgins, interview.
8. Marie Zadravec, R.N., interview by the author, Fallbrook, CA, May 2002.
9. Steven Hickman, interview by the author, San Diego, CA, Jun 2003.

Chapter Three

1. Geneé Jackson, interview by the author, San Diego, CA, Jul 2003.
2. The Americans with Disabilities Act establishes a clear and comprehensive prohibition of discrimination on the basis of disability.
3. Michael Wrobel, Ph.D., interview by the author, San Diego, CA. Dec 2002.
4. Jackson, interview.

Chapter Four

1. Margaret Elizondo, M.D., interview by the author, San Diego, CA, Jan 2003.
2. Malcolm Robinson, M.D., interview by the author, San Diego CA, Sep 2002.
3. Douglas A. Drossman, M.D., interview by the author, San Diego, CA, Nov 2002.
4. Marie Zadravec, R.N., interview by the author, Fallbrook CA, May 2002.
5. Zadravec, interview.
6. Sydney Cassell, M.D., interview by the author, San Diego CA, May 2003.
7. Robinson, interview.
8. Drossman, interview.
9. Roopa Chari, M.D., interview by the author, Del Mar, CA, Jun 2003.
10. Jill Van Meter, L.Ac., interview by the author, Encinitas, CA, Jun 2003.
11. Cheri Reeder, R.N., interview by the author, San Diego, CA, May 2003.
12. Geneé Jackson, Ph.D., interview by the author, San Diego, CA, Jul 2003.

13. Artemio G. Pagdan, M.D., interview by the author, San Diego, CA, Jun 2003.
14. Roger Jahnke. *The Healer Within* (San Francisco: Harper, 1997), 6.
15. G. H. Holt, "See Me, Feel Me, Touch Me, Heal Me," in *Life* v19 1996, 35.
16. Jackson, interview.
17. Vijaya Pratha, M.D., interview by the author, La Jolla, CA, Jun 2003.

Chapter Five

1. *What is Chinese Medicine and How Does it Work?,* brochure (Boulder CO: Blue Poppy Press, Inc., 1996).
2. Richard Gold, Ph.D., interview by the author, San Diego, CA, May 2003.
3. Daniel Kalish, D.C., interview by the author, Del Mar, CA, Jun 2003.
4. H. Ginakes, D.C., interview by the author, La Jolla, CA, Jun 2003.
5. Cynthia Leeder, D.C., interview by the author, San Diego, CA, Jun 2003.
6. Susan Cameron, D.C., interview by the author, San Diego, CA, May 2003.
7. Steven Hickman, Ph.D., interview by the author, San Diego, CA, Jun 2003.
8. Joel Stein, "The Science of Meditation: Just Say Om," in *Time,* Aug 4, 2003, 48.
9. Diane Roberts, interview by the author, San Diego, CA, May 2003.
10. Lori Baker, interview by the author, San Diego, CA, Apr 2003.
11. Christine Issel, interview by the author, San Diego, CA, May 2003.
12. Debra Peterson, C.M.T., interview by the author, San Diego, CA, Jul 2003.
13. Karen Jolley, C.M.T., interview by the author, San Diego, CA, Jun 2003.
14. Kevin Klatt, H.H.P., interview by the author, San Diego, CA, Jun 2003.

Chapter Six

1. Joanne Mason,R.N. interview by the author, San Diego, CA, May 2003.
2. Hollie Ketman,L.P.N., interview by the author, Eugene OR., Mar 2003.
3. Douglas Drossman, M.D., interview by the author, San Diego CA, May 2002.
4. Margaret Elizondo, M.D., interview by the author, San Diego, CA, Jan 2003.
5. Malcolm Robinson, M.D., interview by the author, San Diego, CA, Sep 2002.
6. Bill McCarberg, M.D., interview by the author, San Diego, CA, May 2003.
7. Elissa Blesch, L.Ac., interview by the author, San Diego, CA, Jun 2003.
8. Geneé Jackson, Ph.D., interview by the author, San Diego, CA, Jul 2003.

Chapter Seven

1. Geneé Jackson, Ph.D., interview by the author, San Diego, CA, Jul 2003.
2. Douglas Drossman, M.D., interview by the author, San Diego, CA, May 2002.
3. Bill McCarberg, M.D., interview by the author, San Diego, CA, May 2003.
4. Bejai Higgins, M.F.T., interview by the author, San Diego, CA, Jun 2002.
5. Michael Wrobel, Ph.D., interview by the author, San Diego, CA, Dec 2002.
6. Jan Yaffe, M.F.T., interview by the author, Del Mar, CA, Dec 2002.
7. Higgins, interview.
8. Marie Zadravec, R.N., interview by the author, Fallbrook, CA, May 2002.
9. Drossman, interview.
10. Jackson, interview.
11. Zadravec, interview.
12. Higgins, interview.
13. Higgins, interview.
14. Jackson, interview.

15. Jackson, interview.
16. Higgins, interview.
17. Jackson, interview.
18. Yaffe, interview.

Chapter Eight

1. Bejai Higgins, M.F.T., interview by the author, San Diego, CA, Jun 2002.
2. Higgins, interview.
3. Douglas Drossman, M.D., interview by the author, San Diego, CA, May 2002.
4. Bill McCarberg, M.D, interview by the author, San Diego, CA, May 2003.
5. Sidney Cassell, M.D., interview by the author, Eugene, OR, Mar 2003.
6. Malcolm Robinson, M.D., interview by the author, San Diego, CA, Sep 2002.
7. McCarberg, interview.
8. Marie Zadravec, R.N., interview by the author, Fallbrook, CA, May 2002.
9. Jan Yaffe, M.F.T., interview by the author, Del Mar, CA, Dec 2002.
10. Geneé Jackson, Ph.D., interview by the author, San Diego, CA, Jul 2003.
11. Lori Weisberg, "The Sick Sense" in *San Diego Union-Tribune,* August 18, 2002, E1, E3.
12. Randolph Schmid, "Some People can Tolerate More Pain. . .,"in *San Diego Union-Tribune,* June 24, 2003, A5.
13. Raelene Paulus, R.N., interview by the author, San Diego, CA, May 2003.
14. Higgins, interview.
15. Yaffe, interview.
16. McCarberg, interview.
17. American Pain Foundation, *Pain Care Bill of Rights,* (Baltimore MD: American Pain Foundation, 2003).
18. Michael Wrobel, PhD., interview by the author, San Diego, CA, Dec 2002.

Chapter Nine

1. Geneé Jackson, Ph.D., interview by the author, San Diego, CA, Jul 2003.
2. Jan Yaffe, M.F.T., interview by the author, Del Mar, CA, Aug 2002.
3. Bejai Higgins, M.F.T., interview by the author, San Diego, CA, Jun 2002.
4. Michael Wrobel, Ph.D., interview by the author, San Diego, CA, Dec 2002.
5. Yaffe, interview.
6. Higgins, interview.

Index